SCHISTOSOMIASIS

Edited by **Mohammad Bagher Rokni**

Schistosomiasis
Edited by Mohammad Bagher Rokni

Published by InTech

Janeza Trdine 9, 51000 Rijeka, Croatia

Publishing Process Manager Dejan Grgur

Technical Editor Teodora Smiljanic

Cover Designer InTech Design Team

Additional hard copies can be obtained from orders@intechopen.com

Schistosomiasis , Edited by Mohammad Bagher Rokni
p. cm.
ISBN 978-953-307-852-6

For EU product safety concerns:
IN TECH d.o.o., Prolaz Marije Krucifikse Kozulić 3, 51000 Rijeka, Croatia,
info@intechopen.com or visit our website at intechopen.com.

Meet the editor

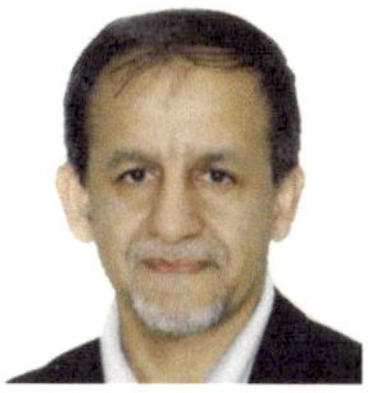

Dr Mohammad Bagher Rokni obtained his BSc in 1979, and his MS and PhD in Medical Parasitology in 1991 and 2002, respectively. He has written 48 papers and contributed to 4 books, as well as taken part in 76 national and international congresses and meetings. Dr Rokni is a Member of the Board of Directors of Iranian Society of Parasitology, Iranian Public Health Association and Iranian Scientific Association of Clinical Laboratory. He is also a member of WHO's Food Borne Disease Burden Epidemiology Reference Group, Vice-president of Eastern Mediterranean Association of Medical Editors (EMAME) Society, Chair of Journal Visibility & Indexing Committee (EMAME), Editor of the Iranian Journal of Public Health and Iranian Journal of Parasitology.

Contents

Preface

Schistosomiasis or blood fluke disease, also know as bilharziasis, is a parasitic disease caused by helminths from a genus of trematodes entitled *Schistosoma*. It is a snail-borne trematode infection. There are three important schistosome species parasitizing in humans: *Schistosoma japonicum, S. mansoni and S. haematobium*, although, out of the 21 currently recognized species, eight have been accounted from humans. *Schistosoma japonicum* and *S. mansoni* cause intestinal and hepatic schistosomiasis, while *S. haematobium*, causes urinary schistosomiasis. Schistosomiasis has been known to man for a long time. There are documentary records, especially of Egyptian origin, which demonstrate that the disease did not only prevail then, but its different clinical manifestations were recognized. Hematuria was the most recognized symptom, and the evidence of this can be found in Egyptian papyri (1500-1800 B.C.). Theodor Bilharz, a German pathologist, was the first researcher to discover the worms in the portal circulation and mention the pathology of the disease.

The importance of schistosomiasis in terms of public health effects has been documented through a variety of scientific methods and reports. The disease is among the *Neglected Tropical Disease* catalogued by the *Global Plan to combat Neglected Tropical Diseases, 2008–2015* and is considered to be the second most socioeconomically devastating parasitic disease by the World Health Organization (WHO), immediately after malaria. It has been reported from Africa and the Americas, to Eastern Mediterranean and the western Pacific. WHO demonstrates that schistosomiasis affects at least 200 million people worldwide, more than 700 million people live in endemic areas and more than 200.000 deaths are reported annually. Most of the cases involved are children. It also estimates that 7.1 million people are infected with *S. mansoni* in the Americas, 95% of which in Brazil. Urinary Schistosomiasis is endemic throughout most of Africa, the Middle East, Madagascar, Reunion, Mauritius and India. According to WHO, it is one of the major public health problems, facing humanity with severe social and economic consequences, leading to the loss of about 4.5 million disability-adjusted life years (DALYs).

Schistosoma parasites are dioecious, with distinct sexual dimorphism between male and female which is in contrast to other trematodes. Freshwater snails play a key role in the evolution cycle of the parasite as intermediate hosts. *Schistosoma japonicum* is transmitted by the amphibian snail *Oncomelania, S. mansoni* by *Biomphalaria,* and *S.*

haematobium by *Bulinus* snails. The evolution cycle starts with the parasites' eggs, which enter the water through urine or faeces of the human host, develop into miracidia, and the latter are attracted to certain snails as intermediate hosts. Inside the snail, the parasite passes the evolution step of sporocyst and after four to seven weeks, cercariae are librated form the snail. The disease occurs when cercariae penetrate the skin of victims swimming in infected waters and after a complicated internal immigration the parasite settles in the final location, which is the host's mesenteric portal system. The lifespan of the parasite is believed to be twenty to thirty years.

Approximately two thirds of the schistosomiasis cases are due to infection caused by *S. haematobium*. The relation between epidermoid carcinoma of the bladder and *S. haematobium* has been demonstrated. Intestinal schistosomiasis usually includeds signs of bloody diarrhea, intestinal polyposis, hepatosplenomegaly and periportal fibrosis. The key role in provoking clinical manifestations is attributed to granuloma. This is shaped by the body's inflammatory reaction to the eggs and larvae. In the blood vessels, attempts at migration through the walls may produce hemorrhages and inflammatory processes. When the eggs are trapped in the intestinal or vesical tissues, they may provoke granuloma, which become calcified and due to long life span of the parasite, the number of them increases repeatedly. In intestinal forms, some of the eggs are transported to the portal venous plexuses and may become trapped in the liver, producing periportal fibrosis.

Parasitological methods (Direct diagnosis) are normally conducted by examination of eggs in the faeces (the Kato-Katz technique) or in 24-hour urine. Detecting the eggs in the intestinal mucosa via biopsy might be effective. At present, the Kato-Katz technique, recommended by the WHO, is the most preferred technique for individual diagnostic instances, as well as for epidemiological investigations. Serological diagnosis methods, including ELISA and indirect immunofluorescence techniques, have been used as well, but serology requires a period of at least six weeks for confirmation. Moreover, some other techniques have been utilized in one way or another, including Vogel-Minning technique, Oliver-Gonzalez technique, and image testing.

According to the usual recommendation, the drug of choice is oral praziquantel, which is prescribed at a dose of 600 mg/12 h, in two doses. The administration of a second dose of praziquantel after 4-6 weeks increases the curation rate to 100%. To prevent resistance, some authors recommend a dose of praziquantel at 60 mg/kg/8 h, for three days. As an alternative treatment for *S. haematobium*, metrifonate or niridazol may be applied.

Due to having a key role in the evolution cycle of the parasite, snail control is among the most emphasized strategies for reduction of trematodes transmission. Some success has been made in some countries, for instance Egypt and Brazil, where the prevalence of infection has been reduced, but apparently this needs more collaboration from involved authorities because of the continuously high level of transmission.

Periodic, focused treatment with praziquantel for all suspected cases, annual checkups for school-age children, programmes to control snail infestation by the drainage and cleaning of all rivers and canals, and improving the public awareness are among the strategies recommended by WHO.

In the wake of InTech Publication invitation, the present book was written by a number of prominent researchers in the field. It is set to present a compendium of all necessary and up-to-date data for all those who are interested, including teachers, researchers and students. The book is recommended to all authorities involved in control and studying of schistosomiasis. Undoubtedly, all critical points and comments are welcome and will be considered by the panel of authors and contributors.

Dr Mohammad Bagher Rokni
Department of Medical Parasitology and Mycology
School of Public Health and Institute of Public Health Research
Tehran University of Medical Sciences
Tehran
Iran

Part 1

Diagnosis

1

Diagnosis of Schistosomiasis in Low Endemic Areas

Amal Farahat Allam
Alexandria University
Egypt

1. Introduction

Schistosomiasis, also known as bilharziasis is caused by snail transmitted parasites of the genus schistosoma that inhabit the human vasculature.[1,2] It is among the most important parasitic diseases worldwide, with a significant socio economic impact[3]. More than 200 million people are infected, and about 200,000 may die from the disease each year. On a global scale, one of thirty individuals has schistosomiasis[4]. About 779 million people live in endemic areas in the Middle East, South America, Caribbean, Southeast Asia and particularly sub-Saharan Africa[4]. Extreme poverty, the unawareness of the risks, the inadequacy or total lack of public health facilities plus the unsanitary conditions in which millions of people lead their daily lives are all factors contributing to the risk of infection[5].

During the past 20 years, much progress in combating the disease has been achieved based on World Health Organization recommendation strategies. Recent years have seen a notable decrease in the prevalence and morbidity of the disease in many endemic countries[6,7]. Many countries of the EMR (Eastern Mediterranean Region) namely Egypt, Iraq, Syria, Libya, Oman and Saudi Arabia have now reached low schistosomiasis endemicity. For instance, the overall prevalence of schistosomiasis in Egypt, was about 40% in (1967) before the national control program started by WHO (EMRO). In 2006, due to different control measures, the overall prevalence fell down to <3%. However there are still hot spot transmission foci with prevalence rate about 10%. Therefore lack of well structured prevention, control and elimination programs could lead to emergence or resurgence of the controlled disease. Schistosomiasis has been eliminated in Iran, Lebanon, Morocco and Tunisia, no new cases were detected over the past few years. Furthermore, WHO adopted a resolution calling on countries in low transmission areas, to sustain successful control activities in order to eliminate schistosomiasis[8] . In these conditions, where elimination of schistosomiasis is aimed for, case detection may pose a problem because the commonly used methods for the assessment of infection may lack necessary sensitivity to accurately determine the prevalence of schistosomiasis or of parasite burden[9,10]. WHO(2001,2006)[11,12] asked for sensitive assays for active surveillance, specially in situations with no or very low transmission.

Notwithstanding the large number of tests for diagnosing schistosomiasis, few have withstood tests of effectiveness, reproducibility, cross reactivity and predictive values (Rabello et al. 2002)[13]. The diagnostic strategies traditionally rely on the detection of parasite eggs in stool (*S. mansoni, S.japonicum*) or urine (*S. haematobium*) , antibody and antigen detection techniques. Lier et al (2008)[14] reported that there is no satisfactory "gold standard" diagnostic test in low intensity infections.

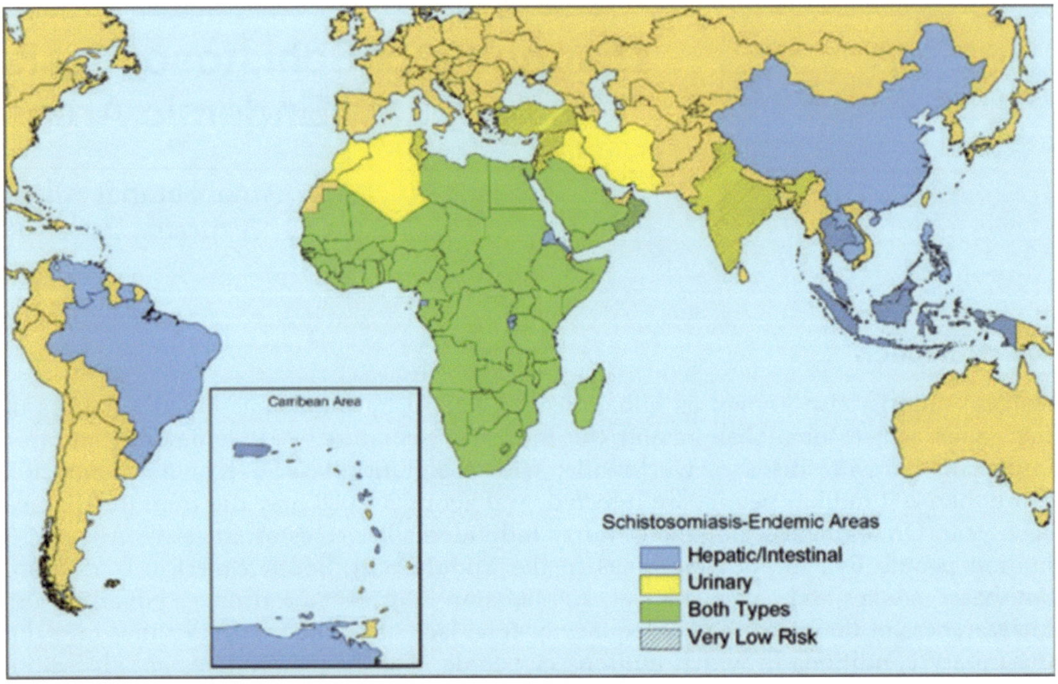

Fig. 1. Map showing Schistosomiasis Endemic Areas

The Kato-Katz technique [15] is currently the most used method for fecal examination because it is quantitative, relatively inexpensive simple and fast. However, due to the small amount of stool examined (less than 50 mg), its sensitivity is logistically prohibitive to monitor regularly or comprehensively low or moderate infections. Due to random distribution effects, the analyzed sample may not contain eggs even if the disease is active. It is thus very difficult to achieve a conclusive confirmation of successful therapy. A significant increase in the sensitivity of the method is gained by microscopic examination of multiple samples, but this is a limiting procedure for field work[16,17].

To overcome the current limitations with respect to diagnosis, the simultaneous use of different diagnostic methods, such as antibody detection followed by stool examination of seropositive individuals, has been applied to monitor the human population and to identify the small number of infected people once morbidity control is achieved. Dias et al. (1989)[18] reported that in low endemic areas for schistosomiasis, serologic prevalence indices have shown to be 2 to 5 times higher than the parasitologic indices. In Pedro de Toledo, the prevalence was 55.5% by the IgG, and it was 22.8%, by Kato-Katz method, with an infection intensity of 58.5 epg. Thus, the serologic prevalence was 2.6 times higher than the parasitologic prevalence. Noya et al(1999)[19] reported that the serologic prevalence by IgG was 33.2%, which was 20 times higher than the parasitologic prevalence of 1.6%, obtained by Kato-Katz method, with an infection intensity of 40.9 epg.

Burlandy- Soares et al (2003)[20] reported that the high difference between serologic and parasitologic prevalence data is undoubtedly due to the low diagnostic sensitivity of the parasitologic methods. Other might be the presence of individuals who have developed immune response to *S. mansoni* antigens after exposure to cercariae, but without development of infection, or have been cured after chemotherapy and still present circulating antibodies. It is a well known fact that immediately after chemotherapy, the levels of specific antibodies rise stimulated by the death of the parasites and fall after. Although the serologic techniques (ELISA, IHA and IFT) are very efficient, they do not constitute part of the diagnostic routine for schistosomiasis, and also they are not commonly used in epidemiologic studies. Moreover, antibody detection methods often cannot distinguish between current and past infection and may also present a high level of cross-reactivity. Blood collection is not easily applicable under field conditions, therefore this method is not recommended for field studies in endemic areas (Gryseels et al.,2006)[21]. However, Kanamura et al (1998)[22] and Burlandy-Soares et al (2003)[20] reported that the introduction of serologic methods in epidemiological studies, identifying potential infection sources, may contribute towards the reduction of residual transmission. This procedure could be included in a national program for the control of *schistosomiasis mansoni.*

Antigen based assays , such as circulating cathodic antigen (CCA) detection in urine and circulating anodic antigen (CAA) in serum, have proven to be a valuable , field applicable method. Unfortunately, in low intensity of infection, most of the positive antigen levels were very close to the cut off value, which is a disadvantage for the epidemiological application of the assay. It was concluded that for the diagnosis of schistosomiasis in low endemic areas, circulating antigen detection should be considered as a complementary tool rather than a substitute for parasitological examination specially that the detection of CCA in urine and CAA in serum supplies additional information to determine more accurately the "true" prevalence of infection[23,24].

To date, Percoll sedimentation technique was established as the technique of choice for diagnosis of *S. mansoni* in low intensity conditions and post treatment[25] . This method always gives better and more consistent estimate than the Kato Katz , and efficiently detects low intensity infections up to 4 eggs /gm. Amongst Kato-Katz negative *Schistosoma mansoni* specimens in a hypoendemic area with a prevalence 0f 5%, Percoll detected 11% positive cases and 7% post treatment. The efficiency of Percoll is based on the fact that it depends on 250 mg feces; one egg in the sediment would mean 4eggs/gm , whilst three Kato slides can diagnose up to 8 epg when only one egg is detected in one of the three slides examined. Moreover, detection of one to two eggs per fecal smear could be missed more easily within the fecal debris of Kato-Katz than the clear fields of the Percoll technique. Similar findings were reported by Eberl et al. (2002)[26], who found that the triple Kato-Katz examination on consecutive samples still missed 7.4% of all patients, whereas low egg numbers were detected efficiently only by Percoll technique.

Pontes et al. (2002)[27] reported the first use of PCR for the diagnosis of *S. mansoni* DNA in fecal samples. PCR methods have shown high sensitivity and specificity for the detection of *S. mansoni* DNA in stool samples, yet PCR gave negative results among few cases considered sure positives by microscopy (tables1,2) . Similar results were obtained by many authors[13,25,28,29,30].

Table (1) shows that the analysis of discordant results revealed that 15 samples were positive only by the PCR and two samples were positive only by Kato Katz technique.

	Kato-Katz faecal examination		
	Positive	Negative	Total
PCR			
Positive	26	15	41
Negative	2	24	26
Total	28	39	67

Kappa index: 0.511 (Gomes et al 2009)[30].

Table 1. Comparative evaluation of the PCR and the Kato-Katz technique for the diagnosis of *Schistosoma mansoni* infection

	Percoll		
	Positive	Negative	Total
PCR			
Positive	2	16	18
Negative	7	52	59
Total	9	68	77

Kappa index = 0.009, P > 0.05 no agreement (Allam et al 2009)[25]

Table 2. Agreement of the Percoll and PCR for the detection of *Schistosoma mansoni* cases negative after Kato–Katz technique

Comparing the results of the 77 cases analyzed by PCR with their results by Percoll revealed that only two patients gave concordant positive results; seven cases positive by Percoll were negative by PCR (Table2).

Pontes et al. (2003)[25] reported that missed cases after PCR were certainly misdiagnosed by the DNA amplification assay due to many factors such as: inhibition of the amplification reaction by fecal compounds and / or DNA degradation during transportation from the field, variation in egg output and uneven distribution in feces.

Oliveira et al.(2010)[31] reported that PCR can be an important tool for detecting *S. mansoni* infection in individuals excreting few eggs in feces. Moreover, the determination of the infection through the detection of *S. mansoni* DNA in stool samples from seropositive individuals represents a new means of confirming the results of IgG-ELISA for schistosomiasis. Therefore, studies in this direction should be encouraged and extended. Also, PCR have shown promise in the detection of parasites in a variety of media. Qualitative techniques have been developed to detect the presence or absence of *S. jabonicum* and avian schistosome cercariae recovered from snail hosts, as well as *S. mansoni* cercariae in water[32].

It was reported that conventional PCR requires several steps after DNA amplification, including electrophoresis or blotting and hybridization, which are limited in the number of samples that can be conveniently analyzed. A multiplex real-time PCR assay for the detection and quantification of *S. mansoni* and Schistosomal DNA in faecal samples was developed and evaluated as an alternative diagnostic method to study the epidemiology of schistosomiasis[33]. Primers and probes targeting the cytochrome c oxidase gene were designed for species-specific amplification and were combined with an internal control. Using positive control DNA extracted from adult Schistosoma worms and negative control samples (n=150) with DNA from a wide range of intestinal microorganisms, the method proved to be sensitive and 100% specific. For further evaluation, duplicate stool specimens with varying *S. mansoni* egg loads were collected in northern Senegal from pre-selected individuals (n=88). The PCR cycle threshold values, reflecting parasite-specific DNA loads in faeces, showed significant correlation with microscopic egg counts both for *S. mansoni* in stool and *S. haematobium* in urine. Although eggs of *S. haematobium* were not observed in stool samples, the presence of *S. haematobium* DNA was detected successfully. The Schistosoma detection rate of PCR (84.1%) was similar to that of microscopy performed on duplicate stool samples (79.5%). The simple fecal sample collection procedure and the high throughput potential of the multiplex real-time PCR provide a powerful diagnostic tool for epidemiological studies on schistosomiasis in remote areas. Moreover, it demonstrates high sensitivity, even in samples containing a single schistosoma egg in stool(33,43).

When comparing the real-time PCR with microscopy-based assays, the PCR is less labour intensive when many samples are to be examined. The PCR method also has the advantage of being less influenced by observer variation/bias as compared to microscopy-based methods.

More recently, Gomes et al (2006)(30) ,Hung et al (2008)(32)and lier et al (2009)(34) established and developed SYBR Green (a fluorescent based technology) and Taq Man probe real time PCR assays for the detection and quantification of schistosomal DNA. They reported that they are potentially useful for quantification of parasite burden in human infection.

Gomes et al (2010)(35) reported development of the PCR-ELISA system for the detection of *Schistosoma* DNA in human feces as an alternative approach to diagnose light infections. The system permits the enzymatic amplification of a specific region of the DNA from minute amounts of parasite material. Using the proposed PCR-ELISA approach for the diagnosis of a population in an endemic area in Brazil, 30% were found to be infected, as compared with the 18% found by microscopic fecal examination. The genus specificity of PCR-ELISA was assessed with purified DNA from *S. mansoni, S. haematobium, S. bovis, S. intercalatum, S. japonicum, S. magrebowiei* and *S. rhodaini* adult worms. Considering the results obtained with the *Schistosoma* PCR-ELISA system based on two levels of intensity of infection (1–100 epg and >100 epg), according to the Kato-Katz stool examination method, the assay revealed the potential to be considered semi-quantitative, as the mean absorbance readings corresponded to the intensity of infection. The high sensitivity of the *Schistosoma* PCR-ELISA system was evidenced by the high number of positive samples in both groups. The advantage of PCR-ELISA as compared to PCR-electrophoresis is that it makes use of standard equipment widely used for the processing of ELISAs, and the reagents used are easy to obtain commercially. Therefore, PCR-ELISA allows for the use of PCR-based DNA diagnosis for routine purposes in laboratories in less developed countries with fewer resources.

Nowadays , we have many sensitive methods for schistosomiasis detection in areas of low endemicity. Percoll sedimentation technique as parasitologic test of choice. Conventional PCR as a molecular technique for detection of schistosoma eggs. It can be used to confirm the results of seropositives through the detection of schistosomiasis in stool samples. Real time PCR assays for detection and quantification of schistosomiasis. PCR ELISA as a semiquantitative technique for diagnosis of low intensity of schistosomiasis.

Thus, as the prevalence and intensity decrease, the benefit of increased sensitivity using the molecular tests must be weighed against additional costs. Although the techniques require a complex laboratory infrastructure and specific funding it may be used by control programs targeting the elimination of schistosomiasis(Lier et al 2009)(34).

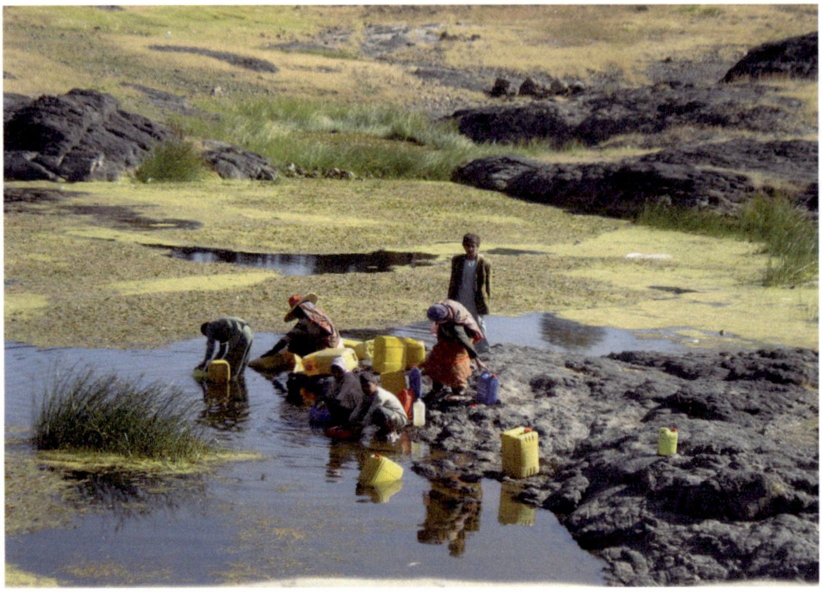

Fig. 2. Can schistosomiasis be eliminated? Fenwick et al(5).

2. References

[1] WHO (2011). Epidemiological records. 86: 73-80.
[2] Lier T, Simonsen GS, Wang T, Lu D, Haukland HH, Vennervald BJ, Hegstad J, and Johansen MV (2009). Real Time Polymerase Chain Reaction for Detection of low intensity *Schistosoms japonicum* infections in China. Am J Trop Med Hyg 81: 428- 432.
[3] World Health Organization (2008). The social context of schistosomiasis and its control: an introduction and annotated bibliography.
[4] Chitsulo L, Loverde P, Engels D (2004). Schistosomiasis. Nat Rev Microbiol 2: 12–13.
[5] Fenwick A et al (2003). Drugs for the control of parasitic diseases: current status and development in schistosomiasis. Trends parasitol 19:509–15.
[6] Lammie PJ, Fenwick A, Utzinger J (2006) A blueprint for success: integration of neglected tropical disease control programmes. Trends Parasitol 22: 313–321.
[7] King CH (2009). Toward the elimination of schistosomiasis. N Engl J Med 360: 106–109.
[8] WHO (2007). Report of inter country meeting on strategy to eliminate schistosomiasis from the Eastern Mediterranean Region. Muscat, Oman . 6-8 November.
[9] Utzinger J, Zhou XN, Chen MG, Bergquist R (2005) .Conquering schistosomiasis in China. Acta Trop 96: 69–96.
[10] World Health Organization (2005) .Report of the scientific working group meeting on Schistosomiasis. Geneva, 14-16 November.
[11] WHO (2001). Report of the World Health Organization informal consultation on schistosomiasis in low transmission areas: control strategies and criteria for elimination. 10-13. WHO/CDS/CPE/SIP/2001.
[12] WHO (2006). World Health Organization Special Programme for Research and Training in Tropical Diseases. TDR home page . at.www. who.int/tdr.

[13] Rabello A, Pontes LA & Dias-Neto E (2002) Recent advances in the diagnosis of Schistosoma infection: the detection of parasite DNA. Mem Inst Oswaldo Cruz 97:171–172.

[14] Lier T, Johansen MV, Hjelmevoll SO, Vennervald, Simonsen GS (2008). Real time PCR for detection of low intensity *Schistosoma japonicum* infections in a pig model. Acta Trop 105-: 74-80.

[15] Katz N, Chaves A & Pellegrino J (1972) A simple device for quantitative stool thick smear technique in Schistosoma mansoni Revista do Instituto de Medicina Tropical de Sao Paulo 14:397–400.

[16] Yu JM, de Vlas SJ, Yuan HC, Gryseels B (1998) Variations in fecal *Schistosoma japonicum* egg counts. Am J Trop Med Hyg 59: 370–375.

[17] Utzinger J, N'Goran EK, N'Dri A, Lengeler C, Xiao S, et al. (2000) Oral artemether for prevention of *Schistosoma mansoni* infection: randomized controlled trial. Lancet 355: 1320–1325.

[18] Dias LCS, Kawazoe U, Glasser CM, Hoshino-Shimizu S, Kanamura HY, Cordeiro JA, Guarata OF, Ishirata GJ (1989). Schistosomiasis mansoni in the municipality of Pedro de Toledo (São Paulo, Brazil) where the *Biomphalaria tenagophila* is the snail host: I. Prevalence in human population. Rev Inst Med Trop 31: 110 -118.

[19] Noya BA, Balzan C, Artega C, Cesari I, Noya O (1999). The last fifteen years of schistosomiasis in Venezuela: features an evolution. Mem Inst Oswaldo Cruz 94: 136-146.

[20] Lanny Cristina Burlandy-Soares Luiz Cândido de Souza Dias, Hermínia Yohko Kanamura, Edward José de Oliveira, Ricardo Mario Ciaravolo (2003). Schistosomiasis mansoni: Follow-up of Control Program Based on Parasitologic and Serologic Methods in a Brazilian Community of Low Endemicity. Mem Inst Oswaldo Cruz 98: 853-859

[21] Gryseels B, Polman K, Clerinx J, Kestens L (2006) Human schistosomiasis. Lancet 368: 1106–1118.

[22] Kanamura HY, Dias LCS, Glasser CM, Silva RM, Patucci RMJ, Chiodelli SG, Addis DG (1998). Detection of IgM antibodies to *Schistosoma mansoni* gut-associated antigens for the study of the dynamics of schistosomiasis transmission in an endemic area with low worm burden. Rev Inst Med Trop São Paulo 40: 225-231.

[23] El-Morshedy H, Kinosien B, Barakat R, Omer E, Khamis N, Deelder AM, Phillips M (1996). Circulating anodic antigen for detection of *Schistosoma mansoni* infection in Egyptian patients. Am J Trop Med Hyg 54: 149-153

[24] Van Dam GJ, Wichers JH, Ferrera TM, Ghati D, Van Amerongen A, Deelder AM (2004). Diagnosis of schistosomiasis by reagent strip test for detection of circulating cathodic antigen. J Clin Microbiol. 42: 5458-5461.

[25] Allam AF, Kader O, Zaki A, Shehab AY, Farag HF (2009). Assessing the marginal error in diagnosis and cure of *Schistosoma mansoni* in areas of low endemicity using Percoll and PCR techniques. Trop Med Int Health 14: 316–321.

[26] Eberl M, Al-Sherbiny M, Hagan P, Ljubojevic S, Thomas AW & Wilson RA (2002). A novel and sensitive method to monitor helminth infections by faecal sampling. Acta Tropica 83: 183- 187.

[27] Pontes LA, Oliveira MC, Katz N, Dias-Neto E&Rabello A (2003). Comparison of polymerase chain reaction and the Kato-Katz technique for diagnosing infection with Schistosoma mansoni. Am J Trop Med Hyg 68:652- 656.

[28] Pontes LA, Dias-Neto E & Rabello A (2002). Detection by polymerase chain reaction of Schistosoma mansoni DNA in human serum and feces. Am J Trop Med Hyg 66: 157–162.

[29] Hamburguer J, Turetski T, Kapeller I & Deresiewi CZR (1991). Highly repeated short DNA sequences in the genome of Schistosoma mansoni recognized by a species specific probe. Mol Biochem Parasitol 44:73–80.

[30] Gomes L I, Marques L HS , Enk M J, Coelho P M Z, Rabello A(2009). Further evaluation of an updated PCR assay for the detection of *Schistosoma mansoni* DNA in human stool samples Mem Inst Oswaldo Cruz 104: 1194-1196

[31] Oliveira LM, Santos HL, Gonçalves MM, Barreto MG, Peralta JM (2010). Evaluation of polymerase chain reaction as an additional tool for the diagnosis of low-intensity Schistosoma mansoni infection. Diagn Microbiol Infect Dis 68:416-21.

[32] Hung YW, Remais J (2008). Quantification and detection of *Schistosoma japonicum* cercariae in water by real time PCR. Plos Neg Trop Dis 11: 337- 348.

[33] Ten Hove RJ, Verweij JJ, Vereecken K, Polman K, Dieye L, van Lieshout L (2008). Multiplex real-time PCR for the detection and quantification of Schistosoma mansoni and S. haematobium infection in stool samples collected in northern Senegal. Trans R Soc Trop Med Hyg 102:179-85.

[34] Lier T, Simonsen GS, Wang T, Lu D, Haukland HH, Vennervald BJ, Hegstad J, and Johansen MV (2009). Real Time Polymerase Chain Reaction for Detection of low intensity *Schistosoms japonicum* infections in China. Am J Trop Med Hyg 81,428-432.

[35] Gomes LI, Marques LHdS, Enk MJ, de Oliveira MC, Coelho PMZ, et al. (2010) Development and Evaluation of a Sensitive PCR-ELISA System for Detection of *Schistosoma* Infection in Feces. PLoS Negl Trop Dis 4(4): e664.

Part 2

Treatment

2

Artenimol-Based Combination Therapy for the Curative Treatment of Schistosomiasis

F. Herwig Jansen and Tinne De Cnodder
Department of Clinical Pharmacology, Dafra Pharma Ltd, Turnhout Belgium

1. Introduction

Recent decades have seen new developments for a number of parasitic diseases, particularly malaria. This has had a major impact and large-scale global health programmes have been developed to alleviate the burden of some of these deadly diseases. Some diseases - such as schistosomiasis - seem to have been ignored internationally. And yet schistosomiasis has a serious impact on public health and the economy. Although the disease can be controlled by praziquantel, elimination programmes are not popular and the disease continues to take its toll on the public. An annual administration of praziquantel could change this markedly and have a pronounced impact on the overall health of the people of Africa. In contrast, malaria programmes are bringing the disease under control; the incidence of malaria has dropped significantly in the last few years. Praziquantel could achieve similar results for schistosomiasis control if it were used in identical health care programmes.

Although praziquantel appears to be an efficacious drug, in recent years problems of resistance have arisen and experts are calling for alternative therapies (Doenhoff et al., 2007). Below is a short review of praziquantel and a discussion on the need for new drugs.

Praziquantel (Figure 1) was discovered and developed by Bayer AG in Germany and co-developed by Merck. Praziquantel has been used since the early 1970s for the treatment of parasitic *Schistosoma* infections (Tchuenté et al., 2004) and for the treatment (to varying degrees of success) of liver flukes, such as *Chlonorchic sinsensis* (Shen et al., 2007). Paragonimiasis is also listed as an indication. One other major indication for praziquantel is its application in the treatment of tapeworms (trematodes and cestodes), such as the various taenias, cysticercosis (Matthaiou DK et al., 2004) and echinococcosis parasites. The WHO considered the drug important enough to add it to its Model List of Essential Medicines.

Absorption and metabolism: Praziquantel is rapidly absorbed (approximately 80%) via the gastrointestinal tract. It undergoes intensive metabolisation during its first pass through the liver so that relatively small amounts enter the systemic circulation. The elimination half-life is short, ranging from 1 to 2 hours. Praziquantel and its metabolites are mainly excreted by the kidneys. After a single oral dose, 70 to 80% is found in urine within 24 hours.

Efficacy: Praziquantel has a particularly dramatic effect on patients with schistosomiasis. Studies have shown that up to 90% of the damage done to internal organs due to schistosomiasis infection could be reversed (http://www.cartercenter.org/health/schistosomiasis/index.html; Tchuenté et al., 2004) within six months of receiving one dose of praziquantel.

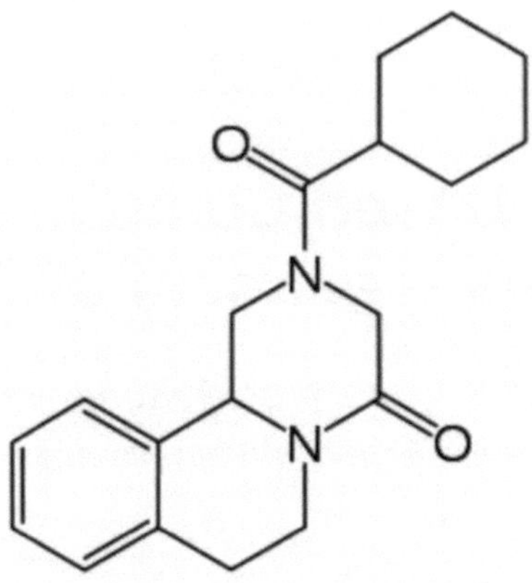

(*RS*)-2-(Cyclohexylcarbonyl) -1,2,3,6,7,11b-
hexahydro-4H-pyrazino (2,1-alpha) isoquinolin-4-on

Fig. 1. Praziquantel: $C_{19}H_{24}N_2O_2$. MW. 312.4

Mode of action: Although the mode of action is not exactly known at present, there is experimental evidence that praziquantel increases the permeability of the membranes of schistosome cells towards calcium ions. The drug thereby induces contraction of the parasites, resulting in paralysis in the contracted state. The dying parasites are dislodged from their site of action in the host organism and may enter systemic circulation. Destruction follows by host immune reaction. Additional mechanisms including focal disintegrations and disturbances of oviposition (laying of eggs) are seen in other types of sensitive parasites (Doenhoff et al., 2008). Others suggest that the drug seems to interfere with adenosine uptake in cultured worms. This effect may have therapeutic relevance given that the schistosome, the taenia and the echinococcus (other praziquantel sensitive parasites) are unable to synthesise *de novo* purines such as adenosine (Angelucci et al., 2007).
Side effects: The majority of side effects develop as a result of host immune reaction due to the release of the contents of the killed parasites. The most frequent side effects are dizziness, headache and malaise. Almost all patients with cerebral cysticercosis experience CNS side effects related to the cell-death of the parasites (headache, worsening of pre-existing neurological problems, seizures, and meningism). Sometimes this requires the administration of corticosteroids. Approximately 90% of patients suffer from abdominal pain or cramps with or without nausea and vomiting. Diarrhoea may develop and may be severe with colic. Increases in liver enzymes are sometimes found during treatment, and urticaria, pruritus and eosinophilia are not uncommon.
Dosage: For schistosomiasis, the dose is 20 mg/kg by mouth every 4-6 hours for one day. An alternative is 40 mg per kg body weight in a single oral dose. For treatment of other worms different dosages might be needed.

2. Need for alternative treatment for schistosomiasis

Although praziquantel maintained its status for many years as a powerful drug for the treatment of various forms of schistosomiasis, reports started coming in about the failure of the drug. Development of resistance was studied experimentally and closely monitored clinically. Resistance could be induced in laboratory experiments, for instance by giving suboptimal doses of the drug to worm infested mice (Ismail et al., 1994, Fallon et al., 1995). Ismail and colleagues confirmed their findings on isolates from Egypt (Ismail et al., 1996). Clinical evidence of resistance came from Senegal and Egypt, expressed as a reduced cure rate in a treated population (Stelma et al., 1995). One strange observation came from northern Senegal, where the cure rate 12 weeks after a single dose of 40 mg per kg was unexpectedly low namely 18% (Gryseels et al., 2001). Fortunately, such a low cure rate was not found elsewhere. Overall it can be concluded that real resistance against praziquantel exists but is not yet dramatic. The mechanism of resistance remains fully unclear.

If resistance against a standard treatment develops it is time to look for new treatments, but very few were found over the years. Oxamniquine is one alternative, but it has never been used on a broad scale for reasons of intrinsic weakness and early resistance development. Others reported that combining oxamniquine with praziquantel had no real advantage over praziquantel alone.

3. Positioning of broad spectrum drugs

Although in general, drugs are developed for the treatment of a single disease, for some indications international experts are calling for the development of broad spectrum drugs that can be used for more than one disease. The treatment of one disease will then have implications on the other disease in the same region. One example would be a drug for malaria that is also able to kill certain helminths. So far, there are very few drugs indeed that can simultaneously destroy plasmodia parasites and devastating worm infections. As a result, such pleas have remained more or less a dream (Hotez et al., 2008). It is not obvious that a particular drug which affects the mechanism of a given disease will also affect the biological factors implicated in another disease. Nevertheless, several examples exist. The classical example is the use of chloroquine to treat malaria and lupus erythematosus (Fischer-Betz and Scheider, 2009). Some anti-folates, such as sulfonamides, have a strong killing effect on bacteria as well as on the parasites that cause toxoplasmosis, not necessarily due to folic acid biosynthesis inhibition. Some single drugs - such as albendazole, paclitaxel and ivermectine - affect various parasites or worms, but do not affect other parasites. It would be of great interest to have a drug that kills malaria parasites while at the same time having an impact on the burden caused by helminthic infections. Is this a dream or can it actually be a practical solution? Leading researchers have advocated moves in this direction. Imagine what it could imply if a strong drug able to kill malaria parasites could simultaneously kill worms, such as *Schistosoma* and hookworms. Such a drug would have a serious impact on disability-adjusted-life years (DALYs) in an African setting. It would definitely reduce the degree of anaemia in the population and therefore have a positive impact on working days lost and on the learning process of schoolchildren.

Such an idea came to the fore when descriptions were published noting that antimalarial drugs derived from artemisinin had a killing effect on some worms, like the *Schistosoma* species. The first to describe such an effect was Chen et al. in 1980 followed by Le et al. in 1982, who found the artemisinins active against *S. japonicum*. Utzinger confirmed this in 2001 (Utzinger et al., 2001). Later, Utzinger wrote that artemether and artesunate in particular were active against all species of schistosomes (Utzinger et al., 2003). Artemether exhibits the highest activity against young liver stages, whereas the invasive stages (cercariae) and the adult worms were found to be less sensitive to this drug. In contrast, the older forms were more vulnerable to praziquantel (Utzinger et al., 2001 and Xiao et al.,

2002). What sort of drugs are these artemisinins and do they have a real place in the treatment of schistosomiasis? And if so, for all species?

4. Artenimol and derivatives in the treatment of malaria: Mechanism of action

Artemisinin was the first substance in the artemisinin derivatives family to be described as being active against malaria. When later the active ingredient dihydroartemisinin (DHA) or artenimol was discovered, also derivatives of DHA like artemether, a methyl ether derivative, and artesunate, a succinic acid ester derivative, were manufactured and studied. Artenimol is the official generic name for a substance generally known as dihydroartemisinin (DHA) (Figure 2a). This compound is the result of a selective borohydride reduction of the lactone function of artemisinin (Figure 2b). Artemisinin, generally referred to as a sesquiterpene lactone (meaning that the drug has a lactone function and contains 15 carbon atoms), is the active ingredient extracted from the plant *Artemisia annua* (sweet wormwood, see boxed text: *The story of artemisinin*). The reduction process creates a reactive place in the molecule permitting derivatisation of the molecule. Artenimol is considered to be the active parent compound of the series of derivates (Jansen and Soomro, 2007; Li et al., 1989).

4.1 Box: The story of artemisinin

During the Vietnam War, the North Vietnamese Army suffered heavily from malaria and appropriate drugs were not available. Vietnamese leader Ho Chi Minh asked for help from his comrades in the People's Republic of China and Mao organised an official research programme. This initiative came at the right time. One of the researchers in traditional Chinese medicine, Xian Weij, had experimented with extracts from a widespread plant called *Artemisia annua*. However, it turned out that this aromatic plant, when cultivated under optimal climatic conditions, contained more crystalline product than plants growing in other areas. When isolated, the crystalline substance turned out to be effective against malaria parasites and was apparently non-toxic. This was the beginning of a strong national programme in China. However, when the drug was ready, the Vietnam War was over. The chemical structure of the crystalline substance ($C_{15}H_{22}O_5$) was determined a few years after the discovery. It turned out that the molecule is small (MW 282.3) but has a complex chemical structure. One of the functions in the molecule, a lactone function, was vulnerable to chemical reaction and a borohydride reduction process yielded a product given the trivial name of dihydroartemisinin. In some models, this molecule had a higher intrinsic activity against malaria parasites. It offered the possibility of making derivatives by etherification or esterification. Thus artemether (a methyl ether) and artesunate (the hemisuccinate ester of DHA) were born. These two drugs revolutionised malaria treatment.

Relatively cheap drugs without side effects could now be used to treat even multiple-drug-resistant malaria, a problem emerging in southeast Asia. A dose of 600 mg administered over 5 days was enough to cure more than 90 percent of all cases. Recrudescence was very low. In order to counter the risk of parasites building up resistance to this class of drugs, the WHO recommended using combination therapies (Artemisinin-based combination therapies or ACTs) and in 2006 the WHO imposed a global ban on the use of artesunate and similar drugs for malaria monotherapy.

As an antimalaria agent, artenimol is 10-15 times more active than artemisinin. For a detailed discussion on the mechanism of action we refer to Krishna et al. (2004) and to

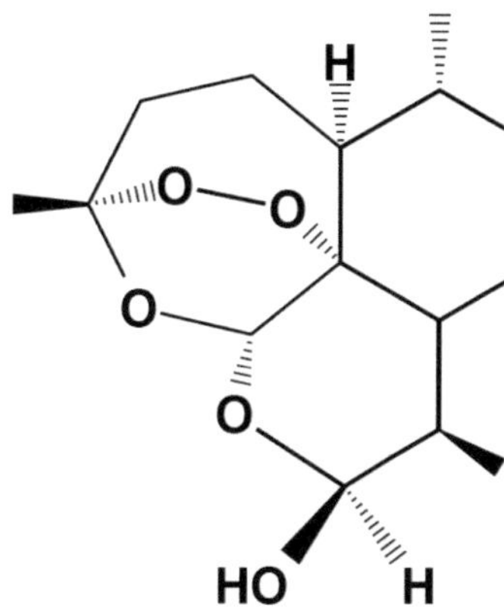

a)

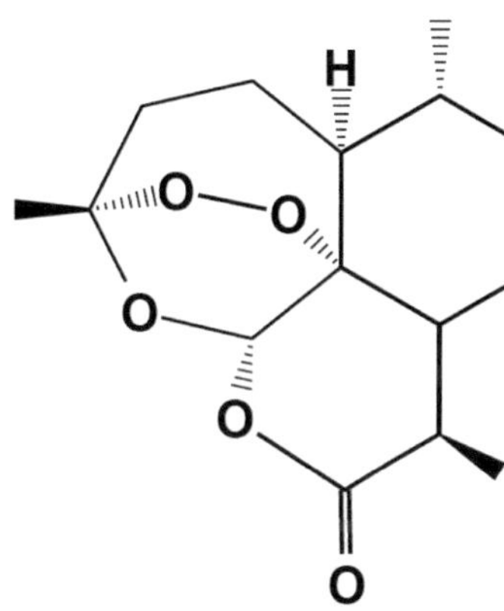

b)

Fig. 2. a) Dihydroartemisinin (artenimol) $C_{15}H_{24}O_5$. MW. 284.3, b) Artemisinin $C_{15}H_{22}O_5$. MW. 282.3.

Jansen and Soomro (2007). Several mechanisms have been put forward to describe the efficacious and fast activity of artemisinin derivates. The first proposed mechanism of action is the activity created by singlet oxygen and of a series of free radicals. This is an obvious approach. The peroxide function in the molecule is carried by an unstable, oxygen-containing, seven-membered ring. Strain on this ring, e.g. occurring when the lactol ring opens (under the influence of alpha-beta flip flop mechanisms of the OH-group), sets singlet oxygen free. Other mechanisms can cause a similar effect and they definitely occur when DHA is absorbed into the parasite. This release of singlet oxygen implies the release of an extremely reactive atomic species that will attack any molecular function in its vicinity that is sensitive to singlet oxygen attack. Non-chemists are very well aware of the strong antibacterial action of hydrogen peroxide and benzoylperoxide gels; they kill all germs. In these preparations, singlet oxygen will be released and the molecules will return to straight water and to benzoic acid, both devoid of any particular killing effect. The resistance of bacteria to this action of peroxide has not been described. Peroxide is also commonly used to bleach hair and tissues. At subcellular level, a large variety of biochemical reactions can be influenced by singlet oxygen. For example, the singlet oxygen sets itself on a double bond of a fatty acid in a membrane, forming an epoxide causing a change in the tertiary structure of a lipid. This is the start of other reactions since e.g. water can create an addition reaction on the peroxide. This results in the formation of vicinal OH groups in the chain leading to the rupture of the molecule. Leaking membranes is the first consequence of such action. At the same time, the artenimol molecule forms a series of other free radicals with or without Fe^{2+} ions and these in turn have alkylating properties leading to more destructive actions. Unfortunately, these properties are not well described and more of a speculative nature. However the destructive activity remains. This was clearly demonstrated in an electron microscopy study on *Plasmodium berghei* parasites. Several years ago, Chinese scientists involved in traditional medicine published a remarkable article. Mice suffering from *P. Berghei* malaria were treated with a single 10 mg/kg dose of artemisinin. At time zero the parasites under the microscopic magnification appear most healthy but 30 minutes later changes were seen in the membranes of the parasite, together with alterations in ribosomal organisation and endoplasmatic reticulum. No changes were observed in the digestive vacuole, but nuclear membrane blebbing developed after one hour and segregation of the nucleoplasm after three hours. Further degenerative changes with disorganisation and death occurred from eight hours onwards. Such a fast and progressive action would indeed fit into a combination of various free radical actions (Ellis et al., 1985).

The inhibition of the SERCA enzyme is another proposed mechanism of action (Eckstein-Ludwig et al., 2003). These investigators show that artemisinins, but not quinine or chloroquine, inhibit the SERCA orthologue (PfATP6) of *Plasmodium falciparum* in Xenopus oocytes, with similar potency to thapsigargin (another sesquiterpene lactone and highly specific SERCA inhibitor). As predicted, thapsigargin also antagonises the parasiticidal activity of artemisinin. Desoxyartemisinin lacks an endoperoxide bridge and is ineffective both as an inhibitor of PfATP6 and as an antimalarial. Chelation of iron by desferrioxamine abrogates the antiparasitic activity of artemisinins and correspondingly attenuates inhibition of PfATP6. Imaging of parasites with BODIPY-thapsigargin labels the cytosolic compartment and is competed by artemisinin. Fluorescent artemisinin labels parasites similarly and irreversibly in a Fe^{2+}-dependent manner. These data provide compelling evidence that artemisinins act by inhibiting PfATP6 outside the food vacuole after activation by iron.

As demonstrated in more recent years, the class of arteminisins is not only active against malaria, but also against cancer cells and schistosomiasis. Artenimol derivates were shown to display remarkable and highly specific cytotoxicity against all human tumour cell lines studied at the Developmental Therapeutics Program of the National Cancer Institute (USA). Cytotoxicity was also shown against radiation- and drug-resistant cancer cell lines. Interestingly, synergism with other common chemotherapeutic therapies was also shown (Efferth et al., 2001). The anti-angiogenesis properties of artenimol derivatives were demonstrated using the chorioallantoic membrane (CAM) assay and the Zebra fish embryo model. Artenimol derivatives were shown to be the first small molecules to display its anti-angiogenic effects on arterial venous and lymphatic vessels (Soomro et al., 2010). In xenografted mice models, artenimol derivatives were shown to reduce tumour size and tumour vascularisation. The multifaceted nature of the action of artenimol derivatives includes protein alkylation, induction of apoptosis, angiogenesis inhibition, oxidative stress and cell cycle regulation (Efferth 2007). At the moment, several published and unpublished case reports and one clinical study prove the tumour-inhibiting activity of artesunate in human cancer. In the world of parasites, artemisinins are active against some blood flukes, the cause of schistosomiasis. The details will be discussed below.

Interestingly, the bioactivity of artemisinin and its semisynthetic derivative artesunate is even broader and includes the inhibition of certain viruses, such as human cytomegalovirus and other members of the Herpesviridae family (e.g., herpes simplex virus type 1 and Epstein-Barr virus), hepatitis B virus, hepatitis C virus, and bovine viral diarrhoea virus (Efferth et al., 2008).

5. Artenimol-based combination drugs for parasitic diseases

The theory behind ACTs is the following: A population of malaria parasites may contain a low number of parasites that is resistant to the drug used to kill them. These resistant parasites can survive and eventually contribute to the spreading of the disease with drug resistant parasites. Even if such a process is slow to develop a real risk, after some years this resistance could have become a clinical reality. If, however, the same population of parasites is treated at the same time with another drug having a totally different mode of action, resistance to this drug could also develop in the same sense as described for the first drug. But the risk that resistant parasites will develop at the same time against two active drugs is very small. In fact, it may be so small that from a practical point of view such resistance does not develop. The ideal combination would consist of two drugs with a different mechanism of action and with more or less similar pharmacokinetic behaviour so that the parasites are exposed for an almost identical period of time to the same drug. Although this theory is attractive, finding such a combination is not easy. In the case of artesunate and artemether, the apparent elimination half-life is about one hour, meaning that after 4 hours almost the full dose given is eliminated from the body. Most of the partner drugs selected for ACTs have a reasonably long elimination half-life. Mefloquine has a mean elimination half-life of 2 to 4 weeks, lumefantrine 3-6 days and amodiaquine, 5.2 ± 1.7 minutes, but its major metabolite has a long elimination half-life. Sulfadoxine-pyrimethamine (SP) has a long but variable elimination half-life ranging from 40 to a few hundred hours. In contrast sulfamethoxypyrazine, an alternative to sulfadoxine has a rather stable elimination half-life of 65 hours and a low protein binding property affecting the dosage possibilities. In the fixed dose combination Co-Arinate^R (Dafra Pharma) the sulfonamide drug sulfalene (sulfamethoxypyrazine), with a rather constant elimination half-life of 65 hours to 85 hours, is combined with pyrimethamine (which has an elimination half-life of 100 hours) and built into a single tablet with artesunate. In spite of the elimination half-life limitation for all ACTs, the various partner drugs are most efficacious when used in combination with artemether or artesunate.

6. Role of artesunate with Fansidar^R and artesunate with Metakelfin^R: for malaria, for infectious diseases

In the late 1960s, new long-acting sulfonamides were being developed. Sulfadoxine was set to replace sulfadimethoxine (Madribon, Roche) as an antimicrobial agent but it was never introduced for reasons of relative toxicity and a wide variation in elimination half-life (varying from 40 to 400h). The combination in an FDC tablet with pyrimethamine offered new possibilities. Roche successively introduced this combination as Fansidar^R in nearly every malaria endemic country, where it became very popular for both curative and prophylactic use. Sulfamethoxypyrazine was the result of one of the first in-depth efforts in the field of structure activity to make a better or optimal molecule based on physicochemical data. The resulting molecule completely fulfilled the theoretical expectations: a long elimination half-life (65-85h), highly soluble in water and a relatively low protein binding (about 60%). Such a molecule would have the property of penetrating all body fluids in adequate concentrations, which was not the case for sulfadoxine. Sulfamethoxypyrazine was successfully introduced in most European countries. The FDC combination with pyrimethamine under the brand name Metakelfin^R was introduced in Africa in the early 1970s. It is still available as a registered European drug in Italy, the licence being held by Pfizer. It was marketed only in a limited number of African countries.

7. Rationale for artenimol and derivatives in the treatment of schistosomiasis

The *in vitro* and *in vivo* evidence that artemether has an effect on *Schistosoma* parasites came from Xiao and Catto in 1989. They showed that the artemisinin related compound is particularly active against the juvenile, 2- to 3- week old, parasites (Xiao and Catto., 1989). Their work was later confirmed in a limited number of *in vivo* and *in vitro* studies conducted on *Schistosoma* species with more artemisinin derivatives (Xiao et al., 2006; Utzinger et al., 2001; Utzinger et al., 2007). Whereas praziquantel showed highest efficacy against adult parasites, artemether and artesunate were found to be more effective against juvenile forms. This might have an impact on the fact that artemether prevents young forms from developing into adult worms of egg-laying capacity. It was speculated that a sequential therapy of artemether and praziquantel could be useful since they address both populations. Moreover, patients usually carry both populations of parasites in high endemic areas. Unfortunately in the experimental studies, high doses of artemether were given to see appropriate effects. Doses of 200 mg/kg are not realistic and cannot be applied to human beings. The meaning of the results obtained is therefore of limited value. Malaria parasites are killed with doses of 2 mg per kg per day for 5 consecutive days in monotherapy; in combination therapies, about 4 mg per kg per day for just 3 days is sufficient.

How does artemisinin affect the *Schistosomas* parasite? Scanning electron microscopy showed that the tegumentum of the parasites was damaged by the schistosomula and this effect lasts a few days. However, the intimate mechanism is not known. The mechanism of action on *Schistosoma* parasites should be compared to the Chinese study in which the researchers used electron microscopy to detect the damage caused by a single oral dose of artesunate in plasmodia causing progressive destruction of membrane systems as explained above (Ellis et al., 1985).

Clinical possibilities were studied with artenimol derivatives against *S. japonicum*. The studies confirmed the theoretical possibility of using these substances as drugs, including as prophylactic drugs. No difference was seen between artemether and artesunate. This is somewhat surprising since not all properties are shared by those compounds. Artemether requires a liver enzyme for its transformation into DHA whereas artesunate will spontaneously generate DHA under the influence of non-specific esterases from the blood. Artesunate and artemether are no longer to be used for the treatment of malaria in monotherapies for fear of malaria parasites developing resistance. Artemisinin-based combinations therapies (ACTs) have replaced the former. The duration of treatment with ACTs is now restricted to 48 hours (sometimes to 72 hours) and the daily dose is increased (doubled) to about 4 mg per kg body weight. In addition, it might be speculated that the ACT partner drug also plays a role in the process of killing the *Schistosomas*. This is of particular importance in areas where both diseases are endemic. It is most likely that patients carrying *Schistosoma* parasites will be treated with an ACT for acute malaria, sometimes several times per year, with a resulting impact on *Schistosoma* carriage too.

8. Clinical efficacy of artesunate and Fansidar^R for *Schistosomiasis haematobium*

New drugs are only meaningful if clinical proof of efficacy can be established. There are few known studies from Africa that investigate the effect of either artesunate or artemether on any of the *Schistosoma* species. Promising results were obtained but the WHO ban on these drugs for malaria monotherapy jeopardised further work. In 2007 two interesting papers were published. The first publication by Boulanger et al., 2007 studied the effect of the ACT artesunate-SP co-blister in *S. haematobium* in children under 6 years old. The children were treated for malaria but they had *S. haematobium* infections at the same time. The results were impressive: Twenty-seven children who entered a clinical trial of antimalaria treatment were excreting *S. haematobium* eggs in their urine on the first day of treatment. Fifteen children received a combination of a single dose of sulfadoxine-pyrimethamine together with three daily doses of artesunate (4 mg/kg); the remaining 12 children received three daily doses of amodiaquine and artesunate. The overall cure rate and reduction in the mean number of excreted eggs at 28 days post treatment were 92.6% and 94.5%, respectively. The authors concluded that "Our findings indicate that artesunate, in addition to being a very effective treatment for uncomplicated malaria, can also sharply reduce the *S. haematobium* loads harboured by pre-school African children".
The publication by Adam et al., 2008 almost coincided with the one published by Boulanger and colleagues. In a small study in eastern Sudan, the effects of the treatment of uncomplicated, *Plasmodium falciparum* malaria with artesunate–sulfamethoxypyrazine–pyrimethamine (AS+SMP) and artemether–lumefantrine (AT+LU) on co-infections with *Schistosoma mansoni* were investigated. Faecal samples from 14 of the 306 patients screened on presentation, at the start of a clinical trial of antimalarial treatment, were found to contain *Schistosoma mansoni* eggs. For the treatment of their malaria, the 14 egg-positive cases, who were aged 6–40 years (mean 13.7 years), were each subsequently treated with three tablets of a fixed combination of AS+SMP, with a 12h- (six patients) or 24h-interval (five patients) between each tablet, or with six doses of AT+LU given over 3 days. When checked 28 and 29 days after the initiation of treatment, all 14 patients were found stool-negative for *Schistosoma* eggs. These results indicate that AS+SMP and AT+LU are apparently very effective treatments not only for uncomplicated, *P. falciparum* malaria but also for *S. mansoni* infections.

9. Clinical efficacy of artesunate and Metakelfin^R (Co-Arinate^R) in the treatment of *Schistosomiasis haematobium* in schoolchildren in Mali

The observations described above led to a multicentre study in which a large population of schoolchildren infected with *S. haematobium* was studied (Sissoko et al., 2009). The objective was to determine the efficacy of the antimalarial artemisinin-based FDC combination therapy artesunate-sulfamethoxypyrazine-pyrimethamine (AS+SMP), administered in doses used for malaria, to treat *Schistosoma haematobium* in school-aged children. The study was conducted in Djalakorodji, a peri-urban area of Bamako, Mali, using a double-blind setup in which AS+SMP was compared with praziquantel (PZQ). Urine samples were examined for *Schistosoma haematobium* on days -1, 0, 28 and 29. Detection of haematuria, and haematological and biochemical exams were conducted on day 0 and day 28. Clinical exams were performed on days 0, 1, 2 and 28. A total of 800 children were included in the trial. The cure rate obtained without viability testing was 43.9% in the AS+SMP group versus 53% in the PZQ group (Chi2 = 6.44, p = 0.011). Egg reduction rates were 95.6% with PZQ in comparison with 92.8% with AS+SMP (p = 0.096). The proportion of participants who experienced adverse events related to the medication was 0.5% (2/400) in AS+SMP treated children compared to 2.3% (9/399) in the PZQ group (p = 0.033). Abdominal pain and vomiting were the most frequent adverse events in both treatment arms. All adverse events were categorised as mild. The study demonstrates that PZQ was more effective than AS+SMP for treating *Schistosoma haematobium*. However, the safety and tolerability profile of AS+SMP was similar to that seen with PZQ. The authors conclude that their findings warrant further investigations to determine the dose/efficacy/safety pattern of AS+SMP in the treatment of *Schistosoma* infections.

10. Clinical efficacy of Co-Arinate[R] on *Schistosomiasis mansoni* in schoolchildren in Kenya

An open-label randomised trial in Rarieda district of western Kenya was conducted with primary investigator Dr C. Obonyo. Schoolchildren (aged 6–15 years) who had *Schistosoma mansoni* infection were enrolled. Children were assigned to receive artesunate (100 mg) with sulfalene (also known as sulfamethoxypyrazine; 250 mg) plus pyrimethamine (12.5 mg) as one dose every 24 h for 3 days (administered as Co-Arinate[R] tablets) or one dose of praziquantel (40 mg/kg per day). The primary efficacy endpoint was the number of participants cured 28 days after treatment. Between October and December, 2009, 212 children were enrolled and assigned to receive artesunate with sulfalene plus pyrimethamine (n = 106) or praziquantel (n = 106). Sixty-nine patients (65%) were cured in the praziquantel treatment group compared with 15 (14%) in the artesunate with sulfalene plus pyrimethamine treatment group (p<0·0001). Adverse events were less common in patients taking artesunate with sulfalene plus pyrimethamine than in those taking praziquantel (22% [n = 23] vs 49% [n = 52], p<0·0001), but no drug-related serious adverse events occurred. The standard treatment with praziquantel is more effective than artesunate with sulfalene plus pyrimethamine in the treatment of children with *S. mansoni* infection in western Kenya (Obonyo et al.,2010).

The results or cure rate in the artesunate-sulfamethoxypyrazine-pyrimethamine group in the two studies above contrast strongly (43.9% versus 14%). Many questions could be raised, in particular about dosage scheme. Whereas Sissoko and colleagues gave the drug as a single dose (as is the case with praziquantel), Dr Obonyo spread the dosing over 48 hours (nearly 3 days). Is the dosing schedule determinant for the contrast in cure rate? Is it the difference in *Schistosoma* species? But why then the excellent results in the study by Adam et al. and in the study by Boulanger et al.? To address this question, a limited additional study described below was conducted by Obonyo and published as an abstract at ASTMH, 2010. Seventy-three children were randomised, receiving either praziquantel 40 mg per kg as a single dose or artesunate-sulfamethoxypyrazine-pyrimethamine in a single dose of 12 mg per kg body weight for artesunate. Cure and egg rate reduction were determined 28 days after treatment. Overall, 25 children (74%) were cured in the praziquantel group compared with 25 (64%) in the AS+SMP group (p = 0.4). Egg reduction rate was comparable (83% vs 96% p = 0.34) after praziquantel and AS+SMP respectively. Adverse events were significantly fewer among AS+SMP recipients (10% versus 29%, p = 0.038) and there were no drug-related serious adverse events. The authors conclude from their second study that there is no difference in response between the two drugs. Unfortunately, overall cure rates remain below expectations since praziquantel has only a 75% cure rate.

In conclusion, it appears that some ACT drugs can be used for the treatment of schistosomiasis, either caused by *haematobium* or *mansoni* species. Dosing schemes seem to be important. Also, it ought to be investigated whether repeated dosing has an additional beneficial impact on the elimination of the parasites. A question not answered in this discussion is the geography of the events. Mali is thousands of miles away from the borders of Lake Victoria in Kenya. Are there different populations with variable sensitivity?

11. Discussion and conclusions

The few clinical studies point to the additional beneficial effect of malaria treatment, administered as an ACT in fixed-dose combination in a population prone to the frequent occurrence of both malaria and schistosomiasis. It remains to be seen whether the broad-scale use of the ACTs will spontaneously impact on the incidence of schistosomiasis. Will this effect be seen with all currently existing ACTs? The following combinations are commonly being used: artesunate in an FDC with amodiaquine: artesunate in a co-blister with SP tablets: and Artemether - lumefantrine FDC tablets:. The last combination is the most widely used product since it is heavily supported by the actions of the Global Fund for the elimination of malaria in Africa. Artesunate with amodiaquine is less popular and causes more side effects, specifically due to amodiaquine. The co-blister with artesunate tablets and SP tablets has now become obsolete and its use is very restricted. This is the current situation in Africa. The FDC Co-Arinate^{R} where the partner drug is sulfamethoxypyrazine with pyrimethamine is most popular in the non-governmental distribution chains.

The variability of the results of ACTs on schistomiasis cure rate is somewhat puzzling. Apparently the dosing scheme has a drastic effect on the treatment outcome because in the limited additional study by Obonyo et al. it could be demonstrated that *S. mansoni* was properly killed when the same dosing regimen as that of Sissoko was followed. At this moment, a large study to confirm these finding is in preparation.

Where do we go from here? From an epidemiological point of view, the following question is raised: Will broad scale malaria treatment with ACTs impact on the incidence and morbidity of schistosomiasis? Time will tell, but additional properly conducted studies ought to be set up to investigate the possibility of further refining treatment regimens with ACTs. If resistance to praziquantel continues to increase, Africa will face a serious new medical problem. The recently published studies do not provide any guarantee of decent efficacy for praziquantel. The fact that this is not the case - as expressed in the studies by Sissoko and Obonyo in which the average resistance to praziquantel is about 35% - is worrying. ACTs as such are not the perfect answer either, but they have some impact. Their optimised dosing scheme could well become a true alternative to the standard drug. In additional, sequential therapy with praziquantel ought to be envisaged.

12. References

Adam I., Elhardello O.A., Elhadi M.O., Abdalla E., Elmardi K.A., Jansen F.H. The anti*Schistosomal* efficacies of artesunate-sulfamethoxypyrazine-pyrimethamine and artemether-lumefantrine administered as treatment for uncomplicated, Plasmodium falciparum malaria. Annals of Tropical Medicine and Parasitology, 2008.

Angelucci F, Basso A, Bellelli A, Brunori M, Pica ML, Valle C. The anti-*Schistosomal* drug praziquantel is an adenosine antagonist. Parasitology 2007 Aug;134(Pt 9):1215-21.

Boulanger D, Dieng Y, Cisse B, Remoue F, Capuano F, Dieme JL, et al., Anti*Schistosomal* efficacy of artesunate combination therapies administered as curative treatments for malaria attacks. Trans R Soc Trop Med Hyg 2007 Feb;101(2):113-6.

Chen DJ, Fu LF, Shao PP, Wu FZ, Fan CZ, Shu H, Ren CS, Sheng XL Studies on anti*Schistosomal* activity of qinghaosu in experimental therapy. Zhong Hui Yi Xue Zha Zhi, 1980, 80 422-428.

Doenhoff MJ, Cioli D, Utzinger J. Praziquantel: mechanisms of action, resistance and new derivatives for schistosomiasis. Curr Opin Infect Dis 2008 Dec;21(6):659-67.

Eckstein-Ludwig U, Webb RJ, Van G, I, East JM, Lee AG, Kimura M, O'Neill,P.M.; Bray,P.G.; Ward,S.A.; Krishna,S. Artemisinins target the SERCA of Plasmodium falciparum. Nature 2003 Aug 21;424(6951):957-61.

Efferth T, Dunstan H, Sauerbrey A, Miyachi H, Chitambar CR. The anti-malarial artesunate is also active against cancer. Int.J.Oncol. 18[4], 767-773. 2001.

Efferth T, Romero MR, Wolf DG, Stamminger T, Marin JJ, Marschall M. The antiviral activities of artemisinin and artesunate. Clin Infect Dis 2008 Sep 15;47(6):804-11.

Efferth T. Willmar Schwabe Award 2006: antiplasmodial and antitumor activity of artemisinin--from bench to bedside. Planta Med 2007 Apr;73(4):299-309.

Ellis DS, Li ZL, Gu HM, Peters W, Robinson BL, Tovey G, et al., The chemotherapy of roden malaria, XXXIX. Ultrastructural changes following treatment with artemisinine of Plasmodium berghei infection in mice, with observations of the localisation of [3H]-dihydroartemisinine in P. falciparum in vitro. Ann Trop Med Parasitol 1985 Aug;79(4):367-74.

Fallon PG, Sturrock RF, Niang AC, Doenhoff MJ. Short report: diminished susceptibility to praziquantel in a Senegal isolate of *Schistosoma* mansoni. Am J Trop Med Hyg 1995 Jul;53(1):61-2.

Fischer-Betz R, Schneider M. [Antimalarials. A treatment option for every lupus patient!?]. Z Rheumatol 2009 Sep;68(7):584, 586-4, 590.

Gryseels B, Mbaye A, de Vlas SJ, Stelma FF, Guisse F, Van LL, et al., Are poor responses to praziquantel for the treatment of *Schistosoma* mansoni infections in Senegal due to resistance? An overview of the evidence. Trop Med Int Health 2001 Nov;6(11): 864-73.

Hotez PJ, Molyneux DH. Tropical anemia: one of Africa's great killers and a rationale for linking malaria and neglected tropical disease control to achieve a common goal. PLoS Negl Trop Dis 2008;2(7):e270.

Ismail M, Metwally A, Farghaly A, Bruce J, Tao LF, Bennett JL. Characterisation of isolates of *Schistosoma* mansoni from Egyptian villagers that tolerate high doses of praziquantel. Am J Trop Med Hyg 1996 Aug;55(2):214-8.

Ismail MM, Taha SA, Farghaly AM, el-Azony AS. Laboratory induced resistance to praziquantel in experimental schistosomiasis. J Egypt Soc Parasitol 1994 Dec;24(3):685-95.

Jansen FH, Soomro SA. Chemical instability determines the biological action of the artemisinins. Curr Med Chem 2007;14(30):3243-59.

Le WJ, You JQ, Yang YQ, Mei Jy, Guo HF, Yang HZ, Zhnag CW. Studies on the efficacy of arthemether in experimental schistosomiasis. 1982 Acta Pharm Sin 17: 187-193.

Lin AJ, Lee M, Klayman DL. Antimalarial activity of new water-soluble dihydroartemisinin derivatives. 2. Stereospecificity of the ether side chain. J Med Chem 1989 Jun;32(6):1249-52.

Matthaiou DK, Panos G, Adamidi ES, Falagas ME (2008). "Albendazole versus Praziquantel in the Treatment of Neurocysticercosis: A Meta-analysis of Comparative Trials". PLoS Negl Trop Dis 2 (3): e194. doi: 10.1371/journal.pntd.0000194. PMC 2265431. PMID 18335068. http://www.plosntds.org/article/info:doi/10.1371/journal.pntd.0000194.

Obonyo CO, Muok EM, Mwinzi PN. Efficacy of artesunate with sulfalene plus pyrimethamine versus praziquantel for treatment of Schistosoma mansoni in Kenyan children: an open-label randomised controlled trial. Lancet Infect.Dis. DOI:10.1016/S1473-3099(10)70161-4. 2010.

Obonyo C.O., Muok E.M., Mwinzi P.N. Efficacy of a single dose of artesunate plus sulfamethoxypyrazine/pyrimethamine versus praziquantel for treatment of *Schistosoma* mansoni in Kenyan children Abstract ASTMH, 2010

Shen C, Kim J, Lee JK, et al., (June 2007). "Collection of Clonorchis sinensis adult worms from infected humans after praziquantel treatment". Korean J. Parasitol. 45 (2): 149–52. doi:10.3347/kjp.2007.45.2.149. PMC 2526309. PMID 17570980.

Sissoko MS, Dabo A, Traore H, Diallo M, Traore B, Konate D, et al., Efficacy of artesunate + sulfamethoxypyrazine/pyrimethamine versus praziquantel in the treatment of Schistosoma haematobium in children. PLoS ONE 2009;4(10):e6732.

Soomro SA, Konkimalla VB, Langenberg T, Mahringer A, Horwedel C, Holenya P, et al., Design of novel artemisinin-like derivates with cytotoxic and anti-angiogenesis properties. Journal of Cellular and Molecular Medicine 2010.

Stelma FF, Talla I, Sow S, Kongs A, Niang M, Polman K, et al., Efficacy and side effects of praziquantel in an epidemic focus of *Schistosoma* mansoni. Am J Trop Med Hyg 1995 Aug;53(2):167-70.

Tchuenté LA, Shaw DJ, Polla L, Cioli D, Vercruysse J (December 2004). "Efficacy of praziquantel against *Schistosoma* haematobium infection in children". Am. J. Trop. Med. Hyg. 71 (6): 778–82. PMID 15642971.

http://www.cartercenter. org/health/schistosomiasis/index.html The Carter Center Schistosomiasis Control Program',

"Intestinal Flukes: Treatment & Medication". http://emedicine.medscape.com/article/ 219662-treatment.

Utzinger J, Chollet J, You J, Mei J, Tanner M, et al., (2001) Effect of combined treatment with praziquantel and artemether on *Schistosoma* japonicum and *Schistosoma* mansoni in experimentally infected animals - Acta Trop 1; 80(1): 9–18.

Utzinger J, Chollet J, You J, Mei J, Tanner M, Xiao S. Effect of combined treatment with praziquantel and artemether on *Schistosoma* japonicum and *Schistosoma* mansoni in experimentally infected animals. Acta Trop 2001 Sep 1;80(1):9-18.

Utzinger J, Keiser J, Shuhua X, Tanner M, Singer BH. Combination chemotherapy of schistosomiasis in laboratory studies and clinical trials. Antimicrob Agents Chemother 2003 May;47(5):1487-95.

Utzinger J, Xiao SH, Tanner M, Keiser J (2007) Artemisinins for schistosomiasis and beyond. Curr Opin Invest Drugs 2007 8(2): 105–116.

Xiao SH, Catto BA (1989) In vitro and in vivo studies of the effect of artemether on *Schistosoma* mansoni. Antimicrob Agents Chemother 33: 1557–62.

Xiao SH, Utzinger J, Chollet J, Tanner M (2006) Effect of artemether administered alone or in combination with praziquantel to mice infected with Plasmodium berghei or *Schistosoma* mansoni or both. - Int J Parasitol 36(8): 957–64.

Xiao S, Yang Y, You Q, Utzinger J, Guo H, Peiying J, et al., Potential long-term toxicity of repeated orally administered doses of artemether in rats. Am J Trop Med Hyg 2002 Jan;66(1):30-4.

3

The Use of Brazilian Medicinal Plants to Combat *Schistosoma mansoni*

Silmara Marques Allegretti, Claudineide Nascimento Fernandes de Oliveira, Rosimeire Nunes de Oliveira, Tarsila Ferraz Frezza and Vera Lúcia Garcia Rehder
Universidade Estadual de Campinas
Brazil

1. Introduction

Human schistosomiasis, which is caused by trematodes of the genus *Schistosoma*, is considered one of the most prevalent and debilitating neglected diseases in tropical and subtropical areas, being endemic to approximately 76 countries and territories and affecting more than 207 million people worldwide. About 800 million people live in infection risk areas and 280,000 die every year due to this disease (Engels et al., 2002, Steinmann et al., 2006).

There are six main species of Schistosoma that can infect humans: *S. mansoni, S. hematobium, S. japonicum, S. intercalatum, S. mekongi* and *S. malayensis*. Among these, only *S. mansoni* is found in Brazil.

S. mansoni schistosomiasis was probably brought to Brazil by the Atlantic slave trade. Afterwards, migration flows spread the disease from the shore to the interior of the country, including areas containing its intermediate hosts, planorbides of the genus *Biomphalaria* (Paraense, 1986, Coura & Amaral, 2004). According to Paraense (1966, 1981), ten species and one subspecies of *Biomphalaria* can be found in the country, three of them being natural intermediate hosts (*B. glabrata, B. tenagophila, B. straminea*) and two having already been experimentally infected (*B. amazonica* and *B. peregrina*).

The life cycle of *S. mansoni* consists of an asexual reproduction stage in the intermediate hosts and a sexual reproduction stage in the definite ones. Under favourable conditions, it lasts 80 days (Katz & Almeida, 2003, Ministério da Saúde, 2005).

Nowadays, there are 25 million people living in endemic areas in Brazil, and 4 to 6 million are infected. It is the most affected country in the Americas (Lambertucci, 2010, World Health Organization [WHO], 2010). According to data provided by Brazil's Ministry of Health, there are cases of the disease in 19 states, from Rio Grande do Norte to Bahia and in the interior of Espírito Santo and Minas Gerais (Ministério da Saúde, 2005). Figure 1 shows the distribution of *S. mansoni* schistosomiasis in Brazil.

A major problem in countries where schistosomiasis is endemic is the control of the disease. In this regard, isolated or combined measures could be taken, such as the control of the intermediate hosts using molluscicides, improvement of basic sanitation and water supply conditions, sanitary education of exposed populations, individual or mass treatment in high-prevalence areas, individual protection against the penetration of cercariae, and development of a vaccine (Coura & Amaral 2004).

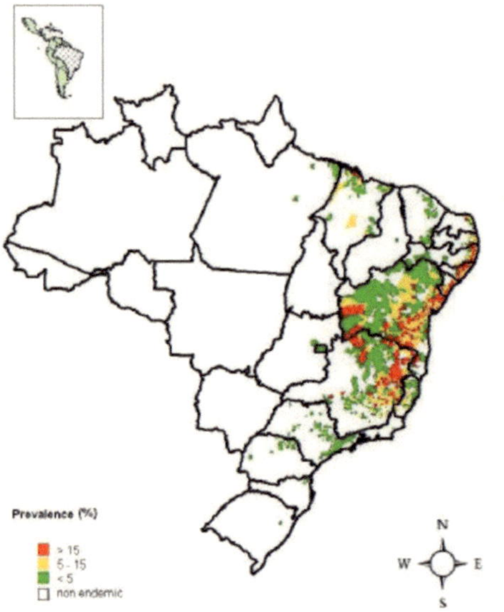

Fig. 1. Distribution of *S. mansoni* schistosomiasis in Brazil. Source: Ministério da Saúde (2005).

However, such control measures have many drawbacks: the wide dissemination of the intermediate hosts, their defence mechanisms against molluscicides, as well as the high costs and low efficiency of that sort of control, the high costs associated with the implementation of adequate sanitary and water supply conditions and the intense contact of rural population with contaminated fresh water, the long time needed for sanitary education, individual or mass treatments can be effective in reducing the morbidity, but they do not prevent reinfections, and patients can develop tolerance and resistance to them, individual protection is unlikely, except for specific groups of exposed people, finally, at the present moment there is no effective vaccine in the treatment for schistosomiasis (Coura & Amaral, 2004).

Despite the fact that the distribution of schistosomiasis has changed along the time, the number of infected people or people at risk of infection has not changed. Not even the efforts carried out for more than a century to control schistosomiasis by means of schistosomicidal drugs have prevented it from being one of the most prevalent diseases in the world (King, 2009). Albeit all the research conducted so far, there are no effective vaccines against parasitic diseases. Therefore, medication treatment is still the most efficient method (Date *et al.*, 2007).

The treatment for *S. mansoni* schistosomiasis is based on the use of praziquantel, a low-cost anthelmintic highly effective against all *Schistosoma* species that may cause infection in humans. Despite its benefits, some deficiences have been reported. As a result, it is necessary to develop new effective schistosomicidal drugs.

Regarding *S. mansoni* schistosomiasis, the World Health Organisation (WHO) points out the need for permanent research on the development of a vaccine (WHO, 1998). Furthermore, current drugs need to be improved, or new ones should be developed. Nevertheless, the

cost for developing safe and effective drugs is extremely high, which leads to a dim perspective on the introduction of new schistosomicides (Cioli et al., 1995). As a result, research with medicinal plants constitutes a very viable alternative.
In this scenario, several studies and researches on natural bioactive products extracted from plants and used against schistosomiasis have been carried out in the search for a new medicine that can replace praziquantel or complement it (Xiao & Catto, 1989, Molgaard et al., 2001, Mahmoud et al., 2002, Mohamed et al., 2005, Shaohong et al., 2005, Penido et al., 2008, Moraes et al., 2010).
Taking into account the great variety of plants that haven't yet been therapeutically studied to combat *S. mansoni* schistosomiasis, in recent years our research group started a multidisciplinary project to perform *in vitro* screening of extracts from native and exotic plants commonly cultivated in Brazil.

2. Chemotherapy against schistosomiasis

It is believed that the use of chemotherapy against schistosomiasis started with Christopherson (1918), who reported a successful treatment for the urinary form of the disease (caused by *S. haematobium*) with tartar emetic. After that, several other antimony compounds were introduced for clinical use (Cioli et al., 1995, Parise-Filho & Silveira, 2001), and they were the most used medicines until the Second World War (Brindley, 1994). However, despite having been the basis of the treatment for schistosomiasis for around 50 years and having been effective against *S. mansoni, S. haematobium* and *S. japonicum*, the clinical use of antimony compounds was suspended on account of their severe side and toxic effects and patients' low tolerance to them (Cunha, 1982, Cioli et al., 1995, Silva, 1997, Cioli, 1998, Novaes et al., 1999).
Before antimony compounds fell into disuse, researches carried out in the 1920's showed activity of emetine and 2,3-dehydroemetine, which were used in the treatment for amoebiasis, against *S. japonicum*. Although emetine has shown a relatively good efficiency, the concentrations needed for activity against *S. japonicum* were two times higher than the required in the treatment for amoebiasis, reaching the toxicity limit. On the other hand, 2,3-dehydroemetine, in spite of being less toxic and having light side effects in comparison with emetine, fell into disuse because of its complicated administration (Blanc & Nosny, 1968, Cioli et al., 1995).
After the Second World War, new drugs were produced, and they were less toxic, more active, free from metals and orally administered (Cunha, 1982, Cioli et al., 1995). Lucanthone (1-{[2-(diethylamino)ethyl]amino}-4-methyl-9*H*-thioxanthen-9-one), or Miracil D, described for the first time in 1932, was the first orally administered schistosomicidal drug introduced in medical practice, being effective against both *S. mansoni* and *S. haematobium*. Its side effects were usually limited to nausea and vomiting, but severe effects on the heart and central nervous system were later reported (Kikuth & Gonnert, 1948).
In 1955, an organophosphate insecticide (2.2,2-trichloro-1-hydroxyenthyl dimethyl phosphonate) was introduced under the general name trichlorphon (Lorenz et al., 1955), later changed to metrifonate. Then, in 1962, the possibility of extending its use to helminths came into consideration, and preliminary studies in humans provided evidence of therapeutic activity against schistosomiasis, ancylostomiasis, ascariasis, trichuriasis and onchocerciasis (Cerf et al., 1962, Davis & Bailey, 1969, Salazar et al., 1969). However, this compound has only proven effective in the treatment for urinary schistosomiasis (Jewsbury

et al., 1977). Therefore, at the present day metrifonate (Bilarcil) is still used in such treatment, but it has to be administered in three doses, and that is its main drawback (Korte et al., 1986, WHO, 1993, Cioli et al., 1995, Berge et al., 2011).

At the beginning of the 1960's, it was reported that a broad-spectrum antimicrobial called nitrofuran, along its derivatives, had shown schistosomicide activity, more specifically, anti-*S. japonicum* effect. Nonetheless, its suboptimal activity, high toxicity, and carcinogenic and mutagenic effects led to its use being stopped, and the same happened to its derivatives, some of which didn't even come to be used in the treatment for human schistosomiasis (Werbel, 1970, Robinson et al., 1970, Hulbert et al., 1973).

A very important moment in the therapeutics of schistosomiasis came after the introduction of niridazole (1-(5-nitro-2-thiazolil)imidazolidin-2-one) in 1964 (Lambert & Stauffer, 1964) and hycanthone (1-*N*-*b*-diethyl-amino-ethyl-amino-4-(hydroxymethyl)-9-thioxanthenone) in 1965 (Rosi et al., 1965). Niridazole (Ambilhar) showed low activity against *S. japonicum*, moderate activity against *S. mansoni* and very high activity against *S. haematobium*, whereas hycanthone (Etrenol), the main metabolite of lucanthone, proved effective against *S. mansoni*, *S. haematobium* and *S. rodhaini*. However, these drugs had some issues, such as the number of doses and various severe side effects (high toxicity in the central nervous system, kidneys and liver, in addition to mutagenic, carcinogenic and teratogenic effects). Furthermore, they were not considered safe enough for being used in large scale in endemic regions. Consequently, they were no longer used in the medication therapy of schistosomiasis (Fontanilles, 1969, Cioli et al., 1995).

At the end of the 1960's, a series of 2-aminomethyl-tetra-hydroquinoline derivatives with schistosomicidal activity were described, the most promising being 2-N-isopropylaminomethyl-7-nitro-l,2,3,4-tetrahydroquinoline, named UK-3883. The hydroxylation of the 6-methyl group by *Aspergillus sclerotiorum* generated UK-4271, later called oxamniquine (Mansil/Vansil) and described for the first time by Richards and Foster in 1969 (Cioli et al., 1993, 1995).

Preclinical assays showed the schistosomicide potencial of oxamniquine against *S. mansoni*, especially males (Foster & Cheetham, 1973).

Clinical assays carried out in Brazil with an orally administered single dose of 15 to 20 mg/kg have shown cure rates up to 90%, as well as good tolerance by patients. These results allowed oxamniquine to be extensively used, and it was included in Brazilian programmes for the control of *S. mansoni* schistosomiasis (Almeida-Machado, 1982, Foster, 1987, Cioli et al., 1993).

Further studies indicated some disadvantages in the use of oxamniquine, though. Since this drug has no cell specificity, which results in undesired peripheral toxicity, there are some side effects on the central nervous system (Davis, 1993, Soyez et al., 1996). It was also observed that oxamniquine showed low activity in the period between the 3rd and the 9th week of infection, which coincided with the egg production stage (Jordan et al., 1993, Frézard & Melo, 1997). Moreover, there were reports of pacients infected with *S. mansoni* who were resistent to the treatment (Cioli et al., 1992).

At the beginning of the 1970's, pyrazinoisoquinoline derivatives were tested as antiparasitic drugs (Andrews, 1981). After many compounds were synthesised, 2-cyclohexylcarbonyl-1,2,3,6,7,1lb-hexahydro-4H-pyrazino[2,1-a]isoquinoline-4-one, first called EMBAY-8440 and then praziquantel (Biltricide/Cysticide/Cesol/Distocid/Pyquiton), was considered the most promising (Cioli et al., 1995). Discovered in 1975 (Andrews et al., 1983, Day et al.,

1992), this drug was initially used against cestodes and limited to veterinary cases (Thomas & Gonnert, 1975).

The first studies with animals infected with *Schistosoma* sp. were performed in 1977, when schistosomicidal activity was detected (Gonnert & Andrews, 1977) and attention was drawn to the large variety of possibilities offered by worms of that genus. Further studies reported activity of praziquantel against *S. haematobium, S. japonicum, S. intercalatum* and *S. matheei,* other species of trematodes (*Opisthorchis sinensis, O. viverrini, Paragonimus* spp., *Fasciolopsis buski, Heterophyes heterophyes* and *Metagonimus yokogawaii*) and cestodes (*Taenia solium, T. saginata, Hymenolepis nana, H. diminuta, Diphyllobotrium latum* and *D. pacificum*) (Webbe & James, 1977, Wegner, 1984, Bouree, 1991, Utzinger et al., 2003, Shuhua, 2005, Jeziorski & Greenberg, 2006, Shaohong et al., 2005).

Preclinical assays have also proven the efficiency of praziquantel in the treatment for 5-6-week infections, but failures were reported in cases of 1 to 5-week infections (Gonnet & Andrews, 1977, Webbe, 1977, Xiao et al., 1985, Sabah et al., 1986).

The first clinical studies took place in 1978 in cooperation with WHO, in endemic regions for *S. mansoni, S. haematobium, S. japonicum* and *S. intercalatum* (Katz et al., 1979, Davis et al., 1979, Ishizaki et al., 1979). In 1984, cure rates of 75% to 85% were reported for *S. haematobium,* 63% to 85% for *S. mansoni,* 80% to 90% for *S. japonicum,* 89% for *S. intercalatum,* and 60% to 80% for simultaneous infections with *S. mansoni* and *S. haematobium* (Wegner, 1984). It was also found out that praziquantel was well tolerated by patients of all ages with different clinical forms of schistosomiasis (Frohberg, 1984, Bassily et al., 1985), having light side effects on them (Cioli et al., 1995). Other studies indicated low toxicity and no mutagenic risks (Frohberg, 1984, Kramers et al., 1991).

Those screenings clearly established praziquantel as the drug of choice in the treatment for schistosomiasis (Cioli & Pica-Mattoccia, 2002). In addition, it was the first anthelmintic to fulfil the requirements of WHO (Silva et al., 2005).

After the development of praziquantel, there was little progress in the therapeutics of *S. mansoni* schistosomiasis.

In 1976, Striebel described the use of amoscanate (4-isothiocyanato-4'-nitrodiphenylamine) against helminthic diseases. At that time its wide activity range was confirmed, as it was used against most *Schistosoma* species, filariae and gastrointestinal nematodes (Bueding et al., 1976). Amoscanate was tested in humans infected with S. japonicum, and the cure rates were as high as 92%. However, this drug fell into disuse in view of hepatotoxicity (Hubei Nithiocyaminum Coodination Research Group, 1980, Cioli et al., 1995).

Also in 1976, a dithiolethione derivative called oltipraz (Barrau et al., 1977), active against *S. mansoni, S. intercalatum* and *S. haematobium* (Leroy et al., 1978, Gentilini et al., 1980, Katz et al., 1984), was synthesised. Preclinical assays confirmed the elimination of *S. mansoni* (Bueding et al., 1982), and clinical assays showed cure rates between 80% and 95% for this species. Photo-onycholysis was the most severe side effect observed, leading to the suspension of the drug in 1984 (Cioli et al., 1995).

Still in 1976, Nelson and Pellegrino (1976) described the schistosomicidal activity of alkylaminoalkanethio-sulfuric acids for the first time. Preclinical assays with *S. mansoni* provided evidence of preferential activity against adult females (Penido et al., 1999), but so far no clinical assays have been carried out.

In 1978, screening of benzodiazepine derivatives showed that some of the compounds of this group have strong schistosomicidal activity, in particular (+)-5-(-o-chlorophenyl)-1,3-dihydro-3-methyl-7-nitro-2H-1,4-benzodiazepine-2-one, which was named Ro 11-3128

(Stohler, 1978). Preclinical studies proved it to be effective against *S. mansoni* and *S. haematobium* (Brickle & Andrews, 1995) and clinical studies confirmed its schistosomicidal activity, but some side effects, including strong sedative effect, have discouraged its development (Pax et al., 1978, Baard et al., 1979).
In the 1980's, derivatives of artemisinin (which is extracted from *Artemisia annua*) were used as anti-*Schistosoma* sp. for the first time by the Chineses, who demonstrated that the administration of this compound in animals experimentally infected with *S. japonicum* reduced their worm burden (Chen et al., 1980).
Such derivatives, which include arteether, artemisone and artelinic acid, among others, have been extensively used in the control of malaria. They are generically known as artemisinins and were developed in the 1970's (Krishna et al., 2008).
In 1982, it was shown that larval stages of *S. japonicum* were susceptible to artemisinins (Le et al., 1982). Further studies confirmed the schistosomicidal activity of both artesunate and artemether, the latter reaching cure rates of 99% (Le et al., 1983, Le et al., 1982). In 1984, such derivatives were proved effective against juvenile stages of *Schistosoma* sp., when treatments carried out with praziquantel fail, thus both artemether and artesunate are potential prophylactic drugs for schistosomiasis (Yue et al., 1984, Lu et al., 2010). Other studies extended the activity of artemisinin derivatives to other *Schistosoma* sp. that infect humans. In particular, assays carried out in Brazil in 1991 showed reduction of parasite burden in mice infected with *S. mansoni* and treated with artemether (Araújo et al., 1991). Since then, outstanding progress has been made in the study of anti-*Schistosoma* sp. activity, especially with artemether and artesunate (Cioli & Pica-Mattoccia, 2002, Xiao et al., 2000, Lu et al., 2010).
Clinical assays with artemether have already been carried out in Ivory Cost (Africa) and have shown less incidence of infections caused by *S. mansoni* and *S. japonicum* (Utzinger et al., 2003, Xiao et al., 2000). In regard to toxicity, it was proved by clinical tests that artemisinins are well tolerated when administered orally (Notprasert et al., 2002).
In some regions of the globe endemic areas for malaria and schistosomiasis overlap, and it is suggested that in such regions the use of artemisinin, intending to treat malaria cases, can reduce the morbidity rate of endemic schistosomiasis (Lescano et al., 2004).
After the first studies on the schistosomicidal activity of artemisinins, another drug had its anti-*Schistosoma* sp. activity researched, namely cyclosporin A, whose anthelmintic activity was discovered by Bueding et al. in 1981. Reduction in the number of worms and suppression of granuloma formation were noted in mice infected with *S. mansoni,* as well as prophylactic effect against this worm (Bout et al., 1986).
In 1984, a series of acridine derivatives showed schistosomicidal activity. *In vivo* studies demonstrated their efficiency against *S. mansoni, S. japonicum* and *S. haematobium* (Stohler & Montanova, 1984). Assays carried out in primates showed cure of the host with the use of some of these derivatives, RO 15-5458/000 being one of them (Coelho & Pererira, 1991). It is a fact that acridine derivatives are an important class of compounds for the development of new drugs with anticonvulsant, antidepressant, analgesic, anti-inflammatory, antiplatelet, antimalarial, antimicrobial, antifungal, vasodilator, antitumour, antiviral, and anti-*Schistosoma* sp. activity (Rollas & Kuçukguzel, 2007).
The most recent researches on new compounds or drugs with schistosomicidal activity have been carried out with: a) inhibitors of cysteine protease, such as K11777, considered a powerful schistosomicide that reduces the pathogenesis of experimental schistosomiasis (Abdulla *et al.,* 2007), b) RNAi, in the attempt to develop drugs or compounds that act as

enzyme silencers, e.g., the compound 4-phenyl-1,2,5-oxadiazole-3-carbonitrile-2-oxide, or furoxan, which acts on thioredoxin-glutathione reductase from *S. mansoni* (Kuntz et al., 2007, Sayed et al., 2008), c) trioxolanes or secondary ozonides (1, 2, 4-trioxolanes), which comprehend a class of synthetic endoperoxides that are cheap, easily synthesised, and similar to artemisinins, having activity on experimental infections with *S. mansoni* and *S. japonicum* (Caffrey, 2007, Xiao et al., 2007), d) mefloquine (antimalarial), which showed schistosomicidal activity against young and adult *S. mansoni* worms (Van Nassauw et al., 2008, Keiser et al., 2009), e) arachidonic acid, which showed schistosomicidal properties against *S. mansoni* and *S. haematobium* (El Ridi et al., 2010), and f) miltefosine (anti-leishmania), which reduced the parasite burden of mice infected with *S. mansoni* (Eissa et al., 2011). At the present moment there are no clinical assays with these compounds.

Research with medicinal plants has gained prominence in recent years. According to WHO, this sort of research should be encouraged because traditional knowledge on biodiversity products is an important tool in the development of new pharmaceutical products intended to combat diseases that affect people in developing countries (WHO, 2002).

Table 1 shows the drugs or compounds used up to this point in the treatment for human schistosomiasis.

YEAR	DRUG/COMPOUND	SPECIES
1918-1927	Tartar Emetic - Antimony Compounds	*S. mansoni, S. haematobium, S. japonicum*
1920	Emetine and 2,3-dehydroemetine	*S. japonicum*
1932	Lucanthone	*S. mansoni, S. haematobium*
1955	Metrifonate	*S. haematobium*
1964	Niridazole	*S. haematobium, S. mansoni, S. japonicum*
1965	Hycanthone	*S. mansoni, S. haematobium, S. rodhaini*
1969	Oxamniquine	*S. mansoni*
1975	Praziquantel	*S. mansoni, S. japonicum, S. haematobium, S. intercalatum, S. mekongi*
1976	Amoscanate	*S. mansoni, S. japonicum*
1976	Oltipraz	*S. mansoni, S. haematobium, S. intercalatum*
1978	Benzodiazepines	*S. mansoni, S. haematobium*
1980	Artemisinin Derivatives	*S. mansoni, S. japonicum, S. Haematobium*

Table 1. Drugs and compounds with schistosomicidal activity that have already been tested in humans. Sources: Cioli et al., 1995, Ribeiro-dos-Santos et al., 2006.

3. Development of tolerance and resistance of *Schistosoma mansoni* to schistosomicidal drugs

In the last 30 years the treatment for schistosomiasis has improved significantly in view of the introduction of praziquantel. Its oral administration in the dose of 40 to 60 mg/kg is efficient in reducing the morbidity, but the results of treatments with this drug have been less promising than expected. The reason is that cases of tolerance and resistance to the treatment for schistosomiasis have been reported for both oxamniquine and praziquantel (Parise-Filho & Silveira, 2001).

Different strains of *S. mansoni* have been found susceptible to treatment, whether they come from the same region or from various individuals within the same community (Parise-Filho & Silverira, 2001).

It has been known since the 1950's that different strains of *S. mansoni* show different responses to treatments carried out with the same medication (Katz, 2008). At that time it was proved that the strain from Egypt was less susceptible to the treatment with Miracil D than the strain from Liberia (Gonnert & Vogel, 1955).

The first cases of resistance to schistosomicidal drugs were actually reported by Katz et al. in 1973 in Brazil, and were related to oxamniquine and hycanthone. In 1978, strains tolerant and resistant to the treatment with praziquantel and oxamniquine were found in Brazil, Egypt, Kenya and Senegal (Dias et al., 1978, Stelma et al., 1995).

In 1987, Kinoti suggested that *S. mansoni* could develop resistance to therapeutic doses of some drugs. At the time, the large variation of susceptibility to drugs among parasites, even among those from the same region, was already known. Studies conducted in Kenya, where the required doses of oxamniquine are higher than in Brazil, suggested the existence of tolerant worms even before the extensive use of chemotherapeutic drugs with schistosomicidal properties (Coles et al., 1987).

In 1994, Fallon and Doenhoff provided an experimental demonstration that subtherapeutic doses of praziquantel, over many generations of parasites, resulted in worms less sensitive to the drug. Such resistance was in fact reported for the first time in Egypt and northern Senegal in 1995, when praziquantel was used in an attempt to control an epidemic of *S. mansoni* schistosomiasis (Fallon et al., 1995, Ismail et al., 1996).

There has been much debate on the possibility of praziquantel becoming less effective due to its potential to generate resistance. Regarding what happened in Senegal, where the cure rates were low (between 18% and 39%, whilst the normal rates are 70% to 90%) (Cioli 2000, Grysseels et al., 2001), some authors suggest that the cure rates were aberrant (Doenhoff et al., 2009). Explanations for such rates included: Rapid reinfections after the treatment, presence of immature forms of the parasite during the treatment, and no prior exposition of the immunological system of the population to *Schistosoma* sp. (Cioli 2000, Grysseels et al., 2001, Harnett & Kusel, 1986, Brindley & Sher, 1987, Doenhoff et al., 1987, Modha et al., 1990). Some authors, however, point out that, since the cure rates in Senegaleses were atipically lower than expected, suspicions of a development of tolerance and resistance to treatment in that region can not be ignored (Danso-Appiah & de Vlas, 2002). Other authors consider that resistance becomes a problem when chemotherapy is massively used aiming to eradicate the disease only by medication, especially when cure rates do not reach 100%. The key in the process is the percentage of surviving worms that will contribute to the resistance of the next generation (Ismail et al., 1999, Liang et al., 2001), because such resistance would favour low cure rates and rapid reinfections after the treatment (Stelma et al., 1995).

Somehow, the extensive use of praziquantel has increased the concern for the development of *Schistosoma* sp. resistant to treatment (Fallon & Doenhoff, 1994). Since there are few other options regarding the treatment for schistosomiasis (Doenhoff et al., 2009), in particular for *S. mansoni* schistosomiasis, it is necessary to search for alternative drugs.

The use of medicinal plants can be a very useful therapeutic alternative because the treatment is efficient and has low operational costs. Furthermore, such plants are easily found in Brazil, a country with a wide variety of native flora (Matos, 1994).

4. Researches with medicinal plants to combat schistosomiasis

Medicinal plants have been one of the most ancient forms of medicinal practice of humankind, having been used in the treatment of many diseases (Akerele, 1993). Based on information gathered along centuries, popular observations on the use and efficiency of medicinal plants have contributed significantly to the disclosure of their therapeutic properties (Maciel et al., 2002, WHO, 2003).

It is estimated that only 17% of all the plants in the world have been studied in one way or another regarding their medicinal use, in most cases, no deep analyses were carried out on their phytochemical and pharmacological properties. Many species are used empirically, with no scientific support on their efficiency and safety. These data show the enormous potential of plants for the discovery of new phytotherapeutic drugs (Cragg et al., 1999, Cordell & Colvard, 2005, Hamburger et al., 1991, Hostettmann, et al., 2003, Guerra, et al., 1999).

Medicinal plants and their derivatives were the basis of drug therapeutics until the middle of the 20th century, when chemical synthesis, initiated at the end of the 19th century, reached a new development stage (Silva & Carvalho, 2004).

In the first half of the 20th century, studies with natural products were temporarily put aside on account of the emergence of new synthetic drugs, obtained from microorganisms that in most cases had no practical use in view of their high toxicity (Devienne et al., 2004). Furthermore, side effects caused by the use of those medicines were more and more frequently. There was no advantage in providing a fast and efficient treatment for a disease and then making another disease appear. Drugs had to be efficient and safe at the same time, as well as affordable (Oliveira & Akisue, 2000).

In fact, there was a revolution in therapeutics at that moment, which led to the development of researches in the pharmacochemical industry with the purpose of synthesising active ingredients with less toxicity. Nevertheless, it did not take too long until the production of new drugs from totally synthetic substances stopped, in view of the high costs involved in their research and development (Devienne et al., 2004).

It should be mentioned that the development of a new drug involves a complex process that may cost aroud 100 to 360 million dolars over a period of 10 to 12 years, representing about 15% of the income of the pharmaceutical industry (Rates, 2001). On the other hand, the development of researches with medicinal plants has much lower costs (Ferreira, 2001). Other estimates show that the world market of pharmaceutical products generates 320 billion dollars per year, of which 20 billion come from active substances derived from medicinal plants (Robbers et al., 1996). These facts have been promoting the interest in medicinal plants and the search for prototypes for the production of new drugs.

A big limiting factor, though, is that most plants under use have not been described in official codes - pharmacopeia -, and there are not even studies on them. In order to introduce the use of medicinal plants in small production centres and prescription pharmacies, there must be investments in the elaboration of related official documents (Toledo et al., 2003). In this regard, the Brazilian government aproved the National Policy for Medicinal Plants and Phytotherapeutic Drugs (PNPMF) by decree n. 5,813 of June 22th, 2006. This policy is an essential part of public policies for health, environment, and social and economic development, and is very important for the implementation of actions capable of promoting improvements in the life quality of Brazilian people (Ministério da Saúde, 2009).

The Brazilian flora consists of about 100,000 species, but only 8% of them had their chemical composition studied. In addition, many active ingredients are still unknown, and it is estimated that only 1,100 species have been examined regarding their therapeutic properties (Anthony et al., 2005, Reis et al., 2007, Varanda, 2006).

According to Rodrigues and West (1995), the study of medicinal plants in tropical countries is very interesting because such species have 3 to 4 times more chemical compounds than plants found in temperate zones.

From the pharmacological viewpoint, it is absolutely necessary that the activities of ingredients or substances isolated from plants be evaluated in preclinical assays. Experimental models are used in the analysis of antiparasitic, anti-inflammatory, antimicrobial, analgesic, antitumour and anticonvulsant effects, among others, as well as in toxicologic evaluation (acute and chronic toxicity), primary and cumulative dermal irritation, ocular irritation, cutaneous sensitivity, and phototoxicity. The development of such studies allows us to reach the end of the multidisciplinary cycle in the research with medicinal plants (Foglio et al., 2006).

According to Githori et al. (2006), plants with antiparasitic activity usually contain saponins, alkaloids, non-protein amino acids, tannins, polyphenols, lignins, terpenes, lactones, glycosides, and phenolic compounds. As a result, many species can be candidates for thorough studies concerning this function. Table 2 describes some species of medicinal plants with confirmed schistosomicidal activities.

Among the several medicinal plants cultivated in Brazil, in this chapter we will focus on four species that for decades have been submitted to biological and pharmacological studies, in view of the fact that their active ingredients have proven effective to combat many diseases. In recent years our research group started a multidisciplinary project intending to carry out *in vitro* screenings of extracts and fractions from these plants against experimental infections in *S. mansoni*. The best results were found for *Artemisia annua, Baccharis trimera, Cordia verbenacea* and *Phyllanthus amarus*.

Scientific Name	Used Part of the Plant	Extract/ Compound	Species	Observations	References
Abrus precatorius	Stem and Roots	Aqueous Extract	*S. mansoni*	*In Vitro* Test - Schistosomulum	Molgaard et al., 2001
Ozoroa insignis	Leaves and Bark of the Roots	Aqueous Extract	*S. mansoni*	*In Vitro* Test - Schistosomulum	Molgaard et al., 2001
Elephantorrhiza goetzei	Barks of the Stem	Aqueous Extract	*S. mansoni*	*In Vitro* Test - Schistosomulum	Molgaard et al., 2001

Scientific Name	Used Part of the Plant	Extract/ Compound	Species	Observations	References
Commiphora molmol	Stem	Myrrh	*S. mansoni e S. haematobium*	–	Sheir et al., 2001, El Baz et al., 2003, Barakat et al., 2005
Nigella sativa	Seeds	Oil, Aqueous, Ethanolic and Chloroform Extracts	*S. mansoni*	*In Vivo* Test with Egyptian strain (Oil), *In Vitro* Test with Miracidia, Cercariae and Adults (Extracts)	Mahmoud et al., 2002, Mohamed et al., 2005, El-Shenawy et al., 2008
Allium sativum	Crushed Scale Leaves	Aqueous Extract, Dry Crude Extract	*S. mansoni*	Egyptian strain, *In Vivo* Test	Riad et al., 2007, Mantawy et al., 2011
Clerodendrum umbellatum	Leaves	Aqueous Extract	*S. mansoni*	Cameroonian strain, *In Vivo* Test	Jatsa et al., 2009
Curcuma longa	–	Curcumin	*S. mansoni*	LE strain,	Magalhães et al., 2009
Zanthoxylum naranjillo	Leaves	Fraction of Ethyl Acetate	*S. mansoni*	*In Vitro* Test	Braguine et al., 2009
Dryopteris sp.	Rhizome	Phloroglucinol	*S. mansoni*	LE strain	Magalhães et al., 2010
Piper tuberculatum	Inflorescence	Piplartine	*S. mansoni*	BH strain, *In Vitro* Test	Moraes et al., 2010
Baccharis dracunculifolia	Leaves	Essential Oil	*S. mansoni*	Native of Brazil, LE strain, *In Vitro* Tests	Parreira et al., 2010
Cratylia mollis	Seeds	Cramoll 1,4	*S. mansoni*	Native of Brazil, BH strain, *In Vivo* Test	Melo et al., 2011
Zingiber officinale	Rhizome	Aqueous Extract	*S. mansoni*	*In Vivo* Test	Mostafa et al., 2011
Ageratum conyzoides L	Leaves	Essential Oil	*S. mansoni*	LE strain, *In Vitro* Test	Melo et al., 2011
Allium cepa	Scale Leaves	Dry Crude Extract	*S. mansoni*	Egyptian strain, *In Vivo Test*	Mantawy et al., 2011

Table 2. Medicinal plants with attested schistosomicidal activity.

4.1 Bioassays – *In vitro* tests

Given the global interest in exploring anthelmintic activities of plants and their products, there is a growing interest in finding the best way to evaluate their bioactivity. Time and financial costs involved in tests require the screening techniques to be sensitive, preferably low-cost and reproducible (Jackson & Coop, 2000).

In general, plants contain a large number of secondary metabolites, which can act individually or in combination to produce direct or indirect effects on the parasites. Accordingly, the first screening stage should reduce the number of substances for the following stage, which consists of the discovery of active compounds, a complex and expensive process. That stage is important because the understanding of the nature of the active compounds, their action mode and their targets in the parasites is what will determine its applicability (Jackson & Coop, 2000, Athanasiadou et al., 2001, Athanasiadou & Kyriazkis, 2004).
In vitro assays are used for screening. *In vitro* tests are a primary screening, considering that a large number of plants can be examined to demonstrate their potential effect (Cabaret et al., 2002, Athanasiadou & Kyriazakis, 2004, Ketzis et al., 2006).
During an *in vitro* test for helminths, the parameter analysed is the viability of adult worms. Motility, oviposition, tegument changes, changes in internal organs, mating, and especially the mortality of such worms can all be observed.

4.2 *In vitro* tests with Brazilian medicinal plants to combat *S. mansoni* schistosomiasis

The plants used in the assays were cultivated and collected at the Experimental Field of the Chemical, Biological and Agricultural Pluridisciplinary Research Centre (CPQBA) - Unicamp - Campinas (-22°54'20"/-47°03'39") - São Paulo - Brazil. In order to obtain the extracts, fractions and isolated compounds the aerial parts of the plants were used. In order to carry out the *in vitro* tests, mated males and females of *S. mansoni* were used. They were kept in RPMI-1640 medium, along with penicillin/streptomycin, in a CO_2 oven at 5% and temperature of 37ºC. The results of these tests showed schistosomicidal activity in the samples during the observation period, which lasted 72 hours.

4.2.1 *Artemisia annua* L.

(Allegretti, S. M., 2011)

Artemisia annua L (Asteraceae), known as Artemisia or Qinghaosu, is indigenous to China and has been used for centuries in Chinese medicine in the treatment for fever crisis (Figure 2). This species was introduced and naturalised in several countries in Europe, northern and central Asia, India, Australia, northern Africa, and South and North Americas (Klayman, 1993, WHO, 2006).
Artemisinin and its derivatives are compounds with low toxicity, no mutagenic effects, and good tolerance, being a primary option in antimalarian therapy in many tropical and subtropical countries, such as China, Thailand, Cambodia, Laos, Vietnam, Brazil, Zaire, Gabon, Madagascar, Ghana, among others (Guo et al., 1998, Xiao, 2002, Jiraungkoorskul et al., 2006). Such compounds have also shown schistosomicidal activity (Jiraungkoorskul et al., 2006, Shaohong et al., 2006, Mitsui et al., 2008).
Our research group has compared the activity of artemisinin and artesunic acid in adult couples of the BH strain of *S. mansoni,* native of Belo Horizonte (-19°55'15"/-43°56'16"), Minas Gerais, Brazil, by means of *in vitro* tests. Twenty-two hours after the addition of the two compounds, death was observed in all concentrations tested. Three replications of the experiment were carried out for each concentration. Worms of negative control groups, i.e., with no addition of compounds or drugs, stayed alive until the end of the experiment. Table 3 shows the mortality of worms within the observation period.

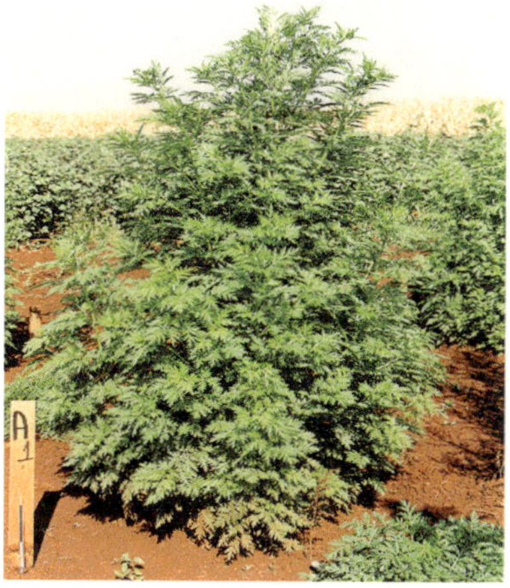

Fig. 2. *Artemisia annua* L. cultivated in the Experimental Field of CPQBA - Unicamp, 2011.

	Time when the mortality rate reached 100%		
	C1(1500μg/mL)	**C2 (1000μg/mL)**	**C3(500μg/mL)**
Artesunic acid	5th hour	5th hour	22nd hour
Artemisinin	20th hour	20th hour	22nd hour
Praziquantel	20th hour	20th hour	22nd hour

Table 3. Activity of artesunic acid, artemisinin and praziquantel in relation to the mortality of *S. mansoni*. Concentrations: C1 = 1500μg/mL, C2 = 1000μg/mL, C3 = 500μg/mL.

It has already been proven that both artemisinin and artesunic acid act in different ways on strains of *S. mansoni*, such as LE, Liberian and Puerto Rico. Tests comparing strains of *S. mansoni* with artesunic acid are still rare in the literature, but in *in vivo* studies we notice that different strains respond differently to the treatment.

All these strains showed differences in the percentage of worm distribution in the hepatic portal system, mortality and oogram change (Araújo et al. 1999, Utzinger et al., 2002, Lu et al., 2004, 2006). Such differences between strains of *S.mansoni* in the vertebrate host are considered a manifestation of the genotypic expression of the trematode (Yoshioka et al. 2002). For the comparison between the activity of artesunic acid and artemisinin against the BH and SJ strains of *S. mansoni* (the latter being native of São José dos Campos, -23°10'46"/-45°53'13", São Paulo, Brazil), experiments in Swiss mice were carried out with further treatments on different days, i.e., on the 30th and 45th days after the infection. Concentrations of 300 and 500 mg/kg were orally administered, divided along five consecutive days. Fifteen days after the administration of the last concentration, the reduction rates of the BH strain worms in the hepatic portal system of mice were compared with negative control group (not treated), and the result was 49% of worm reduction for artesunic acid (with 300 and 500 mg/kg) in treatment carried out after 30 days of infection. However, no reduction was found for artemisinin in neither concentration, tested under the same conditions. In treatments carried out after 45 days of infection, there was worm reduction of 41% with the use of artesunic acid, 500 mg/kg, but no reduction was found in the group treated with artemisinin in the same concentration and on the same day.

In regard to the same strain, eggs eliminated in the feces were reduced at even 100% with the use of artesunic acid, 300 mg/kg, administered after 30 days of infection, but no similar results were found in similar treatments with artemisinin. Oviposition reduction of 100% was also observed with artesunic acid, in treatment carried out on the 45th day of infection in both concentrations, whereas artemisinin reached 81% of oviposition reduction on the same day, in the 300mg/kg concentration.

Better results were achieved with the SJ strain concerning worm reduction: maximum of 49% in treatments with 500 mg/kg of artesunic acid, administered after 30 days of infection, and 30% with artemisinin, in the same concentration and period. In treatments carried out after 45 days of infection worm reduction reached 76% with 300 mg/kg of artesunic acid, whereas no reduction was found with the use of artemisinin in the same period in either concentration.

Regarding oviposition, 500 mg/kg of artesunic acid provided a reduction of 99% when administered after 30 days of infection, whilst the same concentration of artemisinin provided a reduction of 89% in the same period. In treatments carried out with 500 mg/kg of artesunic acid after 45 dias, the reduction rate reached 98%, but no reduction was found in treatments with artemisinin.

These results showed that artesunic acid had better activity regarding the parameters in question (worm and oviposition reduction) for both strains under study. In addition, the use of artesunic acid showed no significant difference between these parameters in treatments carried on the 30th and 45th days of infection for both strains. Regarding artemisinin, we could observe that the SJ strain of *S. mansoni* showed higher worm and oviposition reduction rates than the BH strain, particularly in treatments after 30 days of infection, which demonstrates the difference between the strains in what refers to treatment response.

4.2.2 *Baccharis trimera* (Less) DC.

(Oliveira, R. N., 2011)

Baccharis trimera (Less) DC. (Figure 3) is a plant native of South and Southeast Brazil, also found in Argentina, Bolivia, Paraguay and Uruguay (Bona et al., 2005, Lorenzi & Matos 2002). This species belongs to the family Asteraceae, which includes around 1,100 genera and 25,000 species distributed worldwide (Moreira et al., 2003). Plants of this family are extensively studied regarding their chemical composition and biological activity because of their outstanding allelopathic, anti-inflammatory, antimutagenic and antimicrobial effects. Some of these species have even made possible the development of new drugs and insecticides, among other products (Verdi et al., 2005).

The genus *Baccharis* has more than 500 species widely distributed in Brazil, Colombia, Chile, Argentina and Mexico (Lorenzi & Matos, 2002). The phytochemistry of this genus has been studied since the beginning of the last century, and so far more than 150 compounds have been isolated and identified (Abad et al., 1999). Flavonoids and terpenoids, such as monoterpenes, sesquiterpenes, diterpenes and triterpenes, are the most frequent compounds (Moreira et al., 2003, Verdi et al., 2005).

The name *Baccharis* (*Bakkharis)* comes from Greek and is an old denomination for some shrub-like plants (Kissmann & Groth, 1999). This plant is popularly known as carqueja and its most distinct characteristic is the presence of cladophylls, which replace leaves as the main photosynthetic organs of the plant, as there are no leaves or they are extremely reduced, with limited physiological function (Barroso, 1976). Carqueja was first used in folk medicine in Brazil by Correa in 1931, who described the use of the infusion of its aerial parts in the treatment for female sterility and male impotence (Lorenzi & Matos, 2002). Nowadays *B. trimera* is mostly consumed in teas, being extensively used in folk medicine on account of its diuretic properties and in the treatment for gastrointestinal and hepatic diseases, as well as for angina, poor blood circulation, diabetes and inflammatory processes (Corrêa, 1984, Moreira et al., 2003, Souza et al., 1991).

A. B.

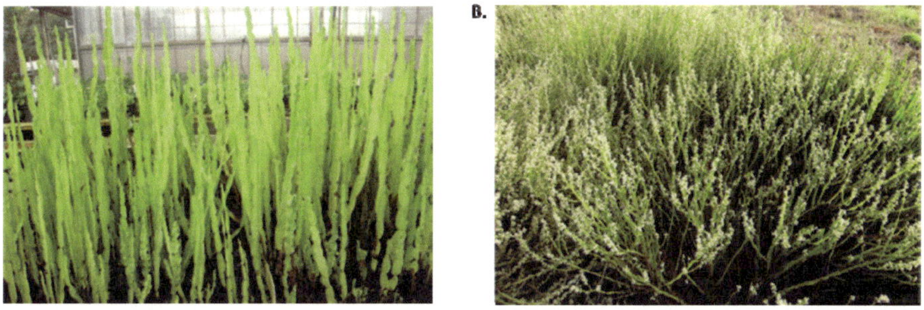

Fig. 3. *Baccharis trimera* (Less) DC. **A.** Seedling, **B.** Inflorescence. Source: Experimental Field of CPQBA- Unicamp, 2011.

From the species *B. trimera* a series of flavonoids have already been isolated, including eupatorin, eupatrin, cirsimaritin, rutin, cirsiliol, genkwanin, eriodictyol, kaempferol, quercetin, luteolin, nepetin, apigenin e hispidulin, 5-OH- 6,7,3,4-OMe flavone, 5,6-OH-7,3',4'-OMe flavone and 5,7,3,4-OH-3-O-rhamnosyl-glycosyl flavone (Borella et al., 2006, Soicke et al., 1987, Verdi et al., 2005).

Several biological studies were conducted intending to confirm the pharmacological properties of *B. trimera*. For instance, the decoction of this plant showed antimicrobial activity (bacteriostatic and bactericidal) in both Gram-positive and Gram-negative bacteria through *in vitro* assays, supporting its use as antiseptic and disinfectant (Avancini et al., 2000).

Among the studies conducted so far we can point out the works carried out with the aqueous extract from *B. trimera*. This extract showed activity on the reduction of gastric lesions induced by stress in mice (Gamberini et al., 1991), on the relaxation of the intestinal smooth musculature in rats (Torres et al., 2003), on the reduction of the blood glucose level in mice, indicating a potential antidiabetic activity (Oliveira et al., 2005), in addition to anti-inflammatory and immunomodulatory effects (Paul et al., 2009).

Hydroalcoholic extract showed antioxidant activity through *in vitro* and *in vivo* tests in neutrophils of mice (Pádua et al., 2010). Another *in vitro* test with the same extract showed antiparasitic activity against amastigote and promastigote forms of *Leishimania* (L) *amazoniesis* and epimastigote forms of *Trypanosoma cruzi* (Luize et al., 2005).

It was also reported that the methanolic extract from *B. trimera* showed antimutagenic activity through *in vitro* assays (Nakasugi & Komai, 1998).

The molluscicidal activity in *Biomphalaria glabrata* (Pulmonata: Planorbidea) was studied from a diterpenic lactone and a flavone isolated from *B. trimera* (Santos-Filho et al., 1980).

The compound neoclerodane diterpene showed inhibitory action on metalloproteases present in the venom of *Bothrops* sp., which demonstrates the antihemorrhagic, antiproteolytic, antimyotoxic and antiedematogenic properties of *B. trimera* (Januário et al., 2004).

Polyphenolic compounds isolated from *B. trimera, B.crispa* and *B.usterii* by means of aqueous extract showed anti-inflammatory and antioxidant activities (Simões, et al., 2005).
In addition to the studies mentioned here, other biological activities *B. trimera* have been demonstrated, as shortly shown in Table 4.

Activity	Extract/ Compound	References
Molluscicidal	Diterpene Lactone and Flavone	Santos-Filho et al., 1980
Antimutagenic	Methanolic Extract	Nakasugi & Komai, 1998
Disinfectant and Antiseptic	Decoction	Avancini et al.,2000
Antiproteolytic, Antihemorrhagic	Chloroform: Methanol	Januário et al., 2004
Antiparasitic, Antiulcer, Antioxidant, Hepatorenal	Hydroalcoholic Extract	Dias et al., 2009, Grance et al., 2009, Luize et al., 2005, Pádua et al., 2010
Hypoglycemic, Anti-inflammatory, Immunomodulatory, Genotoxicity, Antigenotoxicity	Aqueous Extract	Barbosa-Filho et al., 2005, Leite et al., 2007, Paul et al.,2009, Rodrigues et al., 2009

Table 4. Major biological activities of *Baccharis trimera* described in the literature.

Among the several biological activities of *B. trimera* mentioned in the literature, we can highlight its anti-inflammatory and hepatorenal activities, which raised the interest of our research group in studying this plant in the treatment for *S. mansoni* schistosomiasis because granulomatous inflammatory responses, the main pathology of the disease, affect many organs, especially the liver. Therefore, we have been carrying out screening of raw extracts and fractions from this plant by *in vitro* assays.
Crude dichloromethane and hydroalcoholic extracts were used so that the schistosomicidal activity of *B. trimera* on the BH strain of *S. mansoni* could be evaluated. Different concentrations - C1 = 130μg/mL, C2 = 91μg/mL, C3 = 48μg/mL and C4 = 24μg/mL - of the extracts were tested on couples of adult worms, five replications being performed for each concentration. At the end of the experiment, i.e., 72 hours later, the following mortality rates were observed:

	Dichloromethane Extract	Hydroalcoholic Extract	Praziquantel	Control
C1 (130 µg/mL)	**100%**	70%	100%	-
C2 (91 µg/mL)	**100%**	70%	100%	-
C3 (48 µg/mL)	**100%**	50%	70%	-
C4 (24µg/mL)	**90%**	30%	60%	-

Table 5. Evaluation of the mortality of couples of *Schistosoma mansoni* submitted to different concentrations of *Baccharis trimera*. Control: Negative Control Group, with no addition of any extract or drug for 72 hours.

Considering these results, we conclude that the dichloromethane extract showed better activity in comparison with the hydroalcoholic one and that male specimens of *S. mansoni* were more susceptible to the activity of the former. Therefore, it can be accepted that *B. trimera* has active compounds against the BH strain of *S. mansoni*.

The effect of the observation period on the mortality of the worms was also analysed. The crude dichloromethane extract proved to be more effective, as the concentrations C1 (130µg/mL) and C2 (91µg/mL) caused the death of 100% of the worms in an observation period of 48 hours (Figure 4).

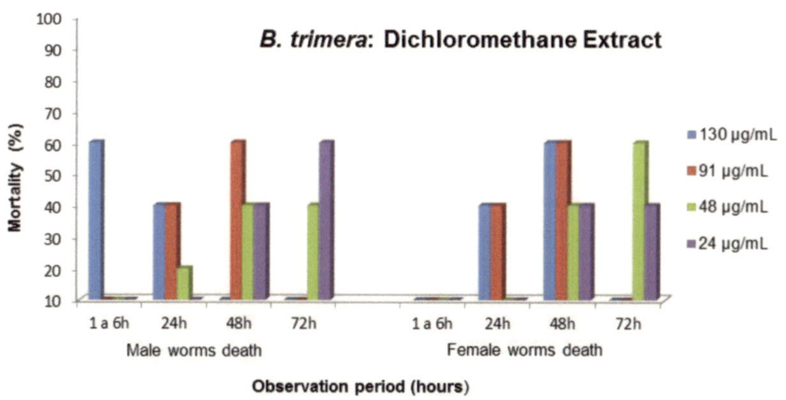

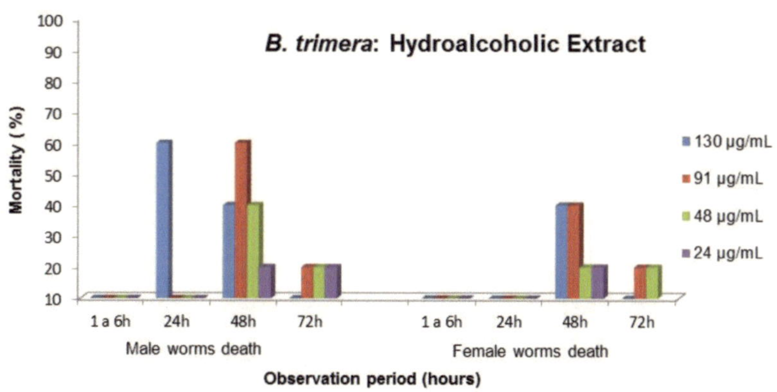

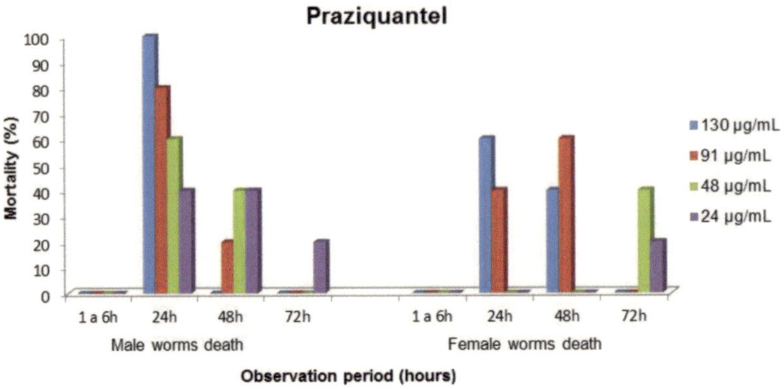

Fig. 4. Activity of the crude dichloromethane and hydroalcoholic extracts from *Baccharis trimera* and praziquantel on the viability of male and female *Schistosoma mansoni* worms in relation to the observation period of 72 hours.

4.2.3 *Cordia verbenacea* DC.

(Frezza, T.F., 2011)

Cordia verbenacea DC (also referred to as *Cordia salicina, Cordia curassavica, Cordia cylindristachia, Lithocardium fresenii, Lithocardium salicinum* and *Lithocardium verbaceum*) is a medicinal plant native of Brazil, commonly known as maggy plant (*erva-baleeira* or *salicina* in Brazilian Portuguese). It belongs to the family Boraginaceae, widely distributed along the Brazilian shore, but found mainly from the shore of São Paulo to Santa Catarina (Carvalho et al., 2004). Species of the genus *Cordia* are found in tropical and subtropical regions in Asia, southern Africa, Australia, Guyana and South America in general (Ficarra et al., 1995). Figure 5 shows a specimen of *C. verbenacea.*

A.

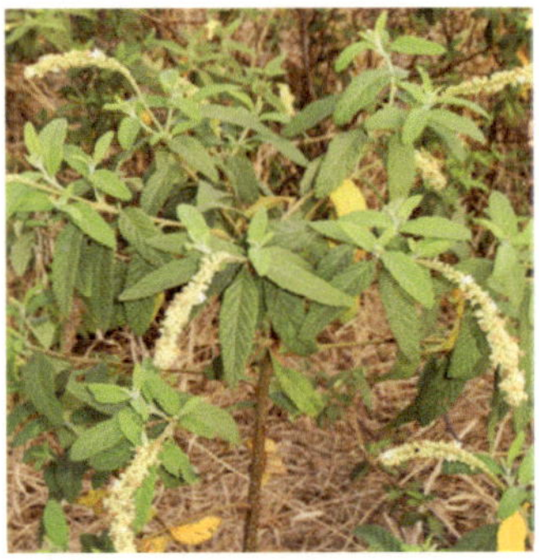

B.

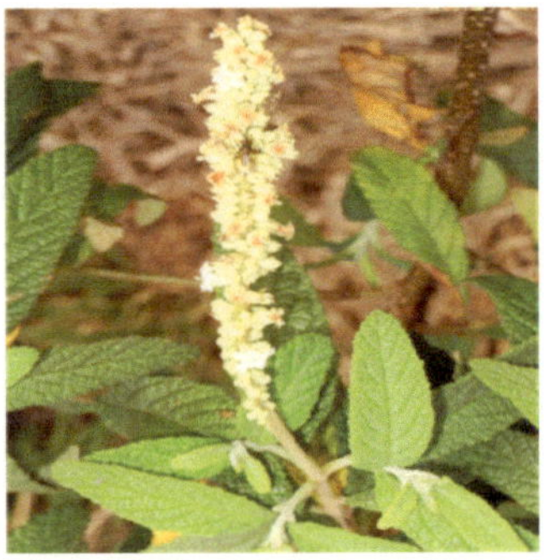

Fig. 5. *Cordia verbenacea.* **A**. Leaves, **B**. Inflorescence. Source: Experimental Field of CPQBA - Unicamp, 2011.

Several compounds are found in the aerial parts of *C. verbenacea,* including tannins, flavonoids and essential oils. Such parts have been used in folk medicine in the form of alcoholic extracts and infusions in view of their antiulcer, antimicrobial, anti-inflammatory and antirheumatic activities, as well as their tonic and analgesic properties (Carvalho et al., 2004, Passos et al., 2007). Since a variety of chemical groups found in extracts from C.

verbenacea allegedly have biological activities, this plant is an important material for pharmaceutical investigation (Michielin et al., 2009). In recent years, the activities of different extracts from *C. verbenacea* have been extensively discussed.

Preclinical studies have shown that the hydroalcoholic extract from *C. verbenacea* has anti-inflammatory activity, either by oral or topical administration, and protects the gastric mucosa (Sertie et al., 2005, Roldão et al., 2008). It also has antioxidant activity (Michielin et al, 2011) and inhibits the growth of Gram-positive and Gram-negative bacteria (Meccia et al., 2009, Michielin et al., 2009).

Its essential oil has antimicrobial activity along with inhibitory activity against the growth of some Gram-positive bacteria in *in vitro* cultures (Carvalho et al., 2004), as well as antialergic activity (Passos et al., 2007) and larvicidal activity against *Aedes aegypti* (Santos et al., 2006). The bioguided isolation of this oil led to the identification of other two active compounds with anti-inflammatory activity, namely alpha-humulene and trans-caryophylllene (Passos et al., 2007).

The anti-inflammatory activity of the essential oil made it possible to develop the first Brazilian phytodrug, Acheflan, an anti-inflammatory drug of topical use.

Different activities have also been reported for other extracts, such as the methanolic extract, which presents effects on oedema formation and reduction of myotoxicity induced by the venom of *Bothrops jararacussu* (Ticli et al., 2005), and the dichloromethane extract, which has shown antiedematogenic activity in *in vivo* assays (Bayeux et al., 2002). The antiparasitic activity of methanolic extracts from *C. verbenacea* has already been tested against *Leishmania* sp. (Braga et al., 2006) and is currently studied by our research group against *S. mansoni*. *C. verbenacea* was chosen by our research group for *in vitro* studies because of its anti-inflammatory properties.

Table 6 provides a summary of the actions of extracts or compounds from *C. verbenacea.*

Activity	Extract/ Compound	Reference
Anti-inflammatory, Protection of the Gastric Mucosa, Antiulcer, Antioxidant, Antimicrobial	Hydroalcoholic Extract	Sertié et al., 1990, Sertié et al., 2005, Passos et al., 2007, Roldão et al., 2008, Meccia et al., 2009, Michielin et al., 2009, Michielin et al., 2011
Anti-inflammatory, Antimicrobial, Antialergic, Larvicidal	Essential Oil	De-Carvalho et al., 2004, Santos et al., 2006, Passos et al., 2007
Reduction of Myotoxicity, Antiparasitic (*Leishmania* sp.)	Methanolic Extract	Ticli et al., 2005,Braga et al.,2007
Antiedematogenic	Dichloromethane Extract	Bayeux et al., 2002

Table 6. Major biological activities of *Cordia verbenacea* described in the literature.

The aqueous fraction, organic fraction (obtained from the ethanolic extract) and essential oil were used for the analysis of the *in vitro* schistosomicidal activity of *C. verbenacea* against the BH strain of *S. mansoni*. Different concentrations of the extracts were tested against couples of adult worms, with five replications carried out for each concentration. At the end of the experiment (72 hours), the following mortality rates were observed:

	Essential Oil	Aqueous Fraction	Organic Fraction	Praziquantel	Control
C1 (400 µg/mL)	30%	30%	**100%**	100%	-
C2 (200 µg/mL)	30%	30%	**100%**	100%	-
C3 (100 µg/mL)	30%	20%	**90%**	90%	-
C4 (50 µg/mL)	20%	10%	**60%**	90%	-

Table 7. Evaluation of the mortality of couples of *Schistosoma mansoni* submitted to different concentrations of *C. verbenacea*. Control: Negative Group Control, with no addition of any extract or drug for 72 hours.

The effect of the observation period on the mortality of the worms was also analysed. We consider that the best extract from *C. verbenacea* was the one that in 24 hours was able to eliminate more worms with higher concentrations (Figure 6).

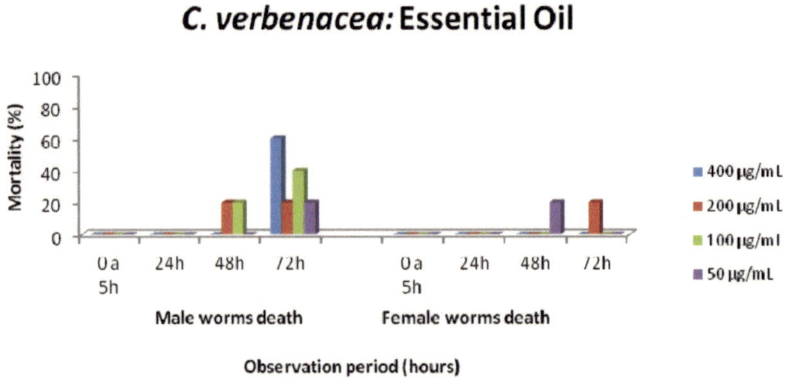

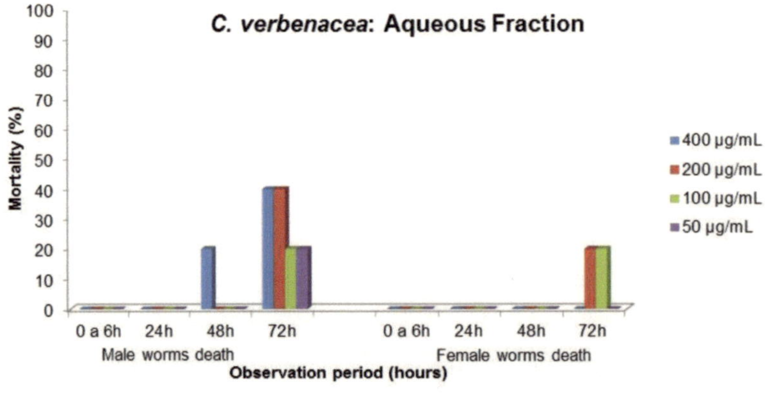

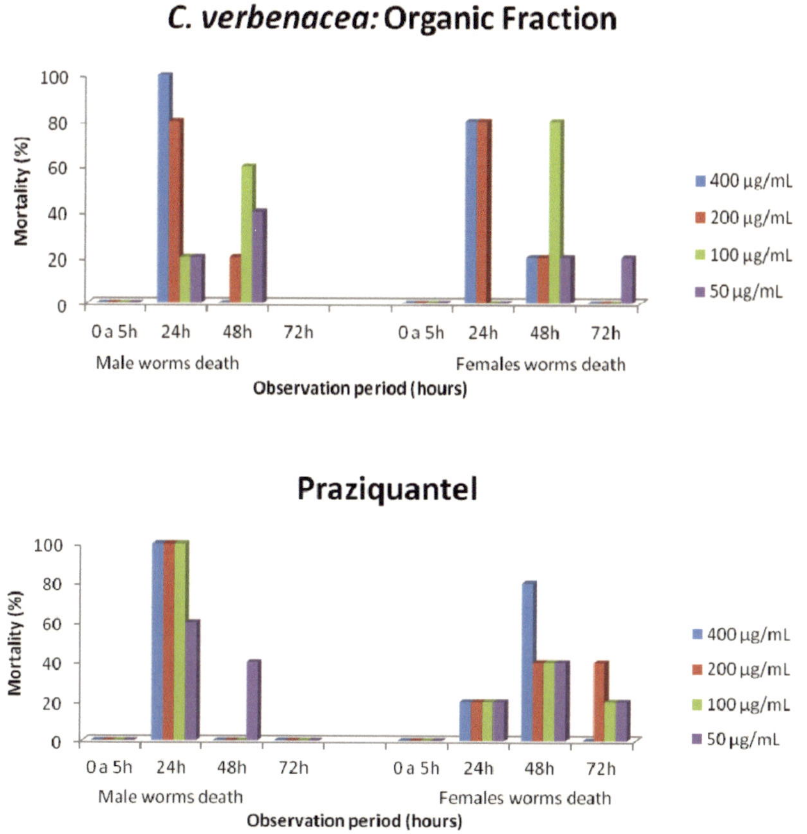

Fig. 6. Activity of the aqueous fraction, essential oil and organic fraction from *Cordia verbenacea* and praziquantel on the viability of male and female *Schistosoma mansoni* worms in relation to the observation period of 72 hours.

4.2.4 *Phyllanthus amarus* L.

(Oliveira, C.N.F., 2011)

Phyllanthus amarus belongs to the family Euphorbiaceae (Calixto et al., 1998), which comprises 317 genera and 8,000 species, grouped into 49 tribes and 5 subfamilies (Torres et al., 2003). Plants belonging to the genus *Phyllanthus* are widely distributed in most tropical and subtropical countries (in both hemispheres) and include between 550 and 750 species. It is believed that there are about 200 species of this genus distributed throughout the Americas, being mostly found in Caribe and Brazil (Calixto et al., 1998, Torres et al., 2003). The name *Phyllanthus* comes from Greek, *phyllon* meaning 'leaf' and *anthos* meaning 'flower', a reference to the flowers produced in branches, resembling compound flowers (Figure 7) (Torres et al., 2003).

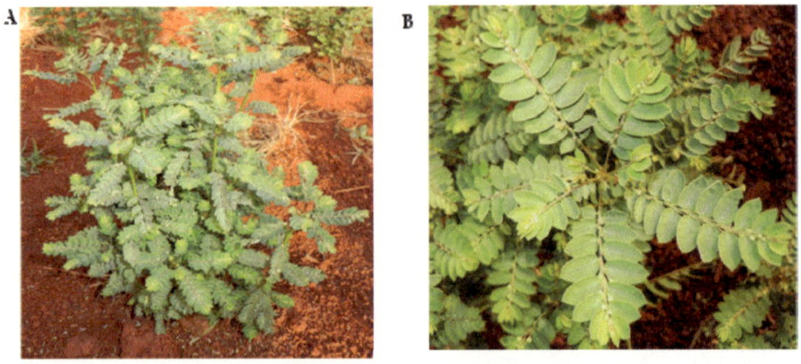

Fig. 7. **A** - Specimen of *Phyllanthus amarus*, **B.** Amplified image. Source: Experimental Field of CPQBA - Unicamp, 2011.

In Brazil, plants of the genus *Phyllanthus* are popularly known as stone-breaker (*quebra-pedra*, *arrebenta-pedra* or *erva-pombinha* in Brazilian Portuguese) and are recognised in folk medicine in Brazil and other countries for their diuretic properties. They are used in the treatment for kidney and bladder disorders, helping in the passage of renal calculi, and also act on intestinal infections, diabetes and hepatitis B (Calixto et al., 1998, Jain et al., 2003, Khatoon et al., 2006, Rajakannan et al., 2003, Torres et al., 2003).

A large variety of species of plants belonging to this genus have been phytochemically and pharmacologically investigated and many molecules have been isolated and identified. Among all the species studied, *P. amarus* has been given special attention. Although many of its compounds are chemically known, the properties of most of these compounds remain unknown. Some pharmacological activities of *P. amarus* have already been confirmed by scientific studies, such as: (1) treatment for hepatitis B, by suppression of the replication of the virus (Thyagarajan et al., 1988), (2) hepatoprotective effect against actions of paracetamol, carbon tetrachloride (CCl4), galactosamine and alcohol (Krithika et al., 2009, Pramyothin et al., 2007) - phyllanthin and hypophyllanthin, which are lignans present in *P. amarus*, are described as having hepatocyte-protective action against carbon tetrachloride (Khatoon et al., 2006), (3) aqueous extracts from *P. amarus* have shown a strong inhibitory action against hepatic carcinoma (Rajeshkumar & Kuttan, 2000), (4) possible antispasmodic effects of the extract on the smooth musculature have been reported because they contribute to the effects on the renal calculi (Kassuya et al., 2003), (5) antibacterial activity of the ethanolic extract (Kloucek et al., 2005), (6) potential anti-inflammatory activity of both the hexane extract and the chemical fraction rich in lignans, obtained from the leaves of *P. amarus*. The anti-inflammatory activity of lignans was evaluated and it was noticed that nirantin is the most active substance of this fraction. Moreover, an analgesic effect has also been reported (Kassuya et al,. 2005, Kassuya et al., 2006), (7) inhibition of gastric lesions with the use of the methanolic extract from *P. amarus* (Raphael & Kuttan, 2003), (8) *in vitro* and *in vivo* inhibition of the replication of the human immunodeficiency virus (HIV) (Notka et al., 2004), (9) hypoglycemic activity, useful in the treatment for diabetes mellitus, with the methanolic extract (Raphael et al., 2002), (10) antiplasmodial activity, demonstrated by the use of the aqueous extract from the leaves and stem of the plant against *Plasmodium berghei* (Dapper et al., 2007), (11) studies on the radioprotective properties of polyphenols (tannins and flavonoids) isolated from *P. amarus* and described by Londhe et al (2009) showed that of all the tested compounds ellagitannin had the best activity, (12) potential antioxidant activity of the aqueous extract in rats (Karuna et al., 2009).

Considering the studies carried out so far, briefly presented in Table 8, the interest for plants of the genus *Phyllanthus* has increased significantly, particularly in regard to their therapeutic potential against many diseases. Many reasons have contributed to this interest, including: their wide distribution in many tropical and subtropical countries, the large number of species in this genus, their extensive therapeutic use in folk medicine, and the great variety of secondary metabolites present in these plants (Calixto et al., 1998).

Activity	Extract/ Compound	Reference
Inhibition of gastric lesions; Hypoglycemic	Methanolic Extract	Raphael & Kuttan, 2003; Raphael et al., 2002
Hepatoprotective	Crude Extract; Phyllantin	Pramyothin et al., 2007; Krithika et al., 2009
Protection of the hepatocytes against carbon tetrachloride (CCl_4)	Phyllantin and Hipophyllantin, which are lignans present in the plant	Khatoon et al., 2006
Inhibition of hepatic carcinoma; Supression of the replication of the virus of hepatitis B; Hepatoprotective; Antisplasmodial (*Plasmodium berghei);* Antioxidant	Aqueous Extract	Rajeshkumar & Kuttan, 2000; Thyagarajan et al., 1988; Pramyothin et al., 2007; Dapper et al., 2007 ; Karuna et al., 2009
In vitro and *in vivo* inhibitory effect of HIV; Antibacterial	Ethanolic Extract	Notka et al., 2004; Kloucek et al., 2005
Anti-inflammatory; Analgesic	Hexane Extract and Chemical Fraction rich in lignans, obtained from the leaves of *P. amarus*	Kassuya et al., 2005; Kassuya et al., 2006
Radioprotective Properties	Ellagitannin, isolated compound	Londhe et al., 2009

Table 8. Major biological activities of *Phyllanthus amarus* described in the literature.

There have been no reports of studies on *P. amarus* applied to the treatment for *S. mansoni* schistosomiasis. Nevertheless, records of anti-inflammatory and hepatoprotective activities of this plant have been found, which has led to the selection of the plant for this study, as the main pathogeny of schistosomiasis is the granulomatous inflammatory response.

An *in vitro* study with the ethanolic extract and fractions obtained from *P. amarus* was carried out so that the schistosomicidal effect of this plant against the BH strain of *S. mansoni* could be verified. Four concentrations - C1= 200µg/mL, C2 = 100µg/mL, C3 = 50µg/mL e C4 = 25µg/mL - of the extracts were tested against couples of adult worms, with five replications carried out for each concentration. At the end of the experiment (72 hours), the mortalities observed are the ones indicated in Table 9.

	Ethanolic Extract	Fraction 1	Fraction 2	Fraction 3	Fraction 4	Praziquantel	Control
C1 (200 μg/mL)	100%	100%	90%	**100%**	100%	100%	-
C2 (100 μg/mL)	100%	100%	40%	**100%**	90%	60%	-
C3 (50 μg/mL)	40%	40%	-	**100%**	30%	80%	-
C4 (25 μg/mL)	20%	20%	10%	**100%**	20%	60%	-

Table 9. Evaluation of the mortality of couples of *Schistosoma mansoni* submitted to different concentrations of *Phyllanthus amarus*. Control: Negative Group Control, with no addition of any extract or drug for 72 hours.

These results show that the fractions had better activity against the worms, taking into account the ones that managed to eliminate them more quickly.

The effect of the observation period on the mortality of the worms was also analysed. We consider that fractions 1 and 4 in C1 (200μg/mL) and fraction 3 in C1, C2 (100μg/mL) and C3 (50μg/mL) were more effective because after 24 hours of observation 100% of the worms were dead (Figure 8).

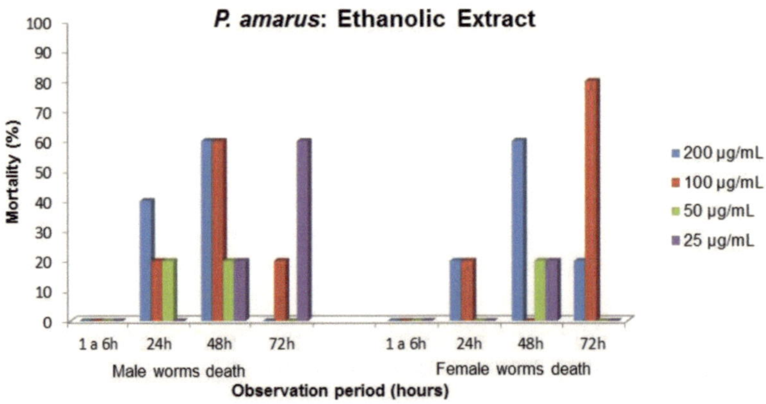

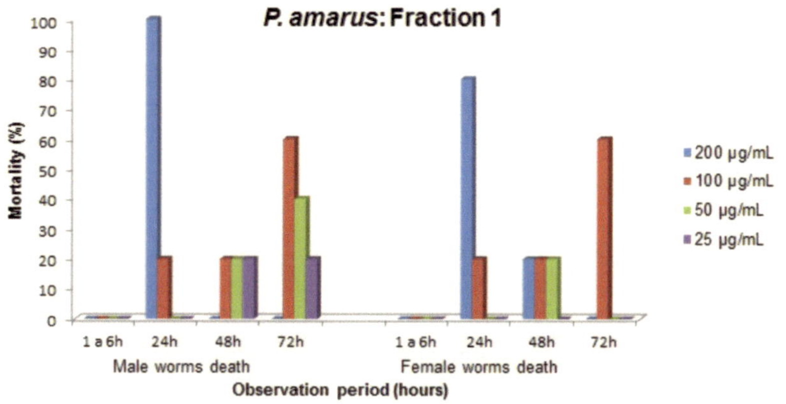
P. amarus: Fraction 1
Mortality (%)
100
90
80
70
60
50
40
30
20
10
0
1 a 6h
24h
48h
72h
Male worms death
1 a 6h
24h
48h
72h
Female worms death
Observation period (hours)
200 µg/mL
100 µg/mL
50 µg/mL
25 µg/mL

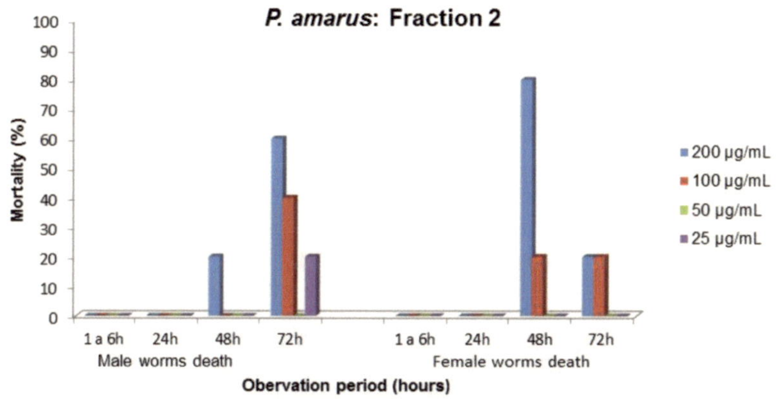
P. amarus: Fraction 2
Mortality (%)
100
90
80
70
60
50
40
30
20
10
0
1 a 6h
24h
48h
72h
Male worms death
1 a 6h
24h
48h
72h
Female worms death
Obervation period (hours)
200 µg/mL
100 µg/mL
50 µg/mL
25 µg/mL

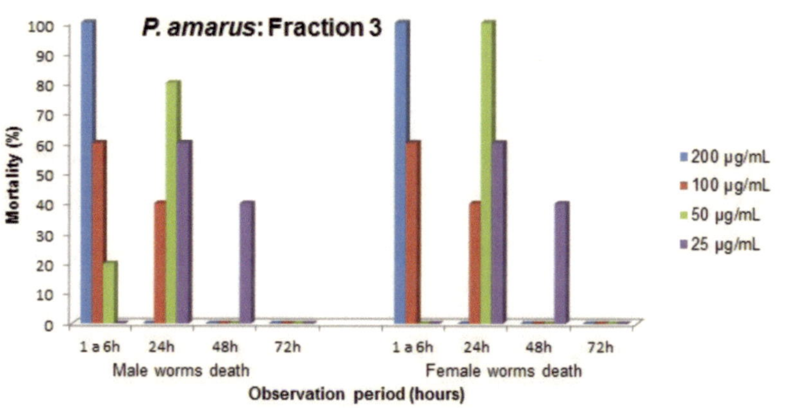
P. amarus: Fraction 3
Mortality (%)
100
90
80
70
60
50
40
30
20
10
0
1 a 6h
24h
48h
72h
Male worms death
1 a 6h
24h
48h
72h
Female worms death
Observation period (hours)
200 µg/mL
100 µg/mL
50 µg/mL
25 µg/mL

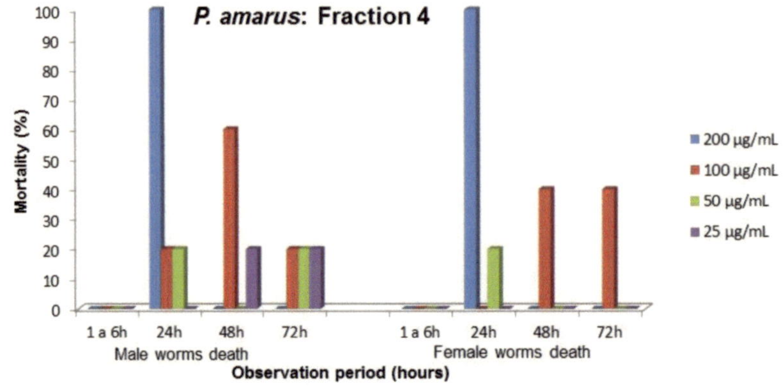

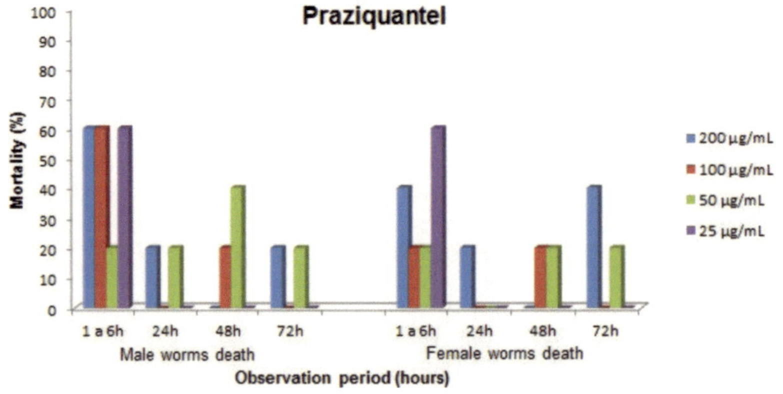

Fig. 8. Activity of the crude ethanolic extract and fractions 1, 2, 3 and 4 of *Phyllanthus amarus* and praziquantel on the viability of male and female *Schistosoma mansoni* worms in relation to the observation period of 72 hours.

As seen in the results of the *in vitro* tests, fraction 3 isolated from the crude ethanolic extract from *P. amarus* showed the best schistosomicidal activity.

5. Conclusion

We can conclude that the species of plants studied by our research group have schistosomicidal activity against *S. mansoni*. It is also worth pointing out that:

- The higher activity of artesunic acid in both *in vitro* and *in vivo* assays in comparison with artemisinin, with higher worm and oviposition reduction rates for both strains studied, which demonstrates that the different responses to the treatment by the two strains have not prevented the compound from working against them,
- *In vitro* assays with *B. trimera* showed better schistosomicidal activity for the crude dichloromethane extract, resulting in the mortality rate of 100% in the three concentrations tested, moreover, it was possible to notice that male *S. mansoni* worms were more susceptible to the action of this extract,

- The higher activity of the organic fraction from *C. verbenacea* in *in vitro* tests on the viability of the worms, killing a larger amount in less time in comparison with other extracts, also showing higher activity against male worms,
- The results of the *in vitro* tests carried out with *P. amarus,* which demonstrated that fraction 3 isolated from the crude ethanolic extract had better schistosomicidal activity because the mortality rate was 100% in all concentrations tested.

Considering the good results obtained so far, our research group will continue the chemical biomonitoring study by means of activity assays, aiming to isolate and identify fractions and compounds responsible for schistosomicidal activities shown by the medicinal plants under investigation.

6. Acknowledgements

The authors are thankful to the FAPESP and CAPES for financial support.

7. References

Abad, M. J., Bermejo, P., Gonzales, E., Iglesias, I., Irurzum, A. & Carrasco, L. (1999). Antiviral activity of Bolivian plant extracts. *Comparative and General Pharmacology,* vol.32, no.4, (April 1999), pp. 499-503. ISSN 0306-3623.

Abdulla, M. H., Lim, K. C., Sajid, M., McKerrow, J. H. & Caffrey, C. R. (2007). Schistosomiasis mansoni: novel chemotherapy using a cysteine protease inhibitor. *PLoS Medicine,* vol. 4, no. 1, (January), pp. 130-138, ISSN 1549-1277.

Akerele, O. (1993). Summary of WHO Guidelines for the Assessment of Herbal Medicines. *Herbal Gram,* vol.28, no. 13, pp.13-19, ISSN 0899-5648.

Almeida-Machado, P. (1982). The Brazilian program for schistosomiasis control. *The American Journal of Tropical Medicine and Hygiene,* vol. 31, no. 1, (January 1982), pp. 76-86, ISSN 0002-9637.

Andrews, P. (1981). A summary of the efficacy of praziquantel against schistosomes in animal experiments and notes on its mode of action. *Arzneimittelforschung,* vol. 31, no. 3a , (no date), pp. 538-541, ISSN 0004-4172.

Andrews, P., Thomas, H., Pohlke, R. & Seubert, J. (1983). Praziquantel. *Medicinal Research Reviews,* vol. 32, no. 2, (April/June 1983), pp. 147-200, ISSN 0198-6325.

Anthony, J. P., Fyfe, L. & Smith, H. (2005). Plant active components - a resource for antiparasitic agents? *Trends in Parasitology,* vol.21, no. 10 (October 2005), pp.462-468, ISSN: 1471-4922.

Araújo, N, Kohn, A. & Katz, N. (1991). Activity of the artemether in experimental *Schistosoma mansoni. Memórias do Instituto Oswaldo Cruz,* vol. 86, Suppl 2, (no date), pp. 185-188, ISSN 0074-0276.

Araújo, N., Kohn, A & Katz, N. (1999). Therapeutic evalution of artesunate in experimental *Schistosoma mansoni* infection. *Revista da Sociedade Brasileira de Medicina Tropical,* vol. 32, no. 1, (January/February 1999), pp. 7-12, ISSN 0037-8682.

Athanasiadou, S., Kyriazakis, I., Jackson, F. & Coop, R. L. (2001) Direct anthelmintic effects of condensed tannins towards different gastrointestinal nematodes of sheep: *in vitro* and *in vivo* studies. *Veterinary Parasitology,* vol. 99, no. 3, (August 2001), pp. 205-219, ISSN 0304-4017.

Athanasiadou, S. & Kyriazakis, I. (2004). Plant secondary metabolites: antiparasitic effects and their role in ruminant production systems. *Proceedings of the Nutrition Society,* vol. 63, no. 4, (November 2004), pp. 631–639, ISSN 0029-6651.

Avancini, C. A. M., Wiest, J.M. & Mundstock, E. (2000). Bacteriostatic and bactericidal activity of the Baccharis trimera *(Less.) D. C. - Compositae decocto, as disinfectant or antisseptic. Arquivo Brasileiro de Medicina Veterinária* e *Zootecnia,* vol.52, no. 3, (June 2000), pp.230-234, ISSN 0102-0935.

Baard, A. P., Sommers, D. K., Honiball, P. J., Fourie, E. D. & Du Toit, L. E. (1979). Preliminary results in human schistosomiasis with Ro 11-3128. *South African Medical Journal,* vol. 55, no. 16, (April 1979), pp. 617-618, ISSN 0256-9574.

Barakat, R., Elmorshedy, H. & Fenwick, A. (2005). Efficacy of myrr in the treatment of human *Schistomiasis mansoni. The American Journal of Tropical Medicine and Hygine,* vol. 73, no. 2, (August 2005), pp. 365-367, ISSN 0002-9637.

Barbosa- Filho, J. M., Tereza, H. C., Vasconcelos, A. A. A., Batista, L. M., Oliveira, R. A. G., Guedes, D. N., Flacão, H. S., Moura, M. D., Diniz, M. F. F. M. & Filho, J. M. (2005). Plants and their active constituents from South, Central, and North America with hypoglycemic activity. *Brazilian Journal of Pharmacognosy,* vol. 15, no. 4, (October /December 2005), pp. 392-413, ISSN 0976-8858.

Barreau, M., Cotrel, C. & Jeanmart, C. (1977). 1,2-Dithiolethiones. *Chemical Abstracts,* vol. 87, no., (no date), pp. 593, ISSN 0009-2258.

Barroso, G.M., (1976). Compositae - Subtribo Baccharidinae Hoffmann - Estudo das espécies ocorrentes no Brasil. *Rodriguésia- Revista do Jardim Botânico do Rio de janeiro,* vol. 28, no. 40, pp. 1-273, ISSN - 2175-7860.

Bassily, S., Farid, Z., Dunn, M., El-Masny & Stek, M. Jr. (1985). Praziquantel for treatment of schistosomiasis in patients with advanced splenomegaly. *Annals of Tropical Medicine and Parasitology,* vol. 79, (December 1979), pp. 629-634, ISSN 0003-4983.

Bayeux, M. C., Fernandes, A. T., Foglio, M. A. & Carvalho, J. E. (2002). Evaluation of the antiedematogenic activity of artemetin isolated from *Cordia curassavica* DC. *Brazilian Journal of Medical and Biological Research,* vol. 35, no. 10, (October 2002), pp. 1229-1232, ISSN 0100-879X.

Berge, S. T., Kabatereine, N., Gundersen, S. G., Taylor, M., Kvalsig, J. D., Mkhize-Kwitshana, Z., Jinabhai, C. & Kjetland, E. F. (2011). Generic praziquantel in South Africa: the necessity for policy change to provide cheap, safe and efficacious schistosomiasis drugs for the poor, rural population. *Southern African Journal of Epidemiology and Infection,* vol. 26, no. 1, (no date), pp. 22-25, ISSN 1015-8782.

Blanc, F. & Nosny, Y. (1968). Le traitement des schistosomes par les inhections de 2-dehydro-emetine. *La Presse Médicale,* vol. 76, no. 1, (no date), pp. 1419-1420, ISSN 0755-4982.

Bona, C. M., Biasi, L. A., Zanette, F. & Nakashima, T. (2005). Propagation of three species of *Baccharis* by cuttings. *Revista Ciência Rural, Santa Maria,* vol. 35, no. 1, (Janeiro/Fevereiro 2005), pp. 223- 226, ISSN 0103-8478.

Borella J. C., Duarte, D. P., Novaretti, A. A. G., Menezes Jr, A., França, S. C., Rufato, C. B., Santos, P. A. S., Veneziani, R. C. S. & Lopes, N. P. (2006). Variabilidade sazonal do teor de saponinas de *Baccharis trimera* (Less.) DC (Carqueja) e isolamento de flavona. *Revista Brasileira de Farmacognosia,* vol. 16, no. 4, (Outubro/Dezembro 2006), pp. 557-561, ISSN 0102-695X.

Bouree, P. (1991). Successful treatment of *Taenia saginata* and *Hymenolepis nana* by single oral dose of praziquantel. *Journal of the Egyptian Society of Parasitology,* vol. 21, no. 2, (August 1991), pp. 303-307, ISSN 0253-5890.

Bout, D. T., Deslée, D. & Capron, A. (1986). Antischistosomal effect of cyclosporin A: cure and Prevention of mouse and rat schistosomiasis mansoni. *Infection and Immunity,* vol. 52, no. 3, (June 1986), pp. 823-827, ISSN 0019-9567.

Braga, F. G., Bouzada, M. L., Fabri, R. L., Matos, M. O., Moreira, F. O. & Coimbra, E. S. (2006). Antileishmanial and antifungal activity of plants used in traditional medicine in Brazil. *Journal of Ethnopharmacology,* vol. 111, no. 2, (May 2007), pp. 396-402, ISSN 0378-8741.

Braguine, C. G., Costa, E. S., Magalhães, L. G., Rodrigues, V., Da Silva Filho, A. A., Bastos, J. K., Silva, M. L., Cunha, W. R., Januário, A. H. & Pauletti, P. M. (2009). Schistosomicidal evaluation of *Zanthoxylum naranjillo* and its isolated compounds against *Schistosoma mansoni* adult worms. *Zeitschrift für Naturforschung,* vol. 64, no. 11-12, (November/December 2009), pp. 793-797, ISSN 1865-7125.

Brickle, Q. D. & Andrews, B. J. (1985). Resistance following drug attenuation (Ro 11-3128 or oxamniquine) of early *Schistosoma mansoni* infections in mice. *Parasitology,* vol. 90, no. 2, (April 1985), pp. 325-338, ISSN 0031-1820.

Brindley, P. J. & Sher, A. (1987). The chemotherapeutic effect of praziquantel against *Schistosoma mansoni* is dependent on host antibody response. *Journal of Immunology,* vol. 139, no. 1, (July 1987), pp. 215–220, ISSN 0022-1767.

Brindley, P. J. (1994). Drug resistance to schistosomicides and other antihelmentics of medical significance. *Acta Tropica,* vol. 56, no. 2-3, (March 1994), pp. 213-231, ISSN 0001-706X.

Bueding, E., Batzinger, R. & Petterson, G. (1976). Antischistosomal and some toxicological properties of a nitrodiphenylaminoisothiocyanate (C 9333-Go/CGP 4540). *Experientia,* vol. 32, no. 5, (May 1976), pp. 604-606, ISSN 0014-4754.

Bueding, E., Hawkins, J. & Cha, Y. N. (1981). Antischistosomal effects of cyclosporin A. *Agents and Actions,* vol. 11, no. 4, (July 1981), pp. 380-383, ISSN 0065-4299.

Bueding, E., Dolan, P. & Leroy, J. P. (1982). The abtischistosomal activity of oltipraz. *Research Communications in Chemical Pathology and Pharmacology,* vol. 37, no. 2, (August 1982), pp. 293-303, ISSN 0034-5164.

Cabaret, J., Bouilhol, M. & Mage, C. (2002). Managing helminths of ruminants in organic farming. *Veterinary Research,* vol. 33, no. 5, (September/October 2002), pp. 625–640, ISSN 0928-4249.

Caffrey, C. R. (2007). Chemotherapy of schistosomiasis: present and future. *Current Opinion in Chemical Biology,* vol. 11, no. 4, (August 2007), pp.433–439, ISSN 1367-5931.

Calixto J.B., Santos A.R., Cechinel-Filho V. & Yunes R.A. (1998). A review of the plants of the genus *Phyllanthus*: their chemistry, pharmacology, and therapeutic potential.

Medicinal Research Reviews, vol. 18, no. 4, (December 1998), pp. 225–258, ISSN 1098-1128.

Carvalho Jr., P. M., Rodrigues, R. F., Sawaya, A. C., Marques, M. O. & Shimizu, M. T. (2004). Chemical composition and antimicrobial activity of the essential oil of *Cordia verbenacea* D.C. *Journal of Ethnopharmacology,* vol. 95, no. 2-3, (December 2004), pp. 297–301, ISSN 0378-8741.

Cerf, J., Lebrun, A. & Dierickx, J. (1962). A new approach to helminthiasis control: the use of an organophosphorus compound. *The American Journal of Tropical Medicine and Hygiene,* vol. 11, no. 1, (July 1962), pp. 514-517, ISSN 0002-9637.

Chen, D. J., Fu, L. F., Shao, P. P., Wu, F. Z., Fan, C. Z., Shu, H., Ren, C. S. & Sheng, X. L. (1980). Studies on antischistosomal activity of qinghaosu in experimental therapy. *Zhong Hui Yi Xue Zha Zhi,* vol. 80, no.1, (no date), pp. 422-428.

Christopherson, J. B. (1918). The successful use of antimony in bilharziosis. Administered as intravenous injections of antimonium tartaratum (tartar emetic). *The Lancet,* vol. 192, no. 4958, (September 1918), pp. 325-327, ISSN 0140-6736.

Cioli, D., Pica-Mattoccia, L. & Moroni, R. (1992). *Schistosoma mansoni*: hycanthone / oxamniquine resistance is controlled by a single autosomal recessive gene. *Experimental Parasitology,* vol. 75, no. 4, (December 1992), pp. 425-432, ISSN 0014-4894.

Cioli, D., Pica-Mattoccia, L. & Archers, S. (1993). Drug resistance in schistosomes. *Parasitology Today,* vol. 9, no. 5, (May 1993), pp. 162-166, ISSN 0169-4758.

Cioli, D., Pica-Mattoccia, L. & Archers, S. (1995). Antischistosomal drugs: past, present ... and future? *Pharmacology and Therapeutics,* vol. 68, no. 1, (no date), pp. 35-85, ISSN 0163-7258.

Cioli, D. (1998). Chemotherapy of schistosomiasis: an update. *Parasitology Today,* vol. 14, no. 10, (October 1998), pp. 418-422, ISSN 0169-4758.

Cioli, D. (2000). Praziquantel: is there real resistance and are there alternatives? *Current Opinion in Infectious Diseases,* vol. 13, no. 6, (December 2000), pp. 659–663, ISSN 0951-7375.

Cioli, D. & Pica-Mattoccia, L. (2002). Praziquantel. *Parasitology Research,* vol. 90, Supp. 1, (June 2003), pp. S3-9, ISSN 0932-0113.

Coelho, P M. Z. & Pereira, L. H. (1991). *Schistosoma munsoni:* preclinical studies with 9-acridanone-hydrazones in *Cebus* monkeys experimentally infected. *Revista do Instituto de Medicina Tropical de São Paulo,* vol. 33, no. 1, (January/February 1991), pp. 50-57, ISSN 0036-4665.

Coles, G. C.; Mutahi, W. T., Kinoti, G. K., Bruce, J. I. & Katz, N. (1987). Tolerance of Kenyan *Schistosoma mansoni* to oxamniquine. *Transactions of the Royal Society of Tropical Medicine and Hygiene,* vol. 81, no. 5, (September/October 1987), pp. 782-785, ISSN 0035-9203.

Cordell, G. A. & Colvard, M. D. (2005). Some thoughts on the future of ethnopharmacologt. *Journal of Ethnopharmacology,* vol. 100, no. 2, (August,2005), pp. 5-14, ISSN: 0378-8741.

Corrêa, M.P., (1984). *Dicionário das plantas úteis do Brasil e das exóticas cultivadas Vol. 1,* 74, Imprensa Nacional, ISBN , Rio de Janeiro, Brazil.

Coura, J. R. & Amaral. (2004). Epidemiological and control aspects of schistosomiasis in brazilian endemic areas. *Memórias do Instituto Oswaldo Cruz,* vol. 99 (Supl I), (July 2004), pp. 13-19, ISSN 0074-0276.

Cunha, A. S. (1982). Avaliação terapêutica da oxamniquine na esquistossomose mansoni humana pelo método do oograma por biópsia de mucosa retal. *Revista do Instituto de Medicina Tropical de São Paulo,* vol. 24, no. 2, (March/April 1982), pp. 88-94, ISSN 0036-4665.

Danso-Appiah, A. & De Vlas, S. J. (2002). Interpreting low praziquantel cure rates of *Schistosoma mansoni* infections in Senegal. *Trends in Parasitology,* vol. 18, no. 3, (March 2002), pp. 125–129, ISSN 1471-4922.

Dapper, D. V., Aziagba, B. N. & Ebong, O. O. (2007). Antiplasmodial effects of the aqueous extract of *Phyllanthus amarus* Schumach and Thonn against *Plasmodium berghei* in swiss albino mice. *Nigerian Journal of Physiological Sciences,* vol. 22, no. 1-2, (June/December 2007), pp. 19-25, ISSN 0794-859X.

Date, A. A., Joshi, M. D. & Patravale, V. B. (2007). Parasitic diseases: liposomes and polymeric nanoparticles versus lipid nanoparticles. *Advanced Drug Delivery Reviews,* vol. 59, no. 6, (July 2007), pp. 505–521, ISSN 0169-409X.

Davis, A. & Bailey, D. R. (1969). Metrifonate in urinary schistosomiasis. Bulletin of the World Health Organization, vol 41, no. 2, (no date), pp. 209-224, ISSN 0042-9686.

Davis, A., Biles, J. E. & Ulrich, A., M. (1979). Initial experiences with praziquantel in the treatment of human infections due to *Schistosoma haematobium*. Bulletin of the World Health Organization, vol. 57, no. 5, (no date), pp. 773-779, ISSN 0042-9686.

Davis, A. (1993). Antischistosomal drugs and clinical pratice, In *Human Schistosomiasis,* Jordan, P., Webbe, G. & Sturrock, R. F, (Eds), 367-404, CAB International, ISBN 0-85198-844-X, Wallingford, United Kingdom.

Day, T. A., Bennett, J. L. & Pax, R. A. (1992). Praziquantel: the enigmatic antiparasitic. *Parasitology Today,* vol. 8, no.10, (October 1992), pp. 342-344, ISSN 0169-4758.

Devienne., K. F., Raddi, M. S. G. & Pozetti, G. L. (2004). From medicinal plants to phytopharmaceuticais. *Brazilian Journal of Medicinal Plant,* vol. 6, no. 3, (April 2004), pp. 11-14, ISSN 1516-0572.

Dias, L. C., Pedro, R. J., Rigo, E., Goto, M. M. & Mafra, G. L. (1978). A human strain of *Schistosoma mansoni* resistant to schistosomicides. *Revista de Saúde Pública,* vol. 12, no. 1, (March 1978), pp. 110, ISSN 0034-8910.

Dias, L. F. T., Melo, E. S., Hernandes, L. S. & Bacchi, E. M. (2009). Atividades antiúlcera e antioxidante *Baccharis trimera* (Less) DC (Asteraceae). *Brazilian Journal of Pharmacognosy*. vol. 19, no. 1B, (January/March 2009), pp. 309-314, ISSN 0102-695X.

Doenhoff, M. J., Sabah, A. A. A., Fletcher, C., Webbe, G. & Bain, J. (1987). Evidence for an immune-dependent action of praziquantel on *Schistosoma mansoni* in mice. *Transactions of the Royal Societyof Tropical Medicine and Hygiene,* vol. 81, no. 6, (November/December 1987), pp. 947–951, ISSN 0035-9203.

Doenhoff, M. J., Hagan, P., Cioli, D., Southgate, V., Pica-Mattoccia, L., Botros, S., Coles, G., Tchuem-Tchuente, L. A., Mbaye, A. & Engels, D. (2009). Praziquantel: its use in control of schistosomiasis in sub-Saharan Africa and current research needs. *Parasitology,* vol. 136, no. 13, (November 2009), pp. 1825-1835, ISSN 0031-1820.

El Baz, M. A., Morsy, T. A., El Bandary, M. M. & Motawea, S. M. (2003). Clinical and parasitological studies on the efficacy of Mirazid in treatment of schistosomiasis haematobium in Tatoon, Etsa Center, El Fayoum Governorate. *Journal of the Egyptian Society of Parasitology*, vol. 33, no. 3, (December 2003), pp. 761-767, ISSN 0253-5890.

El Shenawy, N. S., Soliman, M. F. M. & Reyad, S. I. (2008). The effect of antioxidant properties of aqueous extract and *Nigella sativa* as anti-schistosomiasis agents in mice. *Revista do Instituto de Medicina Tropical de São Paulo,* vol. 50, no.1, (January-February 2008), pp.29-36, ISSN 0036-4665

El Ridi, R., Aboueldahab, M., Tallima, H., Salah, M., Mahana, N., Fawzi, S., Mohamed, S. H. & Fahmy, O. M. (2010). *In vitro* and *in vivo* activities of arachidonic acid against *Schistosoma mansoni* and *Schistosoma haematobium*. *Antimicrobial Agents and Chemotherapy,* vol. 54, no. 8, (August 2010), pp. 3383-3389, ISSN 0066-4804.

Eissa, M. M., El-Azzouni, M. Z., Amer, E. I. & Maddour, N. M. (2010). Miltefosine, a promising novel agent for schistosomiasis mansoni. International Journal for Parasitology, vol. 41, no. 1, (2011), pp. 235-242, ISSN 0020-7519.

Engels, D., Chitsulo, L., Montresor, A. & Savioli, L. (2002). The global epidemiological situation of schistosomisais and new approaches to control and research. *Acta Tropica,* vol. 82, no. 2, (May 2002), pp. 139-146, ISSN 0001-706X.

Fallon, P. G. & Doenhoff, M. J. (1994). Drug-resistant schistosomiasis: resistance to praziquantel and oxamniquine induced in *Schistosoma mansoni* in mice is drug especific. *American Journal of Tropical Medicine and Hygiene,* vol. 53, no. 1, (July 1994), pp. 61-62, ISSN 0002-9637.

Fallon, P. G., Sturrock, R. F., Niang, A. C. & Doenhoff, M. J. (1995). Short report: diminished susceptibility to praziquantel in a Senegal isolate of *Schistosoma mansoni*. *American Journal of Tropical Medicine and Hygiene,* vol. 53, no. 1, (July 1995), pp. 61-62, ISSN 0002-9637.

Ficarra, R., Ficarra, P. & Tommasini, S. (1995). Leaf extracts of some cordia species analgesic and anti-inflammatory activities as well as their chromatographic analysis. *Farmaco,* vol. 50, no. 4, (April 1995), pp. 245-256, ISSN 0014-827X.

Foglio, M. A., Queiroga, C. L., Souza, I. M. O. & Ferreira, R. A. (2006). Plantas Medicinais como Fonte de Recursos Terapêuticos: Um Modelo Multidisciplinar. *MultiCiência,* vol.7, no.1, (October 2006), pp. 1-8, ISSN 1806-2946.

Fontanilles, F. (1969). Risks versus benefits in antischistosomal therapy. *Annals of the New York Academy of Sciences,* vol. 160, no. 2, (October 1969), pp. 811-820, ISSN 0077-8923.

Foster, R. & Cheetham, B. L. (1973). Studies with the schistosomicide oxamniquine (UK – 4271). I: activity in rodents and in vitro. *Transactions of the Royal Society of Tropical Medicine and Hygiene,* vol 67, no. 5, (no date), pp. 674-684, ISSN 0035-9203.

Foster, R. (1987). A review of clinical experience with oxamniquine. *Transactions of the Royal Society of Tropical Medicine and Hygiene,* vol. 81, no. 1, (no date), pp. 55-59, ISSN 0035-9203 .

Frohberg, H. (1984). Results of toxicological studies on praziquantel. Arzneimittelforschung, vol. 34, no. 9, (no date), pp. 1137-1144, ISSN 0004-4172.

Frézard, F. & Melo, A. L. (1997). Evaluation of the schistosomicidal efficacy of lipossome - entrapped oxamniquine. *Revista do Instituto de Medicina Tropical de São Paulo,* vol. 39, no. 2, (March/April 1997), pp. 97-100, ISSN 0036-4665.

Getilini, M., Duflo, B., Richard-Lenoble, D., Bricker, G., Danis, M., Niel, G. & Meunier, Y. (1980). Assessment of 35972 (oltipraz) a new antischistosomal drug against *Schistosoma haematobium, Schistosoma mansoni,* and *Schistosomu intercalatum.* Acta *Tropica,* vol. 37, no. 3, (September 1980), pp. 271-274, ISSN 0001-706X.

Gonnert, R. & Andrews, P. (1977). Praziquantel, a new broad-spectrum antischistosomal agent. *Parasitology Research,* vol. 52, no. 2, (no date), pp. 129-150, ISSN 0932-0113.

Gonnert, R. & Vogel, H. (1955). Dependence on host and parasite strain of the successful therapy of experimental schistosomiasis. *Zeitschrift fur Tropenmedizin und Parasitologie,* vol. 6, no. 2, (June 1955), pp. 193-195, ISSN 0044-359X.

Grance, S. R. M., Teixeira, M. A., Leite, R. S., Guimarães, E. B., Siqueira, J. M., Filiu, W. F. O., Vasconcelos, S. B. S. & Vieira, M. C. (2008). *Baccharis trimera*: Effect on hematological na biochemical parameters and hepatorenal evalution in pregnant rats. *Journal of Ethnopharmacology,* vol. 117, no.1, (April 2008), pp. 28-33, ISSN 0378-8741.

Gragg, G. M. & Newman, D. J. (1999). Discovery and Development of Antineoplasic Agentsfrom Natural Sources. *Cancer Investigation,* vol.17, no. 2, pp. 153-163, ISSN 1532-4192.

Gryseels, D., Mbaye, A., De Vlas, Stelma, F. F., Guisé, F., Van Lieshout, L., Fave, D., Diop, M., Ly, A., Tchen-Tchuenté, L. A., Engels, D. & Polman, K. (2001). Are poor responses to praziquantel for the treatment of Schistosoma mansoni infections in Senegal due to resistance? An overview of the evidence. *Tropical Medicine and International Health,* vol. 6, no. 11, (November 2001), pp. 864–873, ISSN 1360-2276.

Guerra, M. P. & Nodari, R. O. (1999). Biodiversidade: Aspectos Biológicos, geográficos, legais e éticos, In: *Farmacognosia: da planta ao medicamento* (3ª edition), Simões, C. M. O., Schenkel, E. P., Gosmann, G., Mello, P. C. J., Mentz, A. L. & Petrovick, P. R. (Eds.), 48, Editora UFRGS, ISBN 85-7025-479-2, Porto Alegre/Florianóplis, Brazil.

Guo, Y., Wu, L. J. & Xu, P. S. (2000). Safety of artesunate in a long term administration in rats. *Chinese Journal of Schistosomiasis Control,* vol. 12, no. 1, (no date), pp. 27-29, ISSN 1005-6661.

Harnett, W. & Kusel, J. R. (1986). Increased exposure of parasite antigens at the surface of adult male *Schistosoma mansoni* exposed to praziquantel *in vitro. Parasitology,* vol. 93, no. 2, (October 1986), pp. 401–405, ISSN 0031-1820.

Hostettmann, K., Queiroz, E. F. & Vieira, P. C. (2003). A importância das plantas medicinais: Princípios ativos de plantas superiores. *Série de textos da Escola de Verão em Química vol. 4,* Edufscar, ISBN 85851173-99-8, São Carlos, Brazil.

Hubei Nithiocyaminum Coordination Research Group. (1980). Clinical studies on 4022 cases of schistosomiasis japonica treated with nithiocyanminun. *National Medical Journal of China,* vol. 60, no. 11, (no date), pp. 679-682, ISSN 0376-2491.

Hulbert, P. B., Bueding, E. & Robinson, C. H. (1973). Structure and antischistosomal activity in the nitrofuran series. Requirement for a 5-nitro-2-furyl-vinyl moiety based on comparison of 3-(s-nitro-2-furryl)-substituted propionic, acrylic, and propiolic acid derivatives? Journal of Medicinal Chemistry, vol. 16, no. 1, (January 1973), pp. 72-78, ISSN 0022-2623.

Ishizaki, T., Kamo, E. & Boehme, K. (1979). Double-blind studies of tolerance to praziquantel in Japanese patients with Schistosoma japonicum infections. Bulletin of the World Health Organization, vol. 57, no. 5, (no date), pp. 787-791, ISSN 0042-9686.

Ismail, M., Metwally, A., Farghaly, A., Bruce, J., Tao, L. F. & Bennett, J. L. (1996). Characterization of isolates of *Schistosoma mansoni* from Egyptian villagers that tolerate high doses of praziquantel. *American Journal of Tropical Medicine and Hygiene,* vol. 55, no. 2, (August 1996), pp. 214-218, ISSN 0002-9637.

Ismail, M., Botros, S., Metwally, A., William, S., Farchally, A., Tao, L. F., Day, T. A. & Bennett, J. L. (1999). Resistance to praziquantel: direct evidence from *Schistosoma mansoni* isolated from egyptian villagers. *American Journal of Tropical Medicine Hygiene,* vol. 60, no. 6, (June 1999), pp. 932-935, ISSN 0002-9637.

Jackson, F. & Coop, R. L. (2000). The development of Anthelmintic resistance in sheep nematodes. *Parasitology,* vol. 120, Suppl 1, (January 2000), pp. 95-107, ISSN 0031-1820.

Jain, N., Shasany, A. K., Sundaresan, V., Rajkumar, S., Darokar, M. P., Bagchi, G. D., Gupta, A. K., Kumar, S. & Khanuja, P. S. (2003). Molecular diversity in *Phyllanthus amarus* assessed through RAPD. *Currrent Science,* vol. 85, no. 10, (no date), pp. 1454-1458, ISSN 0011-3891.

Januario, A. H., Santos, S. L., Marcussi, S., Mazzi, M. V., Pietro, R. C. L., Sato, D. N., Ellena, J., Sampaio, S. V., Franca, S. C. & Soares, A. N. (2004). Neo-clerodane diterpenoid, a new metalloprotease snake venom inhibitor from *Baccharis trimera* (Asteraceae): anti-proteolytic and anti-hemorrhagic properties. *Chemico-Biological Interactions,* vol.150, no. 3, (December 2004), pp. 243-251, ISSN: 0009-2797.

Jatsa, H. B., Ngo Sock, E. T., Tchuem Tchuente, L. A. & Kamtchouing, P. (2009). Evaluation of the in vivo activity of different concentrations of *Clerodendrum umbellatum* poir against *Schistosoma mansoni* infection in mice. *African Journal of Traditional, Complementary and Alternative Medicines.* Vol. 6, no.3, (May 2009), pp. 216-221, ISSN 0189-6016.

Jewsbury, J. M., Cooke, M. J. & Weber, M. C. (1977). Field trial of metrifonate in the treatment and prevention of schistosomiasis infection in man. Annals of Tropical Medicine and Parasitology, vol. 71, no. 1, (March 1977), pp. 67-83, ISSN 0003-4983.

Jeziorski, M. C. & Greenberg, R. M. (2006). Voltage-gated calcium channel subunits from platyhelminths: potential role in praziquantel action. *International Journal of Parasitology,* vol. 36, no., (May 2006), pp. 625-632, ISSN 0020-7519.

Jiraungkoorsul, W., Sahaphomg, S., Sobhon, P., Riengrojpitak, S. & Kangwanrangsan, N. (2006). *Schistosoma mekongi*: the *in vitro* effect of praziquantel and artesunate on the adult fluke. *Experimental Parasitology,,* vol. 113, no. 1, (May 2006), pp. 16-23, ISSN 0014-4894.

Karuna, R., Reddy, S.S., Baskar, R. & Saralakumari, D. (2009). Antioxidant potential of aqueous extract of *Phyllanthus amarus* in rats. *Indian Journal of Pharmacology,* vol. 41, no. 2, (April 2009), pp. 64-67, ISSN 1998-3751.

Kassuya, C. A., Silvestre, A. A., Rehder, V. L. & Calixto, J. B. (2003). Anti-allodynic and anti-edematous properties of the extract and lignans from Phyllanthus amarus in models of persistent inflammatory and neuropathic pain. *European Journal of Pharmacology*, vol. 478, no. 2-3, (October 2003), pp. 145-153, ISSN 0014-2999.

Kassuya, C. A., Rehder, V. L. G., Melo, L. V., Silvestre, A. A. & Calixto, J. B. (2005). Anti-inflammatory properties of extracts, fractions and lignans isolated from *Phyllanthus amarus*. *Planta Medica*, vol. 71, no. 8, pp. 721-726, ISSN 0032-0943.

Kassuya, C. A., Silvestre, A. A., Menezes de Lima, O., Jr., Marotta, D. M., Rehder, V. L. G. & Calixto, J. B. (2006). Antiinflammatory and antiallodynic actions of the lignan niranthin isolated from *Phyllanthus amarus* evidence for interaction with platelet activating factor receptor. *European Journal of Pharmacology*, vol. 546, no. 1-3, (September 2006), pp. 182-188, ISSN 0014-2999.

Katz, N., Dias, E. P., Araújo, N. & Souza, C. P. (1973). Estudo de uma cepa humana de *Schistosoma mansoni* resistente a agentes esquistossomicidas. *Revista da Sociedade Brasileira de Medicina Tropical*, vol. 7, no. 1, (no date), pp. 381-387, ISSN 0037-8682.

Katz, N., Rocha, R. & Chaves, A. (1979). Preliminary trials with praziquantel in human infections due to Schistosoma mansoni. Bull.etin of the World Health Organizatiom, vol. 57, no. 5, (no date), pp. 781-785, ISSN 0042-9686.

Katz, N., Rocha, R. & Chaves, A. (1984). Assessment of oltipraz in schistosomiasis mansoni clinical trials. Revista do Instituto Brasileiro de Medicina Tropical de São Paulo, vol. 26, no. 3, (May/June 1984), pp. 147-151, ISSN 0036-4665.

Katz, N. & Almeida, K. (2003). Esquistossomose, xistosa, barriga d'água. Ciência e Cultura, vol. 55, no. 1, (January/March 2003), 38-41, ISSN 0009-6725.

Katz, N. (2008). Terapêutica experimental da esquistossomose mansoni, In: Schistosoma mansoni & esquistossomose uma visão multidisciplinar, CARVALHO, O. S., COELHO, P. M. Z. & LENZI, H. L. (eds), 825-870, Fiocruz, ISBN 978-857541-150-6, Rio de Janeiro, Brazil.

Keiser, J., Chollet, J., Xiao, S. H., Mei, J. Y., Jiao, P. Y., Utzinger, J. & Tanner, M. (2009). Mefloquine - an aminoalcohol with promising antischistosomal properties in mice. PloS Neglected Tropical Diseases, vol. 3, no. 1, (January 2009), pp. 1-11, ISSN 1935-2735.

Ketzis, J. K., Vercruysse, J., Stromberg, B. E., Larsen, M., Athanasiadou, S. & Houdijk, J. G. M. (2006). Evaluation of efficacy expectations for novel and non-chemical helminth control strategies in ruminants. *Veterinary Parasitology*, vol. 139, no. 4, (July 2006), pp. 321–335, ISSN 0304-4017.

Kikuth, W. & Gonnert, R. (1948). Experimental studies on the therapy of schistosomiasis. Annals of Tropical Medicine and Parasitology, vol. 42, no. 3-4, (December 1948), pp. 256-267, ISSN 0003-4983.

King, C. H. 2009. Parasites and poverty: the case of schistosomiasis. Acta Tropica, vol. 113, no. 2, (February 2010), pp. 95-104, ISSN 0001-706X.

Kinoti, G. K. (1987). The significance of variation in the susceptibility of Schistosoma mansoni to the antischistosomal drug oxamniquine. Memórias do Instituto Oswaldo Cruz, vol. 2, Suppl. 4, (no date), pp. 151-156, ISSN 0074-0276.

Khatoon, S., Rai, V., Rawat, A. K. S. R. & Mehrota, S. (2006). Comparative pharmacognostic studies of three *Phyllanthus* species. *Journal of Ethnopharmacology*, vol. 104, no. 1-2, (March 2006), pp. 79-86, ISSN 0378-8741.

Klayman, D. L. (1993). *Artemisia annua*: from weed to respectable antimalarial plant, In: *Human Medicinal Agents from Plants,* KINGHORN, A. D. & BALANDRIN, M. F. (eds), 242-255, American Chemical Society, ISBN 0-8412-2705-5, Washington, United States.

Kloucek, P., Polesny, Z., Svobodova, B., Vlkova, E. & Kokoska, L. (2005). Antibacterial screening of some Peruvian medicinal plants used in Callería District. *Journal of Ethnopharmacology*, vol. 99, no. 2, (June, 2005), pp. 302-312, ISSN 0378-8741.

Korte, R., Schimidt-Ehry, B., Kielmann, A. A. & Brinkmann, U. K. (1986). Cost and effectiveness of different approaches to schistosomiasis control in Africa. Tropical Medicine and Parasitology, vol. 37, no. 2, (June 1986), pp. 149-152, ISSN 0177-2392.

Kramers, P. G. N., Gentile, J. M., Gryseels, B. J. M., Jordan, P., Katz, N., Mott, K. E., Mulyihill, J. J., Seed, J. L. & Frohberg, H. (1991). Review of the genotoxicity and carcinogenicity of antischistosomal drugs: is there a case for a study of mutation epidemiology? Report of a task group on mutagenic antischistosomals. Mutation Research, vol. 257, no. 1, (January 1991), pp. 49-89, ISSN 1383-5742.

Krishna, S., Bustamante, L., Haynes, R. K. & Staines, H. M. (2008). Artemisinins: their growing importance in medicine. Trends in Pharmacological Sciences, vol. 29, no. 10, (October 2008), pp 520-527, ISSN 0165-6147.

Krithika, R., Mohankumar, R., Verma, R. J., Shrivastav, P. S., Mohamed, I. L., Gunasekaran, P. & Narasimhan, S. (2009). Isolation, characterization and antioxidative effect of phyllanthin against CCl4-induced toxicity in HepG2 cell line. *Chemico-Biological Interactions*, vol. 181, (July 2009), pp. 351-358, ISSN 0009-2797.

Kuntz, A. N., Davioud-Charvet, E., Sayed, A. A., Califf, L. L., Dessolin, J., Armer, E. S. & Williams, D. L. (2007). Thioredoxin glutathione reductase from *Schistosoma mansoni*: an essential parasite enzyme and a key drug target. *PLoS Medicine*, vol. 4, no. 6, (June 2007), pp. 1071-1086, ISSN 1549-1277.

Lambert, C. R. & Stauffer, P. (1964). Chemotherapy of experimental *Schistosoma mansoni* infections with a nitrothiazole derivate, CIBA 32, 644-Ba. *Annals of Tropical Medicine and Parasitology*, vol. 58, no. 1, (September 1964), pp. 292-303, ISSN 0003-4983.

Lambertucci, J. R. (2010). Acute schistosomiasis mansoni: revisited and reconsidered. *Memórias Instituto Oswaldo Cruz*, vol. 105, no. 4, (July 2010) pp. 422-435, ISSN 0074-0276.

Le, W. J., You, J. Q., Yang, Y. Q., Mei, J. Y., Guo, H. F., Yang, H. Z. & Zhang, Z. W. (1982). Studies on the efficacy of artemether in experimental schistosomiasis. *Acta Phamaceutica Sinica*, vol. 17, no.3 , (March 1982), pp. 187-193, ISSN 0513-4870.

Le, W. J., You, J. Q. & Mei, J. Y. (1983). Chemotherapeutic effect of artesunate in experimental schistosomiasis. *Acta Pharmaceutica Sinica*, vol. 18, no. 8, (August 1983), pp. 619-621, ISSN 0513-4870.

Leite, C. E., Lunardelli, A., Castaman, T. A., Paul, E. L. & Oliveira, J. R. (2007). Extrato Aquoso de *Baccharis trimera* (Asteraceae) diminui a inflamação e o Dano Celular em

Pleurisia induzida por Veneno de *Dirphia* sp. (Saturniidae). *Revista Brasileira de Análises Clínicas*, vol, 39, no. 1, pp. 29-32, ISSN0370-369X.

Leroy, J. P., Barreaneau, M., Cotrel, C., Jeanmart, C., Messer, M. & Benazet, F. (1978). Laboratory studies of 35 972 RP, a new schistosomicidal compound. In: *Current Chemotherapy*, Siegenthaler, W. & Liithy, R. (eds.), 148- 150, American Society for Microbiology, ISBN 0-914826-16-6, Washington, United States.

Lescano, S. Z., Chieffi, P. P., Canhassi, R. R., Boulos, M. & Amato-Neto, V. (2004). Atividade antiparasitária do artemether na esquistossomose mansônica experimental. *Revista de Saúde Pública*, vol. 38, no. 1, (February 2004), pp. 71-75, ISSN 0034-8910.

Liang, Y. S., Coles, G., Doenhoff, M. J. & Vaughan, R. S. (2001). *In vitro* responses of praziquantel-resistant and susceptible *Schistosoma mansoni* to praziquantel. *International Journal for Parasitology*, vol. 31, no. 11, (September 2001), pp. 1227-1235, ISSN 0020-7519.

Londhe, J. S., Devasagayam, T. P. A., Foo, L. Y. & Ghaskadbi, S. S. (2009). Radioprotective Properties of Polyphenols from *Phyllanthus amarus* Linn. *Journal of Radiation Research*, vol. 50, no. 4, (May 2009), pp. 303-309, ISSN 0449-3060

Lorenz, W., Henglein, A. & Schrader, G. (1955). The new insecticide 0,0-dimethyl-2,2,2-trichloro-l-hydroxyethylphosphonate. *Journal of the American Chemical Society*, vol. 77, no. 9, (May 1955), pp. 2553-2554, ISSN 0002-7863.

Lorenzi H. & Matos, F. J. A. (2002). Plantas *Medicinais no Brasil: nativas e exóticas cultivadas*, Instituto Plantarum, ISBN 8586714-18-6, Nova Odessa, Brazil.

Lu, S. H., Yan, X. L., Li, S. W., Shi, J. F., Liu, X., Yan, X. H., Yan, M. J., Lou, L. J., Kumagai, T., Wen, L. Y. & Otha, N. (2004). Prophylatic effect of artesunate against experimental infection of *Schistosoma mansoni. Chinese Journal of Parasitology and Parasitic Diseases*, vol. 22, no. 1, (February 2004), pp. 20-23, ISSN 1000-7423.

Lu, G., Hu, X., Huang, C., Lu, Y., Wu, L., Lihua, L., Xu, J. & Yu, X. (2010). Effect of artmether, hemin and Fe3+ on recombinant lactate dehydrigenase from *Schistosoma japonicum. Asian Pacific Journal of Tropical Medicine*, vol. 3, no. 12, (December 2010), pp. 930-933, ISSN 1995-7645.

Luize, P. S., Tiuman, T. S., Morello, L. G. (2005). Effects of medicinal plant extracts on growth of *Leishmania (L.) amazoniensis* and *Trypanosoma cruzi. Brazilian Journal of Pharmaceutical Sciences*, vol. 41., no.1 (March 2005), pp. 85-94, *ISSN:* 1984-8250.

Maciel, M. A., Pinto, A. C., Veiga Jr., Grynberg, N. F. & Echevarria, A. (2002). Plantas Medicinais: a necessidade de estudos multidisciplinares. *Química Nova*, vol.25, no. 3, (Maio/Junho 2002), pp. 429-438, ISSN 0100-4042.

Magalhães, L. G., Machado, C. B., Morais, E. R., Moreira, E. B. C., Soares, C. S., Silva, S. H., Da Silva Filho, A. A. & Rodrigues, V. (2009). *In vitro* schistosomicidal activity of curcumin against *Schistosoma mansoni* adult worms. *Parasitology Research*, vol. 104, no. 5, (April 2009), pp. 1197-1201, ISSN (electronic) 1432-1955.

Magalhães, L. G., Kapadia, G. J., Tonuci, L. R. S., Caixeta, S. C., Parreira, N. A., Rodrigues, V. & Da Silva Filho, A. A. (2010). *In vitro* schistosomicidal effects of some phloroglucinol derivates from *Dryopteris* species against *Schistosoma mansoni* adults worms. *Parasitology Research*, vol. 106, no. 2, (January 2010), pp. 395-401, ISSN 1432-1955.

Mahmoud, M. R., El-Abhar, H. S. & Salesh, S. (2002). The effect of *Nigella sativa* oil against the liver damage induced *Schistosoma mansoni* infection in mice. *Journal of Ethnopharmacology*, vol. 79, no. 1, (January 2002), pp. 1-11, ISSN 0378-8741.

Mantawy, M.M., Ali, H. F. & Rizk, M. Z. (2011). Therapeutic effects of *Allium sativum* and *Allium cepa* in *Schistosoma mansoni* experimental infection. *Revista do Instituto de Medicina Tropical de São Paulo,* vol. 53, no. 3, (May-June 2011), pp.155-163, ISSN 0036-4665.

Matos, F. J. A. (1994). *Farmácias vivas: sistema de utilização de plantas medicinais. Projeto para pequenas comunidades*, 4ª edition, EUFC, ISBN 8572820086, Fortaleza, Brazil.

Meccia, G., Rojas, L. B., Velasco, J., Diaz, T., Usubillaga, A., Arzola, J. C. & Ramos, S. (2009). Chemical composition and antibacterial activity of the essential oil of *Cordia verbenacea* from the Venezuelan Andes. *Natural Product Communications*, vol. 4, no. 8, (August 2009), pp. 1119–1122, ISSN 1934-578X.

Melo, C. M. L., Lima, A. L. R., Beltrão, E. I. C., Cavalcanti, C. C. B., Melo-Júnior, M. R., Montenegro, S. M. L., Coelho, L. C. B. B., Correia, M. T. S. & Carneiro-Leão, A. M. A. (2011). Potential effects of Cramoll 1,4 lectin on murine *Schistosomiasis mansoni*. *Acta Tropica*, vol. 118, no. 2, (May 2011), pp. 152-158, ISSN 0001-706X.

Melo, N. I., Magalhaes, L. G., Carvalho, C. E., Wakabayashi, K. A. L., Aguiar, G. P., Ramos, R. C., Mantovani, A. L. L., Turatti, I. C. C., Rodrigues, V., Groppo, M., Cunha, W. R., Veneziani, R. C. S. & Crotti, A. E. M. (2011). Schistosomicidal Activity of the Essential Oil of *Ageratum conyzoides* L. (Asteraceae) against Adult *Schistosoma mansoni* Worms. *Molecules*, vol. 16, (January 2011), pp. 762-773, ISSN 1420-3049.

Michielin, E. M. Z., Salvador, A. A., Riehl, C. A. S., Smânia-Jr. A., Smânia, E. F. A. & Ferreira, S. R. S. (2009). Chemical composition and antibacterial activity of *Cordia verbenacea* extracts obtained by different methods. *Bioresource Technology,* vol. 100, no. 24, (December 2009), pp. 6615-6623, ISSN 0960-8524.

Michielin, E. M. Z., Wiesse, L. P. L., Ferreira, E. A., Pedrosa, R. C. & Ferreira, S. R. S. (2011). Radical-scavenging activity of extracts from *Cordia verbenacea* DC obtained by different methods. *Journal of Supercritical Fluids,* vol. 56, no. 1, (February 2011), pp. 89-96, ISSN 0896-8446.

Ministério da Saúde. (2005). Guia de vigilância epidemiológica - série A - normas e manuseios técnicos, 6ª edition, Editora MS, ISBN 85-334-1047-6, Brasília, Brazil.

Ministério da Saúde. (2009). *Programa Nacional de Plantas Medicinais e Fitoterápicos,* Editora MS, ISBN 978-85-334-1597-3, Brasília, Brazil.

Mitsui, Y., Miura, Y. & Aoki, Y. (2008). In vitro effects of artesunate on the survival of worm pairs and egg production of Schistosoma mansoni. Journal of Helminthology, vol. 83, no. 1, (March 2009), pp. 7-11, ISSN 0022-149X.

Modha, J., Lambertucci, J. R., Doenhoff, M. J. & Mclaren, D. J. (1990). Immune dependence of schistosomicidal chemotherapy: an ultrastructural study of *Schistosoma mansoni* adult worms exposed to praziquantel and immune serum in vivo. *Parasite Immunology,* vol. 12, no. 3, (May 1990), pp. 321–334, ISSN 0141-9838.

Mohamed, A. M., Metwally, N. M. & Mahmoud, S. S. (2005). *SATIVA* seeds against *Schistosoma mansoni* different stages. *Memórias do Instituto Oswaldo Cruz,* vol. 100, no. 2, (April 2005), pp. 205-211, ISSN 0074-0276.

Moraes, J., Nascimento, C., Lopes, P. O. M. V., Nakano, E., Yamaguchi, L. F., Kato, M. J. & Kawano, T. (2011). *Schistosoma mansoni*: *In vitro* schistosomicidal activity of piplartine. *Experimental Parasitology*, vol. 127, no. 2, (February 2011), pp. 357-364, ISSN 0014-4894.

Mostafa, O. M. S., Eid, R. A. & Adly, M. A. (2011). Antischistosomal activity of ginger (*Zingiber officinale*) against *Schistosoma mansoni* harbored in C57 mice. *Parasitology Research, in press*, (February 2011), ISSN 1432-1955.

Molgaard, P., Nielsen, S. B., Rasmussen, D. E., Drumond, R. B., Makaza, N. & Andreassen, J. (2001). Anthelmintic screening of Zimbabwean plants traditionally used against schistosomiasis. *Journal of Ethnopharmacology*, vol. 74, no. 3, (March 2001), pp. 257-264, ISSN 0378-8741.

Moraes, J., Nascimento, C., Lopes, P. O. M. V., Nakano, E., Yamaguchi, L. F., Kato, M. J. & Kawano, T. (2010). *Schistosoma mansoni*: *in vitro* schistosomicidal activity of piplartine. *Experimental Parasitoogy*, vol. 127, no. 2, (February 2011) pp. 357-364, ISSN 0014-4894.

Nelson, D. L. & Pellegrino, J. (1976). Experimental chemotherapy of schistosomiasis XI - Active derivatives of aminoethanethiosulfuric acids. *Revista do Instituto de Medicina Tropical de São Paulo*, vol. 18, no. 4, (July/August 1974), pp. 365-370, ISSN 0036-4665.

Nontprasert, A., Pukrittayames, S., Dondorp, A. M., Clemens, R., Looareesuwan, S. & Whitw, N. J. (2002). Neuropathologic toxicity of artemisinin derivatives in a mouse model. *American Journal of Tropical Medicine and Hygine*, vol. 67, no. 4, (October 2002), pp. 423-429, ISSN 0002-9637.

Notka, F., Meier, G. & Wagner, R. (2004). Concerted inhibitory activities of *Phyllanthus amarus* on HIV replication *in vitro* and *ex vivo*. *Antiviral Research*, vol. 64, no. 2, (November 2004), pp. 93-102, ISSN 0166-3542.

Novaes, M. R. C. G., Souza, J. P. & Araújo, H. C. (1999). Síntese do anti-helmíntico praziquantel , a partir da glicina. Química *Nova*, vol. 22, no. 1, (January/February 1999), pp. 5-10, ISSN 0100-4042.

Pádua, B. C., Silva, L. D., Rossini jr.J.V., Humberto, J. L., Chaves, M. M., Silva, M. E., Pedrosa, M. L., Costa. D. C. (2010). Antioxidant properties of *Baccharis trimera* in the neutrophils of Fisher rats. *Journal of Ethnopharmacology*, Vol. 129, no. 3, (June 2010), pp. 381- 386, ISSN: 0378-8741.

Paraense, W. L. (1966). *Biomphalaria amazonica* and *B. cousini*, two new species of Neotropical planorbid mollusc. *Revista Brasileira de Biologia*, vol. 26, no. 2, (July 1966), pp. 115-126, ISSN 0034-7108.

Paraense, W. L. (1981). Biomphalaria occidentalis n. sp. from South America. Memórias dos Intituto Oswaldo Cruz, vol. 76, no. 2, (June 1981), pp. 199-211, ISSN 0074-0276.

Paraense, W. L. (1986). Distribuição dos caramujos no Brasil, In: Moderno conhecimentos sobre esquistossomose mansônica no Brasil, REIS, F. A., FARIA, I. & KATZ, N. (eds), pp. 117-128, Academia Mineira de Medicina, Belo Horizonte, Brazil.

Parreira, N. A., Magalhães, L. G., Morais, D. R., Caixeta, S. C., Sousa, J. P. B., Bastos, J. K., Cunha, W. R., Silva, M. L. A., Nanayakkara, N. P. D., Rodrigues, V. & Silva Filho, A. A. (2010). Antiprotozoal, Schistosomicidal, na Antimicrobial Activities of the

Essential Oil from the Leaves of *Baccharis dracunculifolia*. *Chemistry & Biodiversity*, vol. 7, no. 4, (April 2010), pp. 993-1001, ISSN 1612-1880.

Parise-Filho, R. & Silveira, M. A. B. (2001). Panorama atual da esquistossomíase no mundo. Brazilian Journal of Pharmaceutical Sciences, vol. 37, no. 2, (may/august 2001), pp. 123-135, ISSN 1516-9332.

Passos, G. F., Fernandes, E. S., Cunha, F. M., Ferreira, J., Pianowski, L. F., Campos, M. M. & Calixto, J. B. (2006). Anti-inflammatory and anti-allergic properties of the essential oil and active compounds from *Cordia verbenacea*. *Journal of Ethnopharmacololy*, vol. 110, no. 2, (March 2007), pp. 323–333, ISSN 0378-8741.

Paul, E. L., Lunardelli, A., Caberlon, E., Oliveira, C. B., Santos, R. C., Biolchi, v., Bastos, C. M., Moreira, K. B., Nunes, F. B., Gosmann, G., Oliveira, J. R. (2009). Anti-inflammatory and immunomodulatory effects of *Baccharis trimera* aqueous extract on induced pleurisy in rats and lymphoproliferation *in vitro*. *Inflammation*,vol.32, no.6, (December 2009), pp. 419–425, *ISSN*: *1573-2576*.

Pax, R., Bennett, J. L. & Fetterer, R. (1978). A benzodiazepine derivative and praziquantel: effects on musculature of Schistosoma mansoni and Schistosoma japonicum. *Naunyn-Schmiedeberg's Archives of Pharmacology*, vol. 304, no. 3, (October 1978), pp. 309-315, ISSN 0028-1298.

Penido, M. L. O., Coelho, P. M. Z. & Nelson, D. L. (1999). Efficacy of a new schistosomicidal agent 2[(methylpropyl)amino]-1-octanethiosulfuric acid against na oxamniquine resistant Schistosoma mansoni isolate. Memórias do Instituto Oswaldo Cruz, vol. 94, no. 6, (November/December 1999), ISSN 0074-0276.

Penido, M. L. O., Coelho, P. M. Z., Mello, R. T., Piló-Veloso, D., Oliveira, M. C., Kusel, J. R. & Nelson, D. L. (2008). Antischistosomal activity of aminoalkanethiols, aminoalkanethiosulfuric acids and the corresponding disulfides. *Acta Tropica,* vol. 108, no. 2-3, (November/December 2008), pp. 249-255, ISSN 0001-706X.

Pramyothin, P., Ngamtin, C., Poungshompoo, S. & Chaichantipyuth, C. (2007). Hepatoprotective activity of *Phyllantus amarus* Schum. et. Thonn. extract in ethanol treated rats: *In vitro* and *in vivo* studies. *Journal of Ethnopharmacology,* vol. 114, no. 2, (November 2007), pp. 169-173, ISSN 0378-8741.

Raphael, K. R., Sabu, M. C. & Kuttan, R. (2002). Hypoglycemic effect of methanol extract of *Phyllanthus amarus* Schumach and Thonn on alloxan induced *diabetes mellitus* in rats and its relation with antioxidant potential. *Indian Journal of Experimental Biology*, vol. 40, no. 8, (August 2002), pp. 905-909, ISSN 0019-5189.

Raphael, K. R. & Kuttan, R. (2003). Inhibition of experimental gastric lesion and inflammation by *Phyllanthus amarus* extract. *Journal Ethnopharmacology*, vol. 87, no. 2-3, (August 2003), pp. 193-197, ISSN 0378-8741.

Rajakannan, V., Sripathi, M. S., Selvanayagam, S., Velmurugan, D., Murthy, D. U., Vishwas, M., Thyagarajan, S. P., Raj, S. S. S. & Fun, H. K. (2003). Phyllanthin from the plant P*hyllanthus amarus*. *Acta Crystallografica*,vol. 59, (January 2003), pp.203-205, ISSN 1600-5368.

Rajeshkumar, N. V. & Kuttan, R. (2000). *Phyllanthus amarus* extract administration increases the life span of rats with hepatocellular carcinoma. *Journal of Ethnopharmacology*, vol. 73, no. 1-2, (November 2000), pp. 215-219, ISSN 0378-8741.

Reis, M. S., Mariot, A. & Steenbock, W. (2007). Diversidade e Domesticação de Plantas Medicinais. In: *Farmacognosia: da planta ao medicamento* (6ª edition), Simões, C. M. O., Schenkel, E. P., Gosmann, G., Mello, P. C., Mentz, A. L. & Petrovick, P. R. (Eds.), 45-74, Editora UFRGS, ISBN 9788570259271, Porto Alegre/Florianópolis, Brazil.

Riad, N. H. A., Fares, N. H., Mostafa, O. M. S. & Mahmoud, Y. I. (2007). The effect of garlic on some parasitological parameters and on hepatic tissue reactions in experimental *Schistosomiasis mansoni. Journal of Applied Sciences Research,* vol.3, no. 10, pp.949-960, ISSN 1819-544X.

Ribeiro-Dos-Santos, G., Verjovski-Almeida, S. & Leite, L. C. (2006). Schistosomiasis - a century searching for chemotherapeutic drugs. *Parasitology Research,* vol. 99, no. 5, (October 2006), pp. 505-521, ISSN 0932-0113.

Richards, H. C. & Foster, R. (1969). A new series of 2-aminomethyltetrahydroquinoline derivatives displaying schistosomicidal activity in rodents and primates. *Nature,* vol., 222, no. 5193, (May 1969), pp. 581-582, ISSN 0028-0836.

Robinson, C. H., Bueding, E. & Fisher, J. (1970). Relationship between structure, conformation and antischistosomal activity of nitroheterocyclic compounds. *Molecular Pharmacology,* vol. 6, no. 6, (November 1970), pp. 604-616, ISSN 0026-895 X.

Rodrigues, C. R. F., Dias, J. H., Mello, R. N., Richter, M. F., Picada, J. N. & Ferraz, A. B. F. (2009). Genotoxic and antigenotoxic properties of *Baccharis trimera* in mice. *Journal of Ethnopharmacology,* vol. 125, no. 1, (August 2009), pp.97-101, ISSN: 0378-8741.

Roldão, E., Witaicenis, A., Seito, L. N., Hiruma-Lima, C. A. & Di Stasi, L. C. (2008). Evaluation of the antiulcerogenic and analgesic activities of *Cordia verbenacea* DC. (Boraginaceae). *Journal of Ethnopharmacology,* vol. 119, no. 1, (September 2008), pp. 94–98, ISSN 0378-8741.

Rollas, S. & Kuçuguzel, S. G. (2007). Biological activities of hydrazone derivatives. *Molecules,* vol. 12, no. 8, (August 2007), pp. 1910-1939, ISSN 1420-3049.

Rosi, D., Peruzzoti, G., Dennis, E. W., Berberian, D. A., Freele, H. & Acher, S. (1965). A new active metabolite of Miracil D. *Nature,* vol. 208, no. 5014, (December 1965), pp. 1005-1006, ISSN 0028-0836.

Sabah, A. A., Fletcher, C., Webbe, G. & Doenhoff, M. J. (1986). *Schistosoma mansoni:* chemotherapy of infections of different ages. *Experimental Parasitology,* vol. 61, no. 3, (June 1986), pp. 294-303, ISSN 0014-4894.

Salazar-Mallen, M., Gonzalez-Barranco, D. & Mitrani-Levy, D. (1969). Trichlorophone in onchocerciaisis, Lancet, vol. 1, no. 7591, (February 1969), pp. 426, ISSN 0140-6736.

Santos, R. P., Nunes, E. P., Nascimento, R. F., Santiago, G. M. P., Menezes, G. H. A., Silveira, E. R. & Pessoa, O. D. L. (2006). Chemical composition and larvicidal activity of the essential oils of Cordia leucomalloides and Cordia curassavica from the Northeast of Brazil. Journal of the Brazilian Chemical Society, vol 17, no. 5, (September/October 2006), pp. 1027-1030, ISSN 0103-5053.

Sayed, A. A., Simeonov, A., Thomas, C. J., Inglese, J., Austin, C. P. & Williams, D. L. (2008). Identification of oxadiazoles as new drug leads for the control of schistosomiasis. *Nature Medicine* , vol. 14, no. 4, (April 2008), pp.407–412, ISSN 1078-8956.

Sertié, J. A. A., Woisky, R. G., Wiezel, G. & Rodrigues, M. (2005). Pharmacological assay of *Cordia verbenacea* V: oral and topical anti-inflammatory activity, analgesic effect and fetus toxicity of a crude leaf extract. *Phytomedicine,* vol. 12, no. 5, (May 2005), pp. 338–344, ISSN 0944-7113.

Shaohong, L., Kumagai, T., Qinghua, A., Xiaolan, Y., Ohmae, H., Yabu, Y., Siwen, L., Liyong, W., Maruyama, H. & Ohta, N. (2005). Evaluation of the anthelmintic effects of artesunate against experimental *Schistosoma mansoni* infection in mice using different treatment protocols. *Parasitology International,* vol. 55, no. 1, (March 2006), pp. 63-68, ISSN 1383-5769.

Sheir, Z., Nasr, A. A., Massoud, A., Salama, O., Badra, G. A., El- Shennawy, H., Hassan, N. & Hammad, S. M. (2001). A safe, effective, herbal antischistosomal therapy derived from myrrh. *The American Journal of Tropical Medicine and Hygiene,* vol. 65, no. 6, (December 2001), pp. 700-704, ISSN 0002-9637.

Shuhua, X. (2005). Development of antischistosomal drugs in China, with particular consideration to praziquantel and the artemisinins. *Acta Tropica,* vol. 96, no. 2-3, (November/December 2005), pp. 153-167, ISSN 0001-706X.

Silva, L. C., Chieffi, P. P. & Carrilho, F. J. (2005). Schistosomiasis mansoni - clinical features. *Gastroenterología y Hepatología,* vol. 28, no. 1, (January 2005), pp. 30-39, ISSN 0210-5705.

Soyez, H., Schacht, E. & Vanderkerden, S. (1996). The crucial role of spacer groups in macromolecular prodrug design. *Advanced Drug Delivery Reviews,* vol. 21, no. 2, (September 1996), pp. 81-106, ISSN 0169-409X.

Steinmann, P., Keiser, J., Bos, R., Tanner, M. & Utzinger, J. (2006). Schistosomiais and water resources development: systematic review, meta-analysis, and estimates of people at risk. *The Lancet Infectious Diseases,* vol. 6, no. 7, (July 2006), pp. 411-425, ISSN 1473-3099.

Stelma, F. F., Talla, I., Sow, S., Kongs, A., Niang, M., Polman, K., Deelder, A. M. & Gryseels, B. (1995). Efficacy and side effects of praziquantel in an epidemic focus of *Schistosoma mansoni. The American Journal of Tropical Medicine and Hygiene,* vol. 53, no. 2, (August 1995), pp. 167-170, ISSN 0002-9637.

Stohler, H. R. (1978). Ro 11-3128 – a novel schistosomicidal compund, In: *Current Chemotherapy,* Siegenthaler, W. & Liithy, R. (eds.), 147-148, American Society for Microbiology, ISBN 0-914826-16-6, Washington, United States.

Syohler, H. R. & Montanova, M. (1984). 9-Acridanoneydrazones, a novel class of broad-spectrum schistosomicidal agents, *Proceedings of International Congress of Tropical Medicine and Malaria,* pp. 16-22, Calgary, Canada, September 16-22, 1984.

Striebel, H. (1976). 4-Isothiocyanato-4'-nitrodiphenylamine (C 9333-GoiCGP 4540), an anthelminthic with an unusual spectrum of activity against intestinal nematodes, filarie and schistosomes. *Cellular and Molecular Life Sciences,* vol. 32, no. 4, (April 1976), pp. 457-458, ISSN 1420-682X.

Thyagarajan, S.P., Thirunalasundari,T., Subramanian, S., Venkateswaran, P.S., Blumberg, B.S. (1988). Effect of *Phyllanthus amarus* on cronic carriers of hepatitis B virus. *The Lancet,* vol. 332, no. 8614, (October 1988), pp. 764-766, ISSN 0140-6736.

Thomas, H., Gonnert, R., Pohlke, R. & Seubert, J. (1975). A new compound against adult tapeworms. *Proceedings of the 7th International Conference of the World Association for the Advancement of Veterinary Parasitology,* p. 50, ISBN 0-12-655365-3, Thessaloniki, Greece, July 14-16, 1975.

Ticli, F. K., Hage, L. I., Camabraia, R. S., Pereira, P. S., Magro, A. J., Fontes, M. R., Stabeli, R. G., Giglio, J. R., Franca, S. C., Soares, A. M. & Sampaio, S. V. (2005). Rosmarinic acid, a new snake venom phospholipase A2 inhibitor from *Cordia verbenacea* (Boraginaceae): antiserum action potentiation and molecular interaction. *Toxicon: Official Journal of the International Society on Toxicology,* vol. 46, no. 3, (September 2005), pp. 318–327, ISSN 0041-0101.

Torres, D. S. C. , Cordeiro, I., Giulietti, A .M. (2003). O Gênero *Phyllanthus* L. (*Euphorbiaceae)* na Chapada Diamantina, Bahia, Brasil. *Acta Botanica Brasilica,* vol. 17, no. 2, (April-June 2003), pp.265-278, ISSN 0102-3306 .

Utzinger, J., Chollet, J., Tu, Z. W., Xiao, S. H. & Tanner, M. (2002). Comparative study of the effects of artemether and artesunate on juvenile and adult *Schistosoma mansoni* in experimentally infected mice. *Transactions of the Royal Society of Tropical Medicine and Hygiene,* vol. 96, no. 3, (May/June 2002), pp. 318-323, ISSN 0035-9203.

Utzinger, J., Keiser, J., Shuhua, X., Tanner, M. & Singer, B. H. (2003). Combination chemotherapy of schistosomiasis in laboratory studies and clinical trials. *Antimicrobial Agents and Chemotherapy,* vol. 47, no. 5, (May 2003), pp. 1487-1495, ISSN 0066-4804

Van Nassauw, L., Toovey, S., Van Op Den Bosh, J. Timmermans, J. P. & Vercruysse, J. (2008). Schistosomicidal activity of the antimalarial drug, mefloquine, in *Schistosoma manconi* - infected mice. *Travel Medicine and Infectious Disease,* vol. 36, no. 5, (September 2008), pp. 253-258, ISSN 1477-8939.

Webbe G. & James, C. (1977). A comparison of the susceptibility to praziquantel of *Schistosoma haematobium, S. japonicum, S. mansoni, S. intercalatum* and *S. mattheei* in hamsters. *Parasitology Research,* vol. 52, no. 2, (January 1977), pp. 169-177, ISSN 0932-0113.

Wegner, D. H. G. (1984). The profile of trematodicidal compound praziquantel. *Arzneimittelforschung,* vol. 34, no. 9B , (no date), pp. 1132-1136, ISSN 0004-4172 .

Werbel, L. M. (1970). Chemotherapy of schistosomiasis. *Topics in Medicinal Chemistry,* vol. 3, no. 1, (no date), pp. 125-169, ISSN 1862-2461.

World Health Organization. (1993). *The control of schistosomiasis – second report of the WHO expert committee - Technical Series no. 830,* World Health Organization, ISBN 92-4-120830-9, Geneva, Switzerland.

World Health Organization. (May 2002). Medicina tradicional: necessidades crecientes y potencial, In: *Policy perspectives on medicines n. 2,* 01.07.2011, Available from http://whqlibdoc.who.int/hq/2002/who_edm_2002.4_spa.pdf.

World Health Organization. (2003). Cómo desarrollar y aplicar una política farmacéutica nacional, In: *Perspectivas políticas de la OMS sobre medicamentos,* 01/07/2011, Available from http://apps.who.int/medicinedocs/pdf/s4871s/s4871s.pdf.

World Health Organization. (2006). *WHO monograph on good agricultural and collection practice (GACP) of Artemisia annua L,* World Health Organization, ISBN 92-4-159443-8, Geneva, Switzerland.

World Health Organization. (February 2010). Schistosomiasis, In: *Media Centre - Fact sheets,* 01.07.2011, Available from http://www.who.int/mediacentre/factsheets/fs115/en/index.html.

Xiao, S. H., Catto, B. A. & Webster, L. T. (1985). Effects of praziquantel on different developmental stages of *Schistosoma munsoni* in vitro and in vivo. *Journal of Infectious Diseases.,* vol. 151, no. 6, (June 1985), pp. 1130-1137, ISSN 0022-1899.

Xiao, S. H. & Catto, B. A. (1989). *In vitro* and *In vivo* studies of the effect of Artemether on *Schistosoma mansoni. Antimicrobial Agents and Chemotherapy,* vol. 33, no. 9, (September 1989), pp. 1557-1562, ISSN 0066-4804.

Xiao, S. H., Hotez, P. J. & Tanner, M. (2000). Artemether, an effective new agent for chemoprophylaxis against schistosomiasis in China: its *in vivo* effect on the biochemical metabolism of the asian schistosome. *Southeast Asian Journal of Tropical Medicine and Public Health,* vol. 31, no. 4, (December 2000), pp. 724-732, ISSN 0125-1562.

Xiao P. (2002). *Modern Chinese Materia Medica Vol. 3,* Chemical Industry Press, ISBN 7502540857, Beijing, China.

Xiao, S. H., Keiser, J., Chollet, J., Utzinger, J., Dong, Y., Endriss, Y., Vennerstrom, J. L. & Tanner, M. (2007). *In vitro* and *in vivo* ctivities of synthetic trioxolanes against major human schistosome species. *Antimicrobial Agents and Chemotherapy,* vol. 51, no. 4, (April 2007), pp. 1440-1445, ISSN 0066-4804.

Yoshioka, L., Magalhães, E. M. Z., Magalhães, L. A. & Linhares, A.X. (2002). Schistosoma mansoni: estudo da patogenia da linhagem Santa Rosa (Campinas, SP, Brasil) em camundongos. Revista da Sociedade Brasileira de Medicina Tropical, vol. 35, no. 3, (May/June 2002), pp. 203-207, ISSN 0037-8682.

Yue, W. J., You, J. Q. & Mei, J. Y. (1984). Effects of artemether on *Schistosoma japonicum* adult worms and ova. *Acta Pharmacologica Sinica,* vol. 5, no. 1, (March 1984), pp. 60-63, ISSN 0253-9756.

Part 3

Control

4

Control of Schistosomiasis

Monday Francis Useh
University of Calabar, Calabar
Nigeria

1. Introduction

Schistomiasis is a disease caused by digenetic trematodes that belong to the family Schistosomatoidae. Five species of Schistosomes are involved in human infection. The three principal agents are *Schistosoma mansoni* and *S. japonicum* which are responsible for intestinal schistosomiasis and *S. haematobium*, the aetiologic agent of urinary schistosomiasis. The other two species responsible for intestinal disease though with low frequency are *S. intercalatum* and *S. mekongi*. The disease affects about 240 million people worldwide while an estimated 779 million people (more than 10% of the world population) are at the risk of infection. About 120 million people infected with schistosomiasis are estimated to be symptomatic while about 20 million develop severe diease.The disability-adjusted life years (DALYs) due to schistosomiasis is about 1.7-4.5 million while between 150,000 to 280,000 people are known to die as a consequence of the disease per year. Africa accounts for 85% of the disease burden (Steinmann *et al.*, 2006; WHO, 2002). Although, schistosomiasis is a rural focal disease typically associated with poor rice farmers and fishermen in the tropics, it is increasingly been reported among Europeans with a history of travel to endemic areas in Africa and Asia. It is transmitted by snails found in cercariae infested fresh water streams. Snails belonging to the species *Bulinus, Biomphalaria* and *Onchomelania* are the vectors of *S. haematobium*, *S. mansoni* and *S. japonicum* respectively.

The cardinal objective in the control of schistosomiasis is the reduction of morbidity and mortality to levels below public health significance. Over the years, emphasis has shifted from the non-realizable goal of eradication to the more realistic goal of morbidity control. In this context, Gemmel *et al* (1986), defined "a control programme" as the "implementation of specific measures by a disease control authority to limit the incidence of the disease". Such implementation may involve specific technical interventions and perhaps legislation to enforce compliance. The success of this type of approach is predicated on an accurate ecological diagnosis, that is, a diagnosis of the human community, its parasitological characteristics, its physico-geographical environmental attributes and man's behavioural attitudes and customs (Davis, 1981).

The enormous morbidity associated with schistosomiasis which ranks it next to malaria in terms of public health significance re-emphasises the need for a coordinated and sustainable means for the control of the disease. There is a consensus of opinion that the control of the disease should be integrated. In this model of control, King (2009) identified the applicable approaches as:

- Population based chemotherapy
- Snail control which involves habitat modification and use of plant and chemical molluscicides,

- Proper treatment of sewage,
- Good environmental engineering designs for the development of irrigation and hydroelectric schemes to limit the availability of breeding grounds for the snail vectors
- Provision of clean and safe piped water and
- Massive health education and mobilization of the population to claim ownership of the programme

In this Chapter, the various methods of control of schistosomiasis listed above are reviewed with special emphasis on those that are accessible, affordable, acceptable and capable of yielding high levels of sensitivity and specificity. Chemotherapy which is the most feasible method of morbidity control of the disease particularly in the short-term is examined in more details. In the process, the hindrances to an effective integrated control approach are identified while recommendations on the way forward are proffered. There is no doubt that vaccination holds the key for the cost effective and sustainable control of infectious diseases including schistosomiasis. The progress made in the identification of probable candidate antigen molecules for the control of schistosomiasis is also examined. The basis of this composite approach is to gradually reduce the morbidity due to schistosomiasis. This is likely to result in the drastic reduction in the number of infected subjects and environmental egg pollution. Where this is sustained, infection would no longer be of public health significance.

2. Control of schistosomiasis

The first control programme for schistosomiasis was initiated in 1913 in Egypt where both local people and stationed soldiers were heavily infected. This was anchored on snail control. The effectiveness of the programme was based on the numbers of snails killed and not reductions in the numbers of infections (Jordan, 2000). Mass treatment with tartar emetic was also an integral part of the process although the results were not encouraging. About the 1930s, sanitation was incorporated in the programme, but still the results were not convincing (Jordan & Rosenfield, 1983). Following the elucidation of the life cycle of Schistosomes by Lieper during the first years of the first world war, snail control and mass treatment became the model of control efforts. Jordan (2000) noted that together with recommendations on a number of environmental control measures, Leiper considered it possible to eradicate the disease without the cooperation of the infected individuals by destroying the snail intermediate host. Blas *et al* (1989) reports that the first control programme that integrated research and systematic monitoring of its effect was implemented in Lyte in the Philippines from 1953 to 1962 with the help of the WHO. The initial objective of the schistosomiasis control was aimed at stopping transmission. This could hardly be achieved and remains elusive even up till today.

The WHO Expert Committee on Epidemiology and Control of Schistosomiasis took a holistic approach at the control of the disease and noted that "comprehensive understanding of the environment, demographic, social, human behavioural and economic factors" in schistosomiasis is essential for the design of control programmes that are successful in the long run (Kloos, 1985). With the advent of praziquantel (PZQ) as a safe and efficacious drug for the treatment of schistosomiasis, the WHO in 1991 reinforced its 1984 recommendation to shift from transmission control (focusing on the prevalence of infection) to morbidity control (laying emphasis on intensity of infection) (Bruun and Aagaard-Hansen, 2008). Morbidity control will not only reduced the number of people infected but it will also drastically reduce environmental contamination with the eggs even when cure is not attained. A drastic reduction of the pollution of the environment with the eggs would also reduce the chances of transmission. Should this occur at a level below public health importance, the probability of eventually elimination of disease is certain with a sustained integrated approach

3. Chemotherapeutic control of schistosomiasis

Of all the methods of control listed above, chemotherapy is the only one that is widely used presently in endemic areas for the control of morbidity due to schistosomiasis. Among the first group of drugs used for the treatment of schistosomiasis included; Antimonials, Niridazole, Hycanthone, Lucanthone, Oxamniquine and albendazole. PZQ is currently used for the treatment of all the species while metrifonate is active against *S. haematobium* only. Recently, artemisinins earlier synthesized for the treatment of malaria infection is being used in some endemic communities to treat schistosomiasis. The WHO (1993) identified four approaches in the administration of chemotherapy programme namely;

i. Mass treatment: treatment of the entire population. This is often limited by availability of finance.
ii. Selective population treatment: treatment of infected persons identified by a diagnostic survey of the whole population
iii. Selective group treatment: treatment of all or infected members of a high risk age or occupational group
iv. Phased treatment: use of the above strategies in a sequence of progressively greater selectivity.

It is recommended that treatment should be administered to schoolchildren who are the most vulnerable group through the school system. The outcome of basing treatment on the school system is bound to give variable results. In an area endemic for urinary schistosomiasis in Nigeria, Useh and Ejezie (1999a) showed that relying on the school system alone to deliver control programme may substantially limit the outcome of control of schistosomiasis. The rates of regular, irregular and non school attendance were 69.1%, 5.1% and 25.8% respectively. Out of school children were more associated (90.7%) with *S. haematobium* infection than those in school (86.8%). The authors recommended a dual method of control that would incorporate the integration of recognized local authorities in areas with moderate school attendance like their study area as lack of treatment of infected out of school children would ensure continuous contamination and re-infection. (See Table 1)

Gender	Regular School Pupils, No(%)	Irregular School Pupils, No(%)	Children Out of School, No(%)	Total
Male	889(76.6)	50(4.3)	222(19.1)	1161
Female	699(61.4)	67(5.9)	372(32.7)	1138
X^2	58.02	2.77	55.86	NA
Odds Ratio	2.020	0.72	0.48	NA
95% CI	1.69-2.42	0.49-1.04	0.4-0.58	NA
P	<0.0001	>0.05	<0.0001	NA

(Adopted from Useh & Ejezie, 1999a)

Table 1. Frequency of school attendance and non-attendance by sex of school-age children in Adim, Nigeria.

This recommendation is supported by a study conducted in Tanzania on the effect of community-directed treatment approach (ComDT) versus the school-based treatment approach on the prevalence and intensity of schistosomiasis and soil-transmitted helminthiasis (STH) among schoolchildren (Massa *et al.*,2009). The prevalence of *S. haematobium* and Hookworm infections were significantly lower in the ComDT approach villages compared to the school-based approach villages (10.6 versus 16.3%, P = 0.005 and 2.9 versus 5.8%, P = 0.01, respectively).

3.1 PZQ

3.1.1 Biochemical properties and pharmacokinetics

PZQ is the drug of choice for the treatment of schistosomiasis. It is a broad spectrum anti-schistosomal which is principally active against the adult stage of all the schistosome species infective to man. It is a 2-cyclohexycarbonyl 1,2,3,6,7,11b-hexahydro-4H-pyrazino(2,1-a Isoquinolin-4one) compound with a melting point at 136-140C. It was developed in the laboratories for Parasitological Research of Bayer AG and Merck KGaA in Germany (Elbert and Darmstadt) in the mid 1970s. It has a molecular mass of 312.411 with a serum half life of 0.8 to 1.5 hours in adults with normal liver and kidney function and is mainly excreted in urine. PZQ is a white crystalline powder with bitter taste. It is stable under normal storage conditions. Although, it is insoluble in water, it is soluble in chloroform, dimethylsulfoxide and ethanol. It is sold as a racemate mixture consisting of equal parts of 'laevo' and 'dextro' isomers, of which only the laevo component displays anti-schistosomal properties.

The recommended dose of PZO is 40 mg/kg body weight. The drug is available as a 600mg tablet. The quality of PZQ (proprietary and generic) currently available in the market is quite high. Thirty four PZQ samples from different manufacturers were collected at the user level in various countries and subjected to quantitative analysis of active ingredient, purity, disintegration and dissolution in accordance with established pharmacopoeial standards. The results showed that most of the samples were of high quality except two samples from the same manufacturer that had no PZQ (Sulaiman *et al.*, 2001). About 90% of the damage done to organ function are known to reverse six months following the administration of PZQ. Although it is exceptionally well tolerated, reported side –effects include abdominal discomfort, nausea, headache, dizziness, drowsiness and pyrexia especially in subjects with high egg counts (Andrews,1981).

3.1.2 Mode of action of PZO

The mode of action of PZQ has been extensively reviewed elsewhere (Doenhoff *et al.*, 2008 & 20009). The exact mechanisms of action of PZQ is still poorly understood. PZQ is known to induce rapid calcium influx that distort the morhoplogy and physiology of schistosome. Jeziorski and Greenberg (2006) showed that the B subunits of voltage-gated Ca^{2+} channels is the prime molecular target of PZQ. It has recently been reported that cytochalasin D abolished the schistosomicicidal activity of PZQ but calcium influx into PZQ exposed schistosomes was not halted. This result therefore raises doubts whether calcium influx is essential in the antischistosomal activity of PZQ (Pica-Mattoccia *et al.*,2008). PZQ induces contraction of schistosomes which manifest in paralysis in the contracted state. Additionally, vacuolation and blebbing near and on the surface of the worm have equally been reported (Pax *et al.*, 1978).

PZQ is known to increase exposure of antigens on the worm surface. It is believed that this in turn renders the worm more susceptible to antibody attack. Doenhoff *et al* (1987) inferred that this drug induced antigen exposure is assumed to account for the synergistic effect between PZQ and the host antibodies in killing worms invivo. Recently, it has been shown that PZQ seems to interfere with adenosine uptake in cultured worms. This may have therapeutical relevance given that the schistosome is unable to synthesize purines such as adenosine *de novo*. It may be assumed that the drug interferes with schistosome's obligate need to acquire adenosine from its host. This is confounding as a relationship between Ca^{2+} channels and adenosine receptors has been demonstrated in cells of some other animals and adenosine can antagonize Ca^{2+} release. This informs the inference drawn by Angelucci *et al* (2007) that PZQ-induced Ca^{2+} influx and adenosine receptor blockade may be connected.

3.1.3 Field studies on the efficacy and effectiveness of PZQ

It is important to understand the difference between efficacy and effectiveness as applicable to anthelminthic drugs in field trials. The WHO (2002) defined efficacy as the "effect of a drug against an infectious agent, in isolation and under ideal conditions" while effectiveness refers to the "effect of the drug against an infective agent under operational conditions". Following from the above, effectiveness may be influenced by factors such as patient compliance with treatment, and by ecological, immunological, or epidemiological factors confounding by ongoing disease transmission. Thus the main markers of effectiveness of large-scale deworming exercise is the general improvement in health status of the population at risk and also taking into consideration other important variables such as cost of drug delivery, accessibility and acceptability of treatment, and sustainability. Efficacy and effectiveness are measured using qualitative and quantitative tests for eggs in faeces or urine. Cure rates and egg reduction rates are used to measure the response to treatment. These indicators are simple and easy to determine under field conditions. It is important to note that the qualityof results derived are dependent on the parasitological techniques used and on the time after treatment at which prevalence and intensity of infection are evaluated.

PZQ has been associated with a cure rate of between 60-90% and sometimes egg reduction rate of up to 95% in different community- based studies. A complete cure of all study participants (100%) has not been achieved. In an endemic community in Nigeria, this author and colleagues have shown that the pre-treatment prevalence of *S. haematobium* of 71% with microhaematuria and proteinuria of 83% and 94% respectively declined to 23%, 27.5% and 19% respectively after two annual treatments with PZQ. As a result of the high cost of the drug and the labour intensive diagnostic methods involved, the authors recommended that chemotherapy should be given at yearly intervals to targeted school-age children (Ejezie *et al.,* 1998). The implication of this recommendation is that the money invested in diagnosis could be used in the procurement of more tablets of PZQ. In this same group of schoolchildren, the educational pass rate improved following the first treatment session from 81.4% to 90.7% but later declined to 84.2% following the second treatment session. The net improvement in school performance was statistically significant (X^2 = 7.2; P= 0.027) (Meremikwu *et al.,* 2000).To buttress their findings, the authors noted that the possibility of enhancement of educational performance as observed in the study should make regular, periodic treatment of children in communities with endemic schistosomiasis a more cost-effective and beneficial public health intervention strategy than was previously assumed. kabatereiene *et al* (2003) reported a cure rate of 69% and egg reduction of 97-99% in individuals treated for *S. haematobium* infection in

Uganda. In a related study in Cameroon, a higher cure rate of 83-88.6% and egg reduction rate of 98% was reported following the administration of a standard dose of PZQ (Tchuente *et al* ., 2003).

There are reports of disappointing cure rates with PZQ. In an area of intense *S mansoni* transmission in northern Senegal, PZQ administered at the standard dose gave a cure rate of 18-36% (Gryseels *et al.,* 1994). Subsequently, the dose was increased without any significant improvement in the efficacy rate (Guisse *et al.,* 1997). However, when treated with oxamniquine, there was a significantly higher cure rate (Stelma *et al.*, 1997). Relatedly, Ismail *et a*l (1999) treated 1607 *S. mansoni*-infected patients in Egypt with PZQ at 40 mg /kg and, after an additional two treatments, the last at 60mg/kg, 1.6% of the patients were still passing viable eggs. It is remarkable that these low cure rates are more associated with *S. mansoni* than *S. haematobium* infection.

In 2001, the World Health Assembly set a target of treating about 75% of schoolchildren infected with schistosomisis and soil-transmitted helminthes. This target is yet to be met. Available data showed that 18,151, 619 and 19,570,971 infected subjects were treated with PZQ in 2008 and 2009. Of this, 14, 498,101 subjects in Africa were treated. This statistics is based only on countries rendering treatment reports to WHO. Were all endemic countries to report, it is likely to be higher as more infected people now have access to PZQ and could afford treatment. Unlike in the 1980s and 1990s, PZQ is now cheap and affordable. The average price is about US$ 0.10/tablet or less (WHO, 2003).

The availability of a dose pole which is based on height for the administration of PZQ is another innovation for the ease of community-based studies unlike the previous situation of measuring the weight of pupils. Weight measurement was limited by the sensitivity of the balance used which in some instances could lead to under or over dosing. Montresor et al (2001) reported on the validation of dose pole using existing data. This validation confirmed 98.6% of school-age children would have received a PZQ dosage between 30 and 60 mg/kg body weight, and that 84.7% would have been between 40 and 60 mg/kg. Corresponding figures for the whole populations (including young children and adults) were 95.5% and 68.2%. The validity of an extended PZQ dosing pole has been tested in Uganda (Sousa-Figuriredo et al., 2010). The extended dose pole was found to be very accurate within Uganda as well as in Zanzibar (prevalence levels of acceptable dosages estimated were 98.6% and 97.6%, respectively). It is thus considered to be a reliable and practical method for determining the dose of PZQ needed to treat schistosomiasis.

3.1.4 Resistance of Schistosomes to PZQ

Drug resistance is defined as "a genetically transmitted loss of susceptibility to a drug in a parasite population that was previously sensitive to the appropriate therapeutic dose" (WHO,1996). Currently, molecular biologic techniques are not available for the detection of resistance of schistosomes to PZQ. The resistance of Schistosomes to PZQ has recently been examined (Botros and Bennett, 2007). It cannot be scientifically ascertained whether cases not cured as encountered in the Senegalese and Egyptian studies were cases of resistance or drug tolerance. It has been noted that PZQ is partially immune dependent. Lack of acquired immunity in Northern Senegal where Schistosome infection was newly introduced may have perhaps accounted for the low cure rate. Remarkably, Fallon and Doenhoff (1994) were the first to point to a possible development of resistance as mice infected with *S. mansoni* were insensitive to PZQ.

In a related study, Fallon *et al* (1997) reported that a parasite line derived from an isolate from Senegal was less susceptible to PZQ than other isolates used as controls. Another supportive evidence can be deduced from the work of Ismail *et al* (1996). Several isolates were established in laboratory- maintained life cycles from eggs passed by uncured patients, and adult worms of these isolates were found to have PZQ ED 2- TO 5- fold higher after PZQ treatment in mice than isolates that had been established from eggs before treatment by patients who had been cured.

PZQ is known to kill the adult worms and not the immature stages. It is possible that the uncured subjects were harbouring the immature stages of the parasite at the point of treatment. As a follow up to this, a protocol was suggested for screening for suspected instances of PZQ resistance; this consisted of administering two doses of the drug, 2-3 weeks apart, so that the second would eliminate any schistosomes that had matured in the interval (Renganathan and Cioli, 2000). The utilization of this protocol in Northern Senegal achieved the expected higher cure rates (Picquet *et al.*,1998).

The issue of schistosome susceptibility or resistance to PZQ is further confounded by the fact that PZQ failed to cure a schistosome infection that was acquired by travelers or military personnel in endemic countries after returning to their non-endemic country of origin (Silva *et al.*, 2005).

It is difficult to dismiss the high rate of uncured subjects in Senegal which were subsequently cured upon the administration of Oxamniquine as not being due to resistance. However, in the absence of a clear scientific tool to detect resistance, there is need for vigorous monitoring of the efficacy of PZQ as it remains a drug of choice for the treatment of schistosome infection in the foreseeable future. Additionally, there is a consensus of opinion that drug manufacturers and researchers should commence a sustained search for an alternative drug to PZQ. Ro 15-5458 is one of such candidate compound discovered about 20 years ago by Hoffman-La Roche (Basel, Switzerland). Administered, at a single dose, it was highly efficacious against both the immature and adult worms (Sulaiman *et al.*, 1989; Pereira *et al.*, 1995). Another prospective candidate compound is 2-(alkylamino)-1-phenyl-1-ethanethiosulfuric acid. It has been attributed with the elimination of a very high population of female schistosomes than male worms in a mouse model. A lot of studies are required before it can be used for the treatment of infected human subjects (Moreira *et al.*, 2007).

3.2 Oxamniquine

3.2.1 Molecular structure and pharmacokinetics

Oxamniquine was first described in the late 1960s. The compound is 6-hydromethyl-2-isopropyl-aminomethyl-7-nitro 1,2,4-tetrahydroquinoline. It is produced by biological processes. The drug is administered as 15mg/kg body weight for adults while children are treated with 20mg/kg given in two doses of 10mg/kg each in an interval of 3-8 hours. It is extensively metabolised through oxidation process. The metabolites are active and excreted in urine. The side effects are mild, transient and well tolerated especially when given after a meal (Utizinger *et al.*, 2003).

3.2.2 Mode of action

Unlike PZQ, the mechanism of action of oxamniquine is fairly well understood. Oxamniquine is only active against *S. mansoni* but not effective against *S. haematobium* and *S.*

japonicum. The active ingredient is tetrahydroquinoline which acts on the adult *S. mansoni* and immature invasive stages, with males more susceptible than the females. Its anticholinergic effect, which increases parasite motility and inhibits nucleic acid synthesis, has no notable effect on the other *Schistosome* species (Secor & Colley, 2005). The mechanism of action of oxamniquine is related to irreversible inhibition of nucleic acid metabolism of the parasite. The drug is activated in a single step, in which the *Schistosoma* enzyme converts the oxamniquine to an ester, and spontaneously dissociates resulting in an electrophilic reactant and alkylation of the Schistosoma DNA. Worm death is associated with the formation of sub-tegumental vesicules in adult parasites. Different responses are observed after therapy, with less specific morphological alteration and hepatic shifts, occurring over a period of six days post treatment (Utzinger *et al.*, 2003).

3.2.3 Application of oxamniquine in *S. mansoni* control programmes

Oxamniquine is not used widely for the control of *S. mansoni* infection particularly in Africa because it is more expensive than PZQ. The fact that it proved more effective than PZQ in an endemic focus in Northern Senegal where PZQ gave an embarrassing low cure rate still recommends its usage. However, the drug is widely used in Brazil and other South American Countries for the control of *S. mansoni* infection. Katz and Coelho (2008) reported that over 12 million doses of the drug were administered in a control programme in Brazil alone.

3.3 Metrifonate

Metrifonate was initially introduced as an insecticide in 1952, but later in 1960, it was used to treat helminth infection. The drug also refer to as trichlorophone is a cheap organophosphorus ester which is only active against *S.haematobium*. It is rapidly absorbed, metabolized and excreted. The metabolic pathway yields DDVP (2,2-dichlorovinyl dimethylphosphate), a cholin esterase inhibitor which is the active compound. The mechanism of action is not known. It is relatively cheap and is not toxic. Metrifonate is administered as 7.5-10 mg/kg body weight, given in three divided doses in two weeks interval. Among the side effects reported following the administration of the drug include abdominal pains, diarrhoea, fatigue and muscular weakness which dissipates within 12 -24 hours (Danso-Appiah *et al.*, 2008). The reasoning behind the widely spread dosage has to do with its inhibitory effects on red cells and plasma cholinesterase.

Metrifonate is not used currently for the treatment of urinary schistosomiasis. Several reasons account for this. One of which is poor compliance by patients as a result of the spacing and multiple dosing. The second reason is reduced level of efficacy. For instance, Mgeni *et a*l (1990) reported a cure rate of 40% and egg reduction rate of 90% in Zanzibar. Lastly the advent of PZQ with its superior efficacy rate and broad spectrum activity meant that it was no longer cost effective and sustainable to rely on metrifonate.

3.4 Artemisinin and its derivatives

3.4.1 Biochemical characteristics and pharmacokinetics

The artemisinins though syntheised for the treatment of malaria is the newest drug used for the treatment of schistosomiasis. Unlike PZQ, which is active against the adult stages of the parasite, artemisinin is active against the immature stage of parasite. It is a sequitterpene lactone with a peroxide group, obtained from the leaves of the plant,

Artemisia annua which are grown in Central Europe, China, USA and Argentina among others. The major derivatives of artemisinin are artesunate, artemether, arteether with dihydroartemisinin as the principal active metabolite. Primarily they are antimalarials, but the anti-schistosomal properties were discovered by Chinese scientists in the 1980s especially for the treatment of *S japonicum* infection (Hommel, 2008). They are well tolerated with only minor side effects.

3.4.2 Mode of action of Artemisinin

The precise mode of action of this drug is not known. Artemether is the most potent. It exhibits the highest level of activity on one to three weeks old liver stages of the parasite. When a dosage of 6mg/kg weight is administered, it kills the schistosomulas during the first 21 days. The invasive and adult stages are less affected and the adult females are more susceptible than the males (Allen *et al.*, 2002). Following treatment, artemether induces severe and extensive tegumental damage and significant reduction in glycogen contents through the inhibition of glycolsis, but the onset of this alteration is slow. It also hinders the development of egg laying adult worm pairs (Xiao et al., 2000).

3.4.3 Efficacy of artemisinin in field studies

Several studies have been carried out to test the feasibility of using artemisinin for the treatment of schistosome infection. The efficacy of oral artemether for prevention of *S mansoni* infection was investigated in Western Cote d'Ivore (Utzinger *et al.*, 2000). The group that received artemether had a significantly lower incidence of *S mansoni* infection (31/128 versus 68/140, relative risk: 0.50 [95% CI 0.35-0.71], P=0.00006). The geometric mean egg output among positive children in the artemether group was significantly lower than in the placebo group (19 vs 32 eggs/g stool, p=0.017). The authors recommended the use of artemether in an appropriate situation as an additional tool for the control of intestinal schistosomiasis. In the same country, the activity of artemether against *S haematobium* infection has also been assessed. The incidence of patent *S. haematobium* infections in artemether recipients was significantly lower than in the placebo recipients (49% vs 65%, protective efficacy: 0.25, 95% CI: 0.08-0.38, P=0.007). The geometric mean intensity in the artemether group was less than half that of the placebo recipients (3.4 versus 7.4 eggs/10ml urine, P<0.001). Heavy *S. haematobium* infections, microhaematuria and macrohamaturia, and the incidence of malaria parasitemia were all significantly lower in artemether patients. The authors concluded that artemether was active against *S haematobium* (N'Goran *et al.*, 2003). Boulanger *et al* (2007) have also associated artesunate combination therapies with high cure rate of *S. haematobium* infection in Senegal. This author and colleagues investigated the efficacy of artesunate in the treatment of urinary schistosomiasis in Nigeria (Inyang-Etoh *et al.*, 2004)(Table 2). When the treated children were re-examined 4 weeks after the second dose of artesunate, 70.1% appeared egg- negative and were therefore considered cured. Post-treatment, the geometric mean egg count for the treated subjects who were not cured was significantly lower than the pre-treatment geometric mean egg count for all the treated subjects, with log^{10}[(eggs/10 ml urine) +1] values of 0.9 versus 1.75 (t=4.45; P<0.05). The artesunate was well tolerated. The authors concluded that their observation of a therapeutic effect of artesunate against *S. haematobium* infection in Nigeria confirmed recent observations from Senegal. Furthermore, it would be more cost effective to treat *S. haematobium* infection in this setting with artesunate than with PZQ.

	Males	Females	All	X^2	P
Subjects Aged <10years					
No. Treated	11	21	32	NA	NA
No. and (%) cured	7(64)	15(71)	22(69)	0.2	>0.05
No and (%) without post-treatment haematuria	10(90)	18(86)	28(88)	1.66	>0.05
No and (%) with post-treatment haematuria	1(9)	3(14)	4(13)	0.09	>0.05
Subjects Aged>10 years					
No Treated	31	24	55	NA	NA
No and (%) cured	20(65)	19(79)	39(71)	1.40	>0.05
No and (%) without post-treatment haematuria	23(74)	20(83)	43(78)	0.65	>0.05
No and (%) with post-treatment haematuria	8(26)	4(17)	12(22)	0.66	>0.05

NA, Not Applicable
(Adopted from Inyang-Etoh, Ejezie, Useh *et al.*,2004)

Table 2. The prevalences of haematuria post-treatment with artesunate and the frequencies of parasitological cure, split by age and gender.

Researchers have administered a combination of PZQ and artesunate on schistosomiasis infected subjects in a bid to derive a synergistic effect. While PZQ acts on the adult worms, artesunate acts on the immature stages of the worm. Borrmann *et al* (2001) investigated the efficacy and tolerability of artesunate, singly or in combination with PZQ, for the treatment of *S. haematobium* infections among 300 schoolchildren in Gabon. Of the children given PZQ + placebo, artesunate + placebo, artesunate + PZQ and placebo alone, 73%, 27%, 81% and 20% appeared cured, respectively. In summary, earlier findings of efficacy of artemisinin derivatives against *S. mansoni* and *S, japonicum* could not be confirmed against *S. haematobium* in the endemic focus. In a related study, conducted in two villages endemic for *S. haematobium* infection in Senegal, De Clercq *et al* (2002) reported that treatment with aretesunate alone gave egg count reduction rates that were high and almost as good as those obtained with PZQ (though the results obtained with PZQ were consistently better). Inyang-Etoh *et al* (2009) assessed the efficacy of a combination of PZQ and artesunate in the treatment of urinary schistosomiasis in Nigeria (Table 3). All treatment regimens were well tolerated. The cure rates were 72.7% in the PZQ plus placebo treated group and 70.5% in the artesunate plus placebo group, while the artesunate plus PZQ group had the highest cure rate (88.6%). The authors concluded that the treatment of urinary schistosomiasis with a combination of PZQ and artesunate is safe and more effective than treatment with either drug alone. The authors were however silent about the element of cost of the combination therapy. It is more expensive to use the combination than using either singly. The element of cost is very crucial in the choice of the appropriate drug to use as it should be affordable by the rural poor who are often afflicted by the disease.

Effect of treatment	PZQ Plus placebo (n=44)	Art Plus placebo (n=44)	Art plus PZQ (N=44)	PZQ without placebo (n=42)	Art without placebo (n=44)	Placebo plus placebo
No (%) cured	32(72.7)	31(70.5)	39(88.6)	31(73.8)	33(75)	4(9.1)
Mean ova reduction rate	79.3	72.3	93.6	76.7	52.1	111.5
Mean ova count before treatment ±SD	66.3±3.7	69.6±2.7	62.2±2.1	42.0±1.7	39.8±1.1	34.1±0.8
Mean ova count after treatment±SD	13.8±0.8	19.3±0.9	4.0±15.2	9.8±0.5	19.1±1.0	72±2.3
Mean haematuria before treatment ±SD	55.9±2.0	50.9±1.9	73.0±2.3	47.6±2.0	61.8±2.2	38.0±1.6
Mean haematuria after treatment ±SD	13.6±1.2	11.1±0.9	8.8±8.7	7.6±0.9	25.7±1.6	59.6±2.2
Mean Proteinuria before treatment±SD	190.9±	177.3±5.1	267.5±5.4	160.2±5.2	191.1±5.2	185.2±5.0
Mean Proteinuria after treatment±SD	65.7±3.3	85.5±3.9	4.0±15.2	24.8±1.9	102.1±4.4	213.9±5.3

(PZQ denotes Praziquantel, Art denotes Artesunate)
Source: Inyang-Etoh, Ejezie, Useh *et al.*, 2009) etc

Table 3. Summary of therapeutic efficacy of PZQ and artesunate administered with placebo or in combination in Nigeria.

Artemisinins were originally snythesised for the treatment of malaria. There is a likelihood of a build up of resistance in malaria endemic areas where the drug is equally used in the treatment of schistosomiasis. It is worth noting that the combination therapy as it were has not given 100% efficacy so far in field studies. This is crucial as all the stages (immature stages and adult) of the parasite are targeted by the two drugs. This brings the issue of resistance once again to the fore. It might not be unreasonable to assume that the residuals not responding to the combination therapy might be pointing to a certain level of resistance. This would also imply that we be circumspect in deploying artesunate to treat schistosomiasis in areas endemic for malaria since it may enhance the development of resistance.

4. Molluscididing in schistosomiasis control

In the early days of schistosomiasis control in Egypt, a lot of emphasis was placed on molluciciding in a bid to interrupt transmission. Although, it is a component of an integrated method of control, it is not used currently in many endemic areas. Rather morbidity control in the short term using chemotherapy is more emphasized. Snail control is achieved by using chemical and plant molluscicides, biological predators and ecological methods. The main objectives of the use of molluscicides is to contribute, preferably in combination with chemotherapy and other feasible control measures, to significant reduction/control of schistosome transmission by cost-effective destruction of snail host populations and in particular, infected snails in selected habitats. The snail population density at transmission sites should be reduced by 95% (WHO, 1992).

The advantages to be derived from mollusciciding are:
1. Rapid interruption of transmission
2. Satisfactory cost efficiency
3. Non-desirability of community participation and utilization of simple application tools
4. Guaranteed safety margins to man and his domestic animals and plants
5. Easy integration with other pesticide control programme

The disadvantages to be derived include the following
1. The need for repeated applications, since eradication of snail host populations is rarely attainable
2. Requirement of technical discernment
3. Effect on schistosomal morbidity, even when snail control measures are efficient and in the absence of chemotherapy is delayed (WHO, 1992).

4.1 Qualities of a good molluscicide

There is currently no perfect molluscicide. It is not easy to develop a molluscicide that is likely to offer all the advantages outlined above. However, the basic requirements have been laid out by the WHO (1965). These include the following:
1. Toxicity to snails at low concentration
2. They must be safe to use in respect of acute and chronic mammalian toxicity
3. If they enter the food chain, they must not produce adverse effects
4. They must be stable in storage for 18 months or longer
5. Acceptable cost and ready availability
6. Particularly specific for snails
7. Low toxicity for non-biota
8. Diversity of formulations
9. Simple means of application and reliable means of measuring concentration in habitat

4.2 Assessment of effectiveness of some chemical molluscicides

A variety of compounds are molluscicidal. Among these include; penta chlorophenate, calcium, copper, lead and tin compounds which have been discarded because of toxicity. The molluscicidal property of copper, irrespective of the method of application has been less than satisfactory, especially in the presence of organic materials, certain kinds of dissolved solids, and at high PH values. Moreover, the cost effectiveness for copper sulphate, inspite of its low price, has been shown to be unacceptably high in comparison with that of niclosamide (McCullough, 1992).

4.2.1 Mode of action of some chemical molluscicides

Poisoning with molluscicides causes the snail either to retract into the shell and expel the haemolymph or to become swollen and remain extended from the shell. The later response is seen particularly with organotins and certain carbamates and suggests lost of water balance control (WHO, 1992). The water balance of gastropods is thought to be under neurosecretory control. N-tritymorpholine has been shown to reduce neurosecrtory control in *B. truncatus*, while long term exposure of the pulmonate, *Indoplanorbis exustus*, to barium chloride and copper sulphate also resulted in diminished neurosecretory activity. In addition, it has been shown that water flux through *B. glabrata* falls in the presence of a number of molluscicides at concentrations around their LC 50 values (McCullough, 1992). It may well be, therefore that molluscicides cause stress on the water-balance system and that this alone is lethal to the snail, or that reduction of the normal water flow through the snail precipitates other functions similar to those describe above.

4.2.2 Effectiveness of some chemical molluscicides

In Japan, an inexpensive compound named B-2 (Sodium 2,5 dichloro-4-bromophenol) has been field tested in liquid and wettable powder formulations against the amphibious *Oncomelania nosophora* (Kajihara *et al.*, 1979). Its residual concentration in soil decreased rapidly and its uptake in rice did not exceed 0.03 mg/L. Its toxicity has limited its wide spread use. The properties of some chemical molluscicides is presented on Table 4.

Niclosamide (marketed as bayluscide) is virtually the sole available molluscicide and in terms of effectiveness and completeness of evaluation. It is the molluscicide of choice (WHO, 1992). It has been a commercial success. The usual formulation of bayuscide (70% wettable powder and 25% emulsifiable concentrate) are both highly effective. In practical use, a concentration of 0.6-1 mg/L is recommended with exposure time of 8 hr (WHO, 1973) or 0.33 mg/L for 24 hr (Barnish and Prentice, 1981). Currently, there is no proven resistance to bayluscide. In a recent study, Dai *et al* (2010) showed that a novel suspension concentrate of niclosamide was toxic against *B. glabrata.* There was no differences in the effect of the suspension concentrate, the wettable powder of niclosamide and the ball-milled pure niclosamide against the adult snail.

The distribution of the snail hosts in their habitat is non-random, reflecting the where about of the food resources (e.g decaying vegetation, algae) and also physical features (e.g sandy/muddy substratum, water flow patterns) which attracts or repulse the mollusks (WHO, 1985). Snail host populations thus tend to be dynamic in space and time. These principles and the observations that low infection rates (e.g less than 1%) in snails may be associated with relatively high infection rates in a local community point to the need to identify potential transmission sites both geographically and seasonally, and to predict the

Physical properties	Niclosamide	Copper Sulphate	Sodium Penta Chlorophenat	Nicotinanilidae Candidate compound Group
Form of Technical material	Crystalline Solid	Crystalline solid	Crystalline Solid	Crystalline Solid
Solubility in Water	230mg/L PH Dependent	316g/L	330g/L	Not known
Toxicity				
Snail, LC 90	3-8	20-100	20-100	5
(mg/L x h)	2-4	50-100	3-300	20-50
Cercaria LC 90				
Formulations	700g/kg wetteble powder, 250/ml/L emulsion concentration	980g/kg pentahudrate crystals	750g/kg flaks 800g/kg pellets 800g/kg triquettes	Not yet formulated

Source: WHO (1973)

Table 4. Properties of Some Available and Candidate Molluscicides

habitats favoured by the snails (Anderson & May, 1979). Klumpp and Chu (1987) stated that in their experience in Iran, Egypt and Ghana, area wide mollusciciding was expensive, wasteful, ecologically unsound and generally ineffective. They concluded on the other hand that focal mollusciciding is a cost effective method in virtually all habitats. However, in endemic areas like the Nile Delta, it is unlikely that even focal/seasonal mollusciciding will contribute significantly to a reduction in schistosomal transmission in the area as a whole. However, in certain affected communities where for example, population-based chemotherapy campaigns may have proved less satisfactory, focal/seasonal mollusciciding, if carried out rigorously could probably play a useful, additional role in disease control.

The efficiency of focal molluscicide treatment against schistosomiasis re-infection in an irrigation scheme and in small dams area in Mali has been undertaken (Werler, 1989). The cost factor alone was sufficient to reject focal molluscicide treatment especially at the Plateau Dagon since transmission starts at the end of the rainy season if there is still water in the dams by then and slows down in the cool dry season. Laboratory evaluation of B-2 in the control of the snail intermediate host of schistosomiasis in South Africa has been conducted (Joubert and Precious, 1991). The authors noted that though B-2 has a marked potential for snail control in South Africa, that niclosamide remains the molluscicides of choice.

There are a lot of problems mitigating against the application of chemical molluscicides particularly in sub-Saharan Africa. It is not likely that community participation would be guaranteed for the purpose of focal mollusciciding in endemic areas. The other problems are high illiteracy rate and cost of procurement of molluscicides.

4.3 Plant molluscicides

During the last two decades several excellent reviews on plant molluscicides have been published (Kloss and McCullough, 1982; Mott, 1987). Some major classes of natural products with recognized molluscicidal activity is presented on Table 5.

In several African countries, plant molluscicides have been identified and tested as a component part of an integrated control programme. Mkoji *et al* (1989) evaluated the molluscicidal activity of *Solanum aculeatum* berries against *Biomphalaria pfeifferi, Bulinus globosus* and *Lymnea natalensis* in Kenya. Fifty (50) mg powder L-1 of sun freeze-dried berries killed over 60% of all the tested snails while 25mg L of the sun dried material killed less than 60% of the test snails whereas similar concentrations of the freeze dried molluscicides produced 60-80% mortality in the snails under similar conditions. These findings suggest that *S. aculeatum* is a potent molluscicide and has the potential for the control of vectors of schistosomiasis and fascioliasis in Kenya. In Egypt, the molluscicidal properties of *Ambrosia maritina* on schistosome snail intermediate host has been assessed. This study was combined with the administration of PZQ. The authors concluded that *A. maritina* offers an alternative community participation approach whereby farmers could grow and apply the plant for themselves so that an area of any size could be treated in a short period of time. *A maritina* was able to reduce populations of *Biomphalaria alexandrina* significantly (Elsawy *et al*., 1989). Latex from the plant *Euphorbia splendens var hislopi*, also known as 'Crown of Christ' have been discovered to have molluscicidal effect on snails of the genus *Bulinus* and *Biomphalaria*. Schall *et al* (1998), obtained a 90% lethal impact on egg masses and embryos of these snails. This is one of the most potent molluscicides.

Class of Compoud	Plant	Family
Triterpenoid Saponins	*Phytolacea Dodecandra*	*Phytolaccacee*
	Hedra helix	*Araliaceace*
	Lonicera nigra	*Caprifoliaceace*
Spirostanol Saponins	*Cornus florids*	*Cornaceace*
	Balanites aegytiaca	*Balaniotaceae*
	Asparagus curillus	*Liliaceae*
Steroid glycoalkaloids	*Solanum mammosum*	*Solanaceae*
Diterpenes	*Wedelia scaberrima*	*Compositae*
	Baccharis trimera	*Compositae*
Sesquiterpenes	*Warburgia ugandensis*	*Canellaceae*
	Warburgia stuhlmannii	*Canellaceae*
	Ambrosia maritime	*Compositae*
	Podachaenium eminens	*Compositae*
Monoterpenes	*Genus Lippia*	*Verbenaceae*
Iridoids	*Olea europaea*	*Oleaceae*
Naphthoquinones	*Diospyres usambarensis*	*Ebenaceae*
Alkenyl phenols	*Anacardium occidentale*	*Anacardiaceae*
Chalcones	*Polygonum senegalense*	*Polygonaceae*
Flavonoids	*Baccharis trimera*	*Compositae*
Tannins	*Acacia nilotica*	*Leguminosae*

(Adopted from Marton and Hostettman, 1985)

Table 5. Major Classes of Natural Products with Recognised Molluscicides Activity

A major issue in the utilization of plants molluscicides is the acceptance and ownership of the initiative by community members. In the absence of this, cultural and religious factors may interplay negatively to hinder control. Community acceptance has been tested by different researchers in different settings. The processing and application of the soap berry plant (*Phytolacca dodecandra*) was tested in Ethiopia, where the plant is known as *endod*. Both occasional spraying and the use of *endod* soap for washing clothes were tested and it appeared that spraying would be the least labour- intensive method of control in that setting. Ndamba *et al* (1989) in a related study in Zimbabwe examined the knowledge, attitude and practice of the locals on both schistosomiasis and the soap berry plant. A large number of the participants accepted that schistosomiasis was a problem but none of them knew the role of snails in the transmission of infection. Although, they did not previously know of the plant as a molluscicides, a higher proportion of the people were willing to grow the plant after a brief explanation of it use.

It appears morbidity control of schistosomiasis anchored chiefly on population based chemotherapy has taken the centre stage in the organization of schistosomiasis control even with the acceptance of an integrated approach to control. The vigor thrown in by researchers in the early 1970s to 1990s in the search and evaluation of plant molluscicides has not been sustained.

4.4 Utilisation of competitor snails

Another approach to the elimination of snail hosts of schistosomiasis is the introduction of competitor snails in the habitat to the prey on the former. The South American snail, *Marisa*

cornuarieta is a noted prey of *B. glabrata* and this has been demonstrated in Puerto Rico (Muller, 1975). Similarly, the fresh water fish, *Astateodromes* is known to prey on mollusks. The Planorbid snail, *Helisoma duryi*, originally endemic in Florida, USA has been suggested as a biological competitor against the intermediate host snails of schistosomiasis. During the past three decades researchers have speculated on the possibility of using this particular snail as a biocontrol agent. Althought the results of some experiments indicated that *H. duryi* could control certain intermediate hosts under laboratory conditions and semi natural environment (Madsen, 1981), a number of field trials were either inconclusive or unsuccessful (Jordan, 1985).
Pointer *et al* (1989) have reported on the use of the parthenogenetic snails, *Thiara granifera* and *T. (Melanoides) tuberculara* to eliminate the intermediate host of *S mansoni- B. glabrata* in the Carribean area. These oriental snails are noted for their capacity to colonise rapidly and densely, many types of habitats while at the same time reducing and even eliminating populations of *Biomphalaria Spp.* In St Lucia, *B glabrata* was apparently eliminated from marshes and streams, 6 to 2 months after the introduction of the competitor. In Martinique, *T tuberculata* was introduced and in just less than 3 years, both *B. glabrata* and *B. straminea* were eliminated from the transmission sites. They concluded that, the Thiarid snails as competitors of pulmonates are favoured by the presence of permanent and stable habitat, preferably shallow, with emergent plants.
Taken alongside other measures, such as mollusciciding and chemotherapy, the goal of eradication of schistosomiasis appears feasible and attainable in the long run. But some posers remain. What would likely be the long term impact between the interaction of schistosomes and competitor snails? Would they become vectors themselves someday? The utilization of this method would remain as a research tool for sometimes.

5. Ecological modification

Habitats can be made unsuitable for snails to exist by alternate flooding and drying of water channels, covering and lining of canals and filling in of marshy areas. Though these methods are likely to be permanently successful, they are expensive. Chenq (1971) reported that in Kiagsu and Chekiang provinces of China, the 10.5 million cases of schistosomiasis estimated to be present by 1955 were claimed to have been reduced by one third using ecological procedures in combination with the storage of night soil before use on the land and a three day treatment campaign with tartar emetic. The reduction in the water level, including complete drainage of the habitat, resulted in the death of the snails through desiccation (Boelee & Laamrani, 2004). Similarly, the ecological benefits to the snails such as, the presence of algae which served as their main source of food are removed. The lining of the canals with cement is another measure that may be adopted. It reduces the accumulation of silt and the growth of the vegetation; this in turn reduces the snail population at the site. Local participation is known to ensure the sustainability of this approach. In Morocco, the cost of control was reduced while the people took responsibility for their environment and health (Boelee & Laamrani, 2004). Strickland (1982) noted that such environmental management led to improved agricultural productivity in endemic areas.

5.1 Modification of the water-related activities of residents of an endemic area

Several studies have confirmed a strong link between the water related activities of residents of schistosome endemic communities and the prevalence and intensity of infection. In

Nigeria, Useh & Ejezie (1999b) showed that intensity of infection was more closely correlated with the number of water contacts (r=0.97) than with the total duration of exposure (r=0.77), emphasizing the importance of specific/multiple activities, and of the surface area of the body submerged in transmission. Although, the authors investigated four fresh water streams, one of them (Culvet) was identified as the main transmission point, with bathing/swimming and fishing as the main activities that predisposed people to infection (see Table 6).

Age (years)	No of Observations	No of Contacts	Mean No of Contacts/person-day	Total Duration (min)	Mean Duration/Contact .day (min)	No and (%) of Subjects infected
5-9	479	489	1.20	4328	8.85	265(55.32)
10-14	559	588	1.05	6831	11.62	402(71.91)
15-19	385	442	1.15	7622	17.24	230(59.74)
20-24	298	318	1.07	7273	22.87	114(38.25)
25-29	172	188	1.09	5153	27.41	36(20.93)
30-39	158	162	1.03	4923	30.39	21(13.29)
>40	85	87	1.02	1095	12.59	8(9.41)
All	2136	2274	1.07	37225	16.37	1076(50.37)

(Adopted from Useh & Ejezie, 1999b)

Table 6. Frequency of water contacts, duration of exposure and prevalence of infection, by age of subjects

The application of the results of a study like this may change the attitude of the residents by encouraging them to avoid activities that expose them to infection. In a Zimbabwe study, Chandiwana and Woolhouse (1991) showed that water contact rates were related to age (highest in 8-10 years old) but not sex, with substantial variation unaccounted for by these variables. Their results provide strong quantitative support for control programmes aimed at heavily infected sites (eg focal mollusciciding) or at the minority of individuals making most water contact (e.g targeted chemotherapy).

The creation of habitats for intermediate hosts of many parasitic diseases including schistosomiasis can be avoided if there is collaboration by Government Departments charged with the supervision of building dams for agricultural purposes and hydro-electric power resources for energy supply. In the absence of this and proper channeling of canals, the government and the residents of such disease endemic areas would need any or combinations of the options outlined above to control the disease in question. The WHO (2000) defined three principles that are fundamental in dealing with the association between water resources development and human health:

- Equity. The benefits of water resources development are not disputed, but the uneven distribution of benefits (including health benefits) and of health risks to vulnerable groups, needs to be addressed in the planning, construction, and operation of such projects
- Economics. Negative health impacts of water resources development represent a hidden cost to the health sector whose resources are, as a rule, already over-stretched
- Sustainability. The economic return from investment in water resources development will suffer substantially from the ill health of local communities, with no sustainability at all in extreme case where dramatic health impacts force people to move away.

Where these principles are taken into consideration and actually put into practice water resources development would not create avenues for infection thereby sustaining the cycle of poverty and disease.

6. Sanitation and water supply

At the global level, the disability-adjusted life years (DALYs) from insufficient water, sanitation and hygiene (including contact with schistosome-infested waters) suggested that 4% of all deaths and 5.7% of the total disease burden can be attributed to these largely preventable conditions. However, with the emphasis placed on morbidity control of schistosomiasis using population-based chemotherapy, there is less focus on interventions related to safe water supply and sanitation, which in theory could contribute to controlling transmission of all helminths and many other infections (Prus *et al.*, 2002). Bruun & Aagaard (2008) noted that the establishment of safe and adequate water supply and sanitation facilities at household and village levels has an effect on domestic utilization patterns, but the relationship to prevalence of schistosomiasis remain complex.

6.1 Sanitation

Sanitation is often considered as too expensive, but it is not known what proportion it would make up compared with sums spent on classical measures for the control of schistosomiasis. Schistosomiasis is transmitted through the contamination of water bodies with the eggs of the parasite via stool or urine. Considering the high reproductive potentials of the parasite, a single miracidium produces thousand of cercariae, thus a small proportion of human waste containing parasite eggs, reaching snail infested water is sufficient to maintain effective transmission in an area (Hotez et al., 2006). The provision of latrine facilities does not imply that they are always used by everybody as intended (Asaolu & Ofoezie, 2003). In a Brazilian town, where facilities were limited, Kvale (1981) showed that there was no significant difference in prevalence between people from households with septic tanks and people from households without such facilities. In a recent study in Brazil, Andrade *et al* (2009) showed that improved sanitation and income are associated with decreased rates of hospitalization for diarrhoea in infants. In a related study in Eygpt, el Katsha & Watt, (1997) showed that overall infection levels were higher in the village without a sewage system. When measured at household level, there was a statistical significant relationship between infection levels and the absence of sewerage connections, but in the better drained village, there was no similar significant correlation. Eventhough only a third of households were connected to the sewerage system in this village, the system had contributed to lowering the water table to the benefit of the general village environment.

Quite often sanitation is viewed and accepted as being very expensive. It has tremendous benefits not only in helping to control schistosomiasis but other endemic tropical diseases particularly those associated with fecal-oral route of transmission. When sanitation is accepted as the traditional way of life, the issue of cost would be grossly reduced. The Governments of endemic areas have the responsibility of the provision of sustained safe disposal of waste and the provision of simple public toilets. What is needed is to educate the people to desist from using faeces as fertilizer and enlightenment on their other actions which may predisposed them to infection

6.2 Water supply

The provision of alternative sources of safe water, such as piped water, wells, water tanks and laundry areas for domestic and recreational uses, contributed to effective reduction in the rate of transmission and re-infection (Kloos et al., 2008). As an experimental control measure to reduce the transmission of *S. mansoni*, an individual household water supply was provided in 400 houses in 5 rural settlements of the Riche Fond Valley, St Lucia (Jordan *et al.*, 1975). This population of about 2000 had previously been dependent for water on infected streams and rivers. Six other settlements in the valley, all provided with limited piped water from public standpipes, served as comparison area. After 2 years the incidence, prevalence and intensity of infection with *S. mansoni* were significantly lower in the household water supply area, whereas all these indices of infection had increased in the comparison area. The authors concluded that an adequate, reliable, and convenient supply of water can reduce the transmission of *S. mansoni* and should be considered as a control measure in other endemic areas. A comprehensive water delivery system consisting of a water outlet to each house, communal laundries, shower facilities, and play pools, coupled with health education were studied to determine the role they could play in the spread of schistosomiasis in St Lucia, West Indies (Jordan, 1988). After a 4 year period, the incidence of new *S mansoni* infections among children aged 2-5 years fell from 19.3% to 4.5% while over the same period in villages served by a standpipe system the incidence fell only slightly from 16.5%- 14%. In a related study in Cameroon, Ndamkou and Ratard (1990) investigated the role of sanitation, water supply and a health centre in the control of schistosomiasis. The authors noted that these parameters were effective in reducing the prevalence of schistosomiasis infection. In a different focus in Cameroon, Tchuem *et al* (2001) studied the impact of installation of a water pump on schistosomiasis transmission. They concluded that schistosomiasis focus evolve dynamically, and demonstrated that changes in water supply, in association with other actions such as repeated chemotherapy, may have a profound effect on disease transmission. A study in Kenya that installed community standpipes and a shower unit at the local school observed that the new water sources had a great influence on some villagers water contact behaviour and very little on the rest of the villagers (Noda *et al.*, 1997). El Kholy *et al* (1989) investigated the effects of borehole wells on water use in a high prevalence area in Kenya, which showed no short-term effect on the transmission of *S. haematobium*, but a significant number of households changed to borehole water for drinking, cooking and dish washing.

A clean source of water would limit the possibility of contacting parasitic, virial and bacterial diseases. Although the importance of this is realized in the Developing world, the governments lack the financial and political will to embark on this. Where borehole water is provided, no mechanism is often in place for the maintenance of the facility. When it malfunctions, the residents resort to infested water bodies and become infected and the cycle of infection continues. There is also the need to take care of the recreational needs of the residents where piped water is available.

7. Health education

Health education is recommended as the entry point for initiating a control programme. Health education is that "aspect of health care directed towards promoting and reinforcing healthy behaviour through full participation of the individuals and communities concerned". It is a voluntary process that encourages people to make informed decisions to improve and maintain their health (WHO, 1990). A systematical approach is required in order to properly educate the residents of schistosomiasis endemic areas to buy into the project. This is achieved through health educational planning which has the ten under listed components:

- A title
- A description of the target population,
- A statement of the problem or need
- A list of programme and educational objective
- A description of the means for community involvement
- An analysis of the factors that will promote or hinder programme success
- A list of appropriate health education strategies
- An outline of the resources available and the need for the programme
- A timetable for action
- A scheme for evaluation

A programme executed after the above consideration would yield excellent results.

Children are known to carry the greatest burden of schistosomiasis and soil transmitted infections. It is on this basis that the WHO recommended that the school system should be the focus in mounting intervention against these disorders. To meet this objective, Bundy and Guyatt (1996) summarized the key points to be taken into consideration when addressing health education in schools. It should be aimed to:

- Create awareness about the existence of the diseases, and build a bridge between scientific understanding of disease and children's perception of the disease in their every day lives
- Foster in children an understanding of what is healthy living, and what they can do to promote and practice this for themselves and their communities
- Give children practical skills in recognition of disease in themselves and their families, and in how to protect themselves and the community against such diseases,
- Encourage children's sense of responsibility for their own health and that of their families in the future.

Kamga *et al* (2003) assessed a health education strategy in the control of urinary schistosomiasis in Cameroon. School children given health education were found to be significantly less infected than those who had no health education. The investigators concluded that health education through the framework of a school could be adopted as a national policy for urinary schistosomiasis control programmes in tropical developing countries, planned with school children as full partners, provided that they received appropriate orientation. Assessing the knowledge, attitude and practice of residents of schistosome endemic areas about schistosomiasis and its control is critical in preventing infection. In Nigeria, Useh and Ejezie (1994) showed that 92% of respondents admitted knowledge of the disease (in their local language), although none of them knew about the aetiologic agent. About 82% of the respondents admitted procuring medication while 15.2% did not seek treatment of any kind. Perception of schistosomiasis and water- contact studies are very valuable in deploying control approaches.

8. Development of a schistosome vaccine

Despite the existence of effective chemotherapeutic agents, progress towards controlling schistosomiasis has been slow. Additionally, the possible development of resistance to PZQ and other compounds, rapid re-infection and the overall economic cost, demand that other approaches be pursued (Coles *et al.*, 1987). Butterworth *et al* (1992) argued that the aim of vaccination is to reduce morbidity. As in the various animal models, immunity in humans appears to be frequently incomplete. "Immune" adults often do become infected, but at lower intensities than "susceptible" children. Several investigations have confirmed that the severity of clinical disease is dependent on intensity of infection rather than simply the presence or absence of infection (Lehman *et al.*,1976 ; Chen and Mott, 1988) implying that even an incomplete immunity may be of considerable value.

An excellent review on the search for a schistosome vaccine was published not too long ago by Wilson and Coulson (2006). These authors rightly chronicled the search for the discovery of candidate vaccine molecules to have transited through mining crude extracts, monoclonal antibody targets, anti-idiotypes, expression library screening and immunogenicity. The early disappointment that was recorded with the vaccination of mice with crude worm extracts or purified components, followed by cercarial challenge (Sadun and Lin,1959 ; Murrell *et al.*, 1975) and utilizing the idea of concomitant immunity (Smithers and Terry, 1969) were equally reviewed. Wilson and Coulson (2006) concluded that the sequencing of *S. mansoni* transriptome and genome and the development of proteomic and microarray technologies has drastically improved the possibilities for identiflying novel vaccine candidates, particularly proteins secreted from or exposed at the surface of schistosomula and adult worms. The parameters of an attenuated schistosome vaccine has been evaluated in the Olive Baboon (Kariuki *et al.*, 2004). Five exposures of baboons to the attenuated schistosome vaccine gave greater protection than three exposures, but this attenuation was not sustained when challenge was delayed. Within the scope of the data collected, faecal and circulating antigen levels did not accurately predict the observed worm burdens. Levels of immunoglobulin G at challenge correlated best with protection, but there was little evidence of a recall response. In a related study in baboons, Coulson and Kariuki (2006) showed that neither a preceding infection, terminated by chemotherapy, nor an ongoing chronic infection affected the level of protection. Whilst IgM responses to vaccination or infection were short-lived, IgG responses rose with each successive exposure to vaccine.

The greatest hope for the discovery of a schistosome vaccine lies in Sh28GST which has already undergone Phases 1 and 2 human trials (Capron *et al.*, 2002). No adverse side effects were recorded in human recipients and high titres of antibodies were elicited in Phase 1 and phase 2 trials (Capron *et al.*, 2005). The results of phase 3 human trials is being awaited. As noted by Curwen *et al* (2004) and Dillion *et al* (2006), current advances in post-genomic techniques are providing new avenues and hope to identify the secreted and surface-exposed antigens that mediate protection. The search must be sustained as vaccination is the most cost-effective and sustainable means of controlling endemic infectious diseases.

9. Conclusion

Schistosomiasis would continue to be relevant as one of the Neglected Tropical Diseases (NTDs) of public health significance in the tropics because of the attitude of the authorities of endemic countries in terms of mobilization of financial resources and political will to fight the disease. The hope of control still lies in an integrated approach. For now, the emphasis in the short term is based on chemotherapy with PZQ. The reduction in the price of PZQ means that millions of infected subjects can afford the drug. The artemisinins have performed well in relation to potency and price to PZQ in the control of all forms of schistosomisasis and is recommended particularly in areas where malaria is not endemic. Although, clinical resistance to PZQ has not been scientifically proven, there is an urgent need to monitor its effectiveness closely as it is likely to remain the drug of choice for the foreseeable future.

The other elements that constitute the integrated approach such as the provision of piped water, health education and elimination of snail hosts of schistosomiasis have not been implemented with the same zeal as population based chemotherapy

10. Recommendation

In order to sustain the fight against schistosomisais, governments of disease endemic areas would have to increase funding to health including schistosomiais. A support programme that would further reduce the cost of PZQ with increase accessibility would go a long away. The activity of PZQ and artemisinins should be closely monitored both in vivo and in vitro for the development of resistance. The search for other potent anti-schistosome drugs should be pursued vigorously. Other key components like the provision of pipe borne water and health education should be put in place by the governments of endemic countries. There should be close collaboration between the Ministries of Health, Agriculture, Water Resources and Power Supply in the construction of Dams for water supply and provision of energy to avoid creating breeding grounds for vectors of diseases.

11. Acknowledgements

I am most grateful to Prof M J. Doenhoff of the University of Nottingham, UK for his encouragement and the materials he readily made available to me. I am also grateful to Prof G. C. Ejezie of the University of Calabar, Nigeria for his support and advice. Lastly, I wish to acknowledge the authors whose works are referenced in this publication. I am grateful to all of you.

12. References

Allen, H. E., Crompton, D. W. T., de Silva, N., LoVerde, P. T. & Olds, G. R. (2002). New policies for using anthelmintics in high risk Group. *Trends in Parasitology,* 18, 381-382

Anderson, R. M. & May, R. M. (1979). Prevalence of Schistosomes infection within molluscan populations. Observed patterns and theoretical predictions. *Parasitology,* 79, 63-64.

Andrade, I. G., Queiroz, J. W., Cabral, J. A. L. & Jeronimo, S. M. B. (2009). Improved sanitation and income are associated with decreased rates of hospitalization for diarrhoea in Brazilian infants. *Transactions of the Royal Society of Tropical Medicine and Hygiene,* 103, 506-511.

Andrews, P. (1981) Preclinical data of praziquantel. A summary of the efficacy of praziquantel against schistosomes in animal experiments and notes on its mode of action. *Arzneim Forsch Res.* 31(1), 538-541.

Angelucci, F., Basso, A., Bellelli, A et al (2007). The antischistosomal drug praziquantel is an adenosine antagonist. *Parasitology,* 134: 1215-1221.

Asaolu, S. O. & Ofoezie, I.E. (2003). The role of health education and sanitation in the control of helminth infections. *Acta Tropica*, 86(2-3): 283-294

Barnish, G. & Prentice, M. A. (1981). Lack of resistance of the snail *Biomphalaria glabrata* after nine years of exposure to bayluscide. *Transactions of the Royal Society of Tropical Medicine and Hygiene*. 75, 106-107

Blas, B. L. et al (2004). The schistosomiasis problem in the Philippines: A review. *Parasitology International*, 53(2): 127-134

Boelee, E. & Laamrani, H (2004). Environmental control of schistosomiasis through community participation in a Morocco oasis. *Tropical Medicine and International Health*, 9(9): 997-1004.

Borrmann, S., Szezale, N., Faucher, J. F., Matsiegui, P. B., Neubauer, R. Binder, R. K., Lell, B. & Kremsner, P. G. (2001). Artesunate and praziquantel for the treatment of *Schistosoma haematobium* infections; a double blind randomized placebo controlled study. *Journal of Infectious Diseases*, 184, 1363-1366.

Botros, S. S. & Bennett, J. L. (2007). Praziquantel resistance. *Expert Opinion on Drug Discovery*, 2(Suppl.1), S35-40.

Boulanger, D. Dien, Y., Cisse, B., Remouse, F., Capuano, F., Dieme, J., Ndiaye, T., Sokhna, C., Trape, J., Greenwood, B. & Simondon, F. (2007). Antischistosomal efficacy of aretesunate combination therapies administered as a curative treatments for malaria attacks. *Transactions of the Royal Society of Tropical Medicine and Hygiene*, 101, 113-116.

Bruun, B & Aagaard-Hansen, J. (2008). *The social context of schistosomiasis and its control- An introduction and annotated bibliography*. UNICEF/UNDP/World Bank/WHO, Switzerland, 19-42

Bundy, D. A. P. & Guyatt, H. L. (1996). School for health: focus on health, education and the school-age child. *Parasitology Today*, 12.8, 1-16

Butterworth, A. E., Dunne, D. W., Fulford, A. J. C., Thorne, K.J. I., Gachuhi, K., Ouma, J. H & Sturrock, R. K (1992). Human immunity to *S. mansoni*: Observations on mechanisms and implications for control. *Immunological Investigations*, 21(5), 391-407.

Capron, A., Capron, M & Riveau, G. (2002). Vaccine development against schistosomiasis from Concepts to clinical trials. *British Medical Bulletin*, 62, 139-148.

Capron, A., Riveau, G., Capron, M. & Trottein, F (2005). Schistosomes: the road from host-parasite interactions to vacines in clinical trials. *Trends in Parasitology*, 21:143-149.

Chandiwana, S. K. & Woolhouse, M. E.J. (1991). Heterogeneities in water-contact patterns and the epidemiology of *Schistosoma haematobium*. *Parasitology*, 103, 363-370

Chen, M. G. & Mott, K. E. (1989). Progress in assessment of morbidity due to schistosomiasis. *Tropical Disease Bulletin*, 86, 1-56

Chenq, T. S. (1971). Schistosomiasis in mainland China. *American Journal of Tropical Medicine and Hygiene*, 20, 26-53

Coles, G. C., Bruce, J. I., Kinotic, G. K., Muttahi, W. T., Dias, J. C. S., Rocha, R. S. & Katz, N. (1987). The potential for drug resistance in schistosomiasis. *Parasitology Today*, 3, 34-38.

Coulson, P.S & Kariuki, T. M. (2006). Schistosome vaccine testing: lessons from the baboon model. *Mem Inst Oswaldo Cruz, Rio de janeiro*, 101(Suppl.1): 369-372.

Curwen, R. S., Ashton, P. D., Johnston, D. A. & Wilson, R. A. (2004). The *S. mansoni* soluble protem: a comparison across four life-cycle stages. *Molecular Biochemistry and Parasitology*,138, 57-66.

Dai, J., Coles, G. C., Wang, W & Liang, Y (2010). Toxicity of a novel suspension concentrate of niclosamide against *B. glabrata*. *Transactions of the Royal Society of Tropical Medicine and Hygiene*, 104, 304-306.

Danso-Appiah, A., Utzinger, J., Liu,J., Olliaro, P. (2008). Drugs for treating urinary schistosomiasis. Cochrane Database System Review, CD000053

Davis, A. (1981). Principles of schistosomiasis control in relation to community health care. *Arneim Forsch* 31(1), 616-618

De Clercq, D., Vercruysse, J., Kongs, A., Verlo, P., Dompnier, J. P. & Faye, P. C. (2002). Efficacy of artesunate and praziquantel in *Schistosoma haematobium* infected school children. *Acta Tropica*, 82, 61-66.

Dillon, G. P., Feltwell, T., Skelton, J. P., Ashton, P. D., Coulson, P. S., Quail, M. A., Nikolaidou-Katsaridou, N, Wilson, R. A. & Ivens, A. C. (2006). Microarray analysis identifies genes preferentially expressed in the lung schistosomulum of *S. mansoni*. *International Journal of Parasitology*,36, 1-8

Doenhoff, M. J., Cioli, D. & Utzinger, J. (2008). Praziquantel: mechanisms of action, resistance and new derivatives for schistosomiasis. *Current Opinions in Infectious Diseases*, 21: 659-667.

Doenhoff, M. J., Hagan, P., Cioli, D., Southgate, V., Pica-Mattocca, L., Botros, S., Coles, G., Tchuem, L. A. Mbaye, A. and Engels, D. (2009). Praziquantel: its use in control of schistosomiasis in sub-saharan Africa and current research needs. *Parasitology*, 136, 1825-1835.

Doenhoff, M. J., Sabah, A. A., Fletcher, C., Webbe, G. & Bain, J. (1987). Evidence for an immune dependent action of praziquantel on *Schistosoma mansoni* in mice. *Transactions of the Royal Society Medicine and Hygiene*. 81, 947-951.

Ejezie, G. C., Udoh, A. E., Meremikwu, M., Odigwe, C. O. & Useh, M. F. (1998). Some effects of annual treatment and re-treatment on morbidity indicators of urinary schistosomiasis. *Mary Slessor Journal of Medicine*, 1, 67-72

El Katsha, S. & Watts, S. (1997). Schistosomiasis in two Nile Delta villages: an anthropological perspective. *Tropical Medicine and International Health*, 2(9), 846-854

El sawy, M. F., Duncan, J., Amer, S., Ruweini, H. E. & Brown, N, (1989). The molluscicidal properties of *Ambrosia maritina* L. (Compositae). A temporal and spatial distribution of *B. alexandrina* in Egyptian village irrigation systems with reference to schistosomiasis control work. *Annals of Tropical Medicine and Parasitology*, 40, 103-106.

Fallon, P. G., Mubarak, J.S., Fookes, R. E., Niang, M., Butterworth, A. E., Sturrock, R. F. & Doenhoff, M. J. (1997). *Schistosoma mansoni*: maturation rate and drug susceptibility of different geographical isolates. *Experimental Parasitology*, 86, 29-36.

Gemmel, M. A., Lawson, B. D. & Roberts, M. G. (1986). Control of echinococcus/hydatidosis: Present status of the world wide progress. *Bulletin of the World Health Organisation*, 64, 313-323

Gryseels, B., Stelma, F. F., Talla, I., Van Dam, G. J., Polman, K., Sow, S., Diaw, M., Sturrock, R. F., Doehring, E., Kardorff, R., Decam, C., Niang, M. & Deelder, A. M. (1994). Epidemiology, immunology and chemotherapy of *Schistosoma mansoni* infection in a recently exposed community in Senegal. *Tropical Geographical Medicine*, 46, 209-216.

Guisse, F., Polman, K., Stelma, F. F., Mbaye, A., Talla, I., Niang, M., Deedler, A. M., Ndir, O & Gryseels, B (1997). Therapeutic evaluation of two different dose regimens of praziquantel in a recent *Schistosoma mansoni* focus in Northern Senegal. *American Journal of Tropical Medicine and Hygiene*, 56(5): 511-514

Hommel, M. (2008). The future of artemisinins: natural, synthetic or recombinant. *Journal of Biology*, 7(10): 38.

Hotez, P.J., Bundy, D. A. P., Beegle, K. et al (2006). Helminth infections: soil transmitted helminth infections and schistosomiasis. In ; *Disease Control Priorities in Developing Countries*, 468-472

Inyang-Etoh, P. C., Ejezie, G. C., Useh, M. F. & Inyang-Etoh, E (2004). Efficacy of artesunate in the treatment of urinary schistosomiasis in an endemic community in Nigeria. *Annals of Tropical Medicine and Parasitology*, 98.5, 491-499.

Inyang-Etoh, P. C., Ejezie, G. C., Useh, M. F. & Inyang-Etoh, E (2009). Efficacy of a combination of praziquantel and artesunate in the treatment of urinary schistosomiasis in Nigeria. *Transactions of the Royal Society of Tropical Medicine and Hygiene*, 103, 38-44

Ismail, M., Metwally, A., Farghaly, A., Bruce, J., Tao, L., and Bennet, J. L. (1996). Characterization of isolates of *Schistosoma mansoni* from Eygptian villagers that tolerate high doses of praziquantel. *American Journal of Tropical Medicine and Hygiene*, 55(2), 214-218

Ismail, M., Botros, S., Metwally, A., William, S., Farghally, A., Tao, L., Day, T.A. & Bennettt, J. L. (1999). Resistance to praziquantel: direct evidence from *Schistosoma mansoni* isolated from Egyptian villagers. *American Journal of Tropical Medicine and Hygiene* 60, 932-935.

Jeziorski, M. C. & Greenberg, R. M. (2006). Voltage-gated calcium channel subunits from platyheminths: potential role in praziquantel action. *American Journal of Tropical Medicine and Hygiene*, 36, 625-632.

Jordan, P. (1985). The St Lucia Project. Cambridge : Cambridge University Press.

Jordan, P. (1988). The Sainst Lucia Project. *World Health Forum*. 9, 104-106.

Jordan, P. (2000). From Katayama to the Dakhla Oasis: the beginning of the control of bilharzia. *Acta Tropica*, 77(1), 9-40.

Jordan, P., Woodstock, L., Unrau, G. O. & Cook, J. A. (1975). Control of *Schistosoma mansoni* transmission by provision of domestic water supplies: a preliminary report of a study in St Lucia. *Bulletin of the World Health Organisation*, 52, 1-20.

Jordan, P & Rosenfield, P. L. (1983). Schistosomiasis control: Past, present and future. *Annual Review of Public Health*, 4:311-334

Joubert, P. H. & Pretorius, S. J. (1991). Laboratory evaluation of B-2 as a molluscicide in the control of the snail intermediate hosts of schistosomiasis in South Africa. *Annals of Tropical Medicine and Parasitology*, 85, 1-7.

Kabatereine, N. B., Kemijumbi, J., Ouma, J. H., Sturrock, R. F., Butterworth, A. E., Madsen, H., Ornbjerg, N., Dunne, D. W. & Vennnervald, B. J. (2003). Efficacy and side effects of praziquantel treatment in a highly endemic *Schistosoma mansoni* focus at Lake Albert, Ugandan, *Transactions of the Royal Society of Tropical Medicine and Hygiene* 97, 599-603.

Kajihara, N., Horimi, R., Minai, M. & Josaka, Y. (1979). Field assessment of B-2 as a new molluscicide for the control of *Onchomelania nosophora*. *Japanese Journal of Medical Science and Biology*, 32, 225-28.

Kariuki, T. M., Farah, I. O., Yole, D. S., Mwenda, J.M., Van Dam, G. J., Deelder, A. M., Wilson, R. A. & Coulson, P. S. (2004). Parameters of attenuated schistosome vaccine evaluated in the olive baboon. *Infection and Immunology*. 72, 5526-5529.

Katz, N & Coelho, P. M. (2008). Clinical therapy of schistosomiasis mansoni: the Brazilian contribution. *Acta Tropica*,108, 72-78

King, C. H. (2009). Towards the elimination of schistosomiasis. *New England Journal of Medicine*, 360(2), 106-109

Kloos, H. (1985). Water resources development and schistosomiasis ecology in the Awash Valley, Ethiopia. *Social Science and Medicine*, 17(9), 545-562.

Kloos, H & McCullough, F. S. (1982). Plant molluscicides. *Journal of Medical Plants*, 46, 195-209.

Kloos, H., Correa-Oliveira, R., Quintes, H. F. O., Souza, M. C.C., Gazzinelli, A. (2008). Socio-economic studies of schistosomiasis in Brazil: an overview. *Acta Tropica*, 108, 194-201

Klump, R. K. & Chu, K. Y (1987). Focal mollusccidіng: an effective way to augment chemotherapy of schistosomiasis. *Parasitology Today*, 3, 74-76.

Kvale, K. M. (1981). Schistosomiasis in Brazil: preliminary results from a case study of a new focus. *Social Science and Medicine. Part D, Medical Geography*, 15(4), 489-500.

Lehman, J. S., Mott, K. E., Morrow, R. H., Muniz, T. M. & Boyer, M. H. (1976). The intensity and effects of infection with *S. mansoni* in a rural community in north East Brazil. *American Journal of Tropical Medicine and Hygiene*, 25, 285-294

Madsen, H. (1981). Prospects for the use of *H. duryi* in biological control of schistosomiasis. Proceedings of the 10th Scandinavian Society of Parasitology, Denmark

Massa, K., Magnussen, P., Sheshe, A., Ntakamulenga, R., Ndawi, B. & Olsen, A (2009). The effect of the community-directed approach versus the school-based treatment approach on the prevalence and intensity of schistosomiasis and soil-transmitted helminthiasis among schoolchildren in Tanzania. *Transactions of the Royal Society of Tropical Medical and Hygiene*, 103, 31-37.

McCullough, F. S. (1992). The role of mollusciciding in schistosomiasis control. WHO/SCHIST/92.107, 1-35.

Meremikwu, M. M., Asuquo, P.N., Ejezie, G. C., Useh, M. F. & Udoh, A. E. (2000). Treatment of *S haematobium* with praziquantel in children: its effect on educational performance in rural Nigeria. *Tropical Medicine*, 39-45.

Mgeni, A. F., Kisumku, U. M., McCullough, F. S., Dixon, H., Yoon, S. S. & Mott, K. E. (1990). Metrifonate in the control of urinary schistosomiasis in Zanzibar. *Bulletin of the World Health Organisation*, 68(6), 721-730

Mkoji, G. M., Njunge, K., Kimarii, G., Tsekp, W. K., Munga, B. N. & Muthaura, C. (1989). Molluscicidal activity of *Solanum aculeatum* berries on *B. pfeifferi, Bulinus globosus* and *Ly. Natalensis. Annals of Tropical Medicine and Parasitology*, 40, 119-120

Montressor, A., Ramsan, M., Chwaya, H. M., Ameir, H., Foum, A., Albonico, M., Gyorkos, T. W. & Saviolo, L. (2001). Extending anthelminthic coverage to non-enrolled school-age children using a simple and low cost method. *Tropical Medicine and International Health*, 6(7), 535-537.

Moreira, L. S. A., Pilo-Veloso, D., Teixeira de Mello, R., Coelho, P. M. Z. & Nelson, D. L. (2007). A study of the activity of 2-(alkylamino)-1-phenyl-1-ethanethiosulfuric acids against infection by *S. mansoni* in a mouse model. *Transactions of the Royal Society of Tropical Medicine and Hygiene, 101*, 385-390.

Mott, K. E. (1987). Plant molluscicides. Edited by K. E. Mott. Published on behalf of the UNDP/World Bank/WHO Special Programme for Research and Training in Tropical Diseases by John Wiley and Sons Ltd, New York

Muller, R. (1975). *Worms and Diseases: A manual of medical helminthology* (1st Edition). Heinemann, London, 7-20.

Murrell, K. D., Dean, D. A. & Stafford, E. E. (1975). Resistance to infection with *S. mansoni* after immunization with worm extracts or live cercarial: role of cyctotoxic antibody in mice and guinea pig. *American Journal of Tropical Medicine and Hygiene*, 24, 955-962

Ndamba, J., Chandiwana, S. K. & Makaza, N. (1989). Knowledge, attitude and practices among rural communities in Zimbabwe in relation to *Phytolacca dedocandra*, a plant molluscicide. *Social Science and Medicine*, 28(12), 1249-1253.

Ndamkou, N. C. & Ratard, R .C. (1990). Are sanitation, water supply and a health centre sufficient to control schistosomiasis? The case of Douloumi, North Cameroon. *Tropical Doctor*. 20, 176-177.

N'Goran, E. K., Utzinger, J., Gnaka, H. N., Yapi, A., N'Guessan, N. A., Kigbafori, S. D., Lengeler, C., Chollet, J., Shuhua, X. & Tanner, M. (2003). Randomized, double-blind, placebo-controlled trial of oral artemether for the prevention of patent *S. haematobium* infections. *American Journal of Tropical Medicine and Hygiene*, 68(1), 24-32.

Noda, S., Shimada, M., Sato, K., Ouma, J. H., Thiongo, F. W., Muhoho, N.D., Sato, A. & Aoki, Y. (1988). Effect of mass chemotherapy and piped water on numbers of *S. haematobium* and prevalence in *B. globosus* in Kwale, Kenya. *American Journal of Tropical Medicine and Hygiene*, 38(3), 487-495.

Pax, R., Bennett, J. L.& Fetterer, R. (1978). A benzodiazine derivative and praziquantel: effects on musculature of *S. mansoni* and *S. japonicum*. *Naunyn-Schiedbergs Arch Pharmacol*, 304, 309-315

Pereira, L. H., Coelho, P.M., Costa, J.O. & Mello, R. T. (1995). Activity of a 9-acridanone-hydrazone drugs detected at the pre-postural phase, in experimental *S. mansoni*. *Mem Inst Oswaldo Cruz*, 90, 425-428

Pica-Mattoccia, L., Orsini, T., Basso, A., Festucci, A., Liberti, P., Guidi, A., Marcatto-Maggi, A. L., Nobre-Santana, S., Troiana, A. R., Cioli, D. & Valle, C. (2008). *Schistosoma mansoni*: lack of correlation between praziquantel-induced intra-worm calcium influx and parasite death. *Experimental Parasitology*, 119,332-335

Picquet, M., Vercruysse, J., Shaw, D. J., Diop, M & Ly, A. (1998). Efficacy of praziquantel against *S. mansoni* in Northern Senegal. *Transactions of the Royal Society of Tropical Medicine and Hygiene*, 92, 90-93

Pointer, J. P. & MucCullough, F. (1989). Biological control of the snail hosts of *S. mansoni* in the Caribean area using *Thiara spp*. *Acta Tropica* Basel 46(3), 147-155.

Pruss, A. et al (2002). Estimating the burden of disease from water, sanitation, and hygiene of global level. *Environmental Health Perspectives*, 110(5), 537-542.

Renganathan, E. & Cioli, D. (1998). An international initiative on praziquantel use. *Parasitology Today*, 14, 390-391.

Sadun, E. H. and Lin, S. S. (1959). Studies on the host parasite relationship to *S. japonicum*. IV. Resistance acquired by infection, by vaccination and by the injection of immune serum, in monkeys, rabbits and mice. *Journal of Parasitology*, 45, 543-548

Schall, V. T., Vasconcellos, M. C., Souza, C. P. & Baptista, D. F. (1998). The molluscicidal activity of "Crown of Christ" (*Euphorbia splendens var hislopii*) latex snails acting as intermediate hosts of *Schistosomiasis mansoni* and *Schistosomiasis haematobium*. *American Journal of Tropical Medicine and Hygiene*, 58, 7-10

Secor, W. E. & Colley, D. G. (2005). Schistosomiasis. Springer Science and Business Media Incoporated, New York, USA.

Silva, I.M., Thiengo., Conceicao, M. J., Rey, L., Lenzi, H. L., Pereira Filho, E et al (2005). Therapeutic failure of praziquantel in the treatment of *S. haematobium* infection in Brazilians returning from Africa. *Mem Inst Oswaldo Cruz*, 100, 445-449.

Smithers, S. R. & Terry, R. J. (1969). Immunity in schistosomiasis. *Annals of NewYork Academy of Science*,160,826-840.

Sousa-Figueiredo, J. C., Pleasant, J., Day, M., Betson, M., Rollinson, D., Montressor, A., Kazibwe, F., Kabatereine, N. B. & Stothard, J. R. (2010). Treatment of intestinal schistosomiasis in Ugandan preschool children: best diagnosis, treatment efficacy and side-effects, and an extended praziquantel dosing pole. *International Health* 2, 103-113.

Stelma, F. F., Sall, S., Daff, B., Sow, S., Niang, M & Gryseels, B. (1997). Oxamniquine cures *S. mansoni* infection in a focus in which cure rates with praziquantel are unusually low. *Journal of Infectious Diseases*,176, 304-307.

Steinmann, P. et al (2006). Schistosomiasis and water resources development: systematic review, meta-analysis and estimates of population at risk. *The Lancet Infectious Diseases*, 6(7),411-425.

Sulaiman, S. M., Ali, H. M., Homeida, M.M & Bennet, J. L. (1989). Efficacy of a new Hoffman-La Roche compound (Ro-15-5458) against *S. mansoni* (Gezira strain, Sudan) in vervet monkeys (*Cercopithecus aethiops*). *Tropical Medicine and Parasitology*, 40, 335-336.

Sulaiman, S. M., Traore, M., Engels, D., Hagan, P & Cioli, D. (2001). Counterfeit Praziquantel. *Lancet*. 358, 666-667.

Strickland, G. T. (1982). Schistosomiasis: eradication or control? *Review of Infectious Diseases*, 4(5), 951-954.

Tchuem, A. L., Tcheunte, J. M., Behnke, F. S., Gilbert, V. R., Southgate, J & Vercruysse, J. (2003). Polparasitism with *Schistosoma haematobium* and soil-transmitted helminth infections among school children in Loum, Cameroon. *Tropical Medicine and International Health*, 8.11, 975-986

Tchuem, A. L.T., Southgate V. R, Webster, B. L., Bont, J. B & Vercruysse, J. (2001). Impact of installation of a water pump on schistomiasis transmission in a focus in Cameroon. *Transactions of the Royal Society of Tropical Medicine and Hygiene*, 95, 255-256

Useh M. F. & Ejezie, G. C. (1994). Urinary schistosomiasis in Cross River State, Nigeria. perception and response to infection by the residents of an endemic area. *Journal of Medical Laboratory Science*,4, 10-14

Useh M. F. & Ejezie, G. C. (1999a). School-based schistosomiasis control programme: a comparative study on the prevalence and intensity of urinary schistosomiasis among Nigerian school-age children in and out of school. *Transactions of the Royal Society of Tropical Medicine and Hygiene*, 93, 387-391

Useh M. F. & Ejezie, G. C. (1999b). Modification of behaviour and attitude in the control of schistosomiasis. 1. observations on water-contact patterns and perceptions of infection. *Annals of Tropical Medicine and Hygiene*, 93(7), 711-720.

Utzinger, J., N'Goran, E. K., N'Dri, A., Lengeler, C., Xiao, S. H. & Tanner, M.(2000).Oral artemether for prevention of *Schistosoma mansoni* infection: randomized controlled trial. *Lancet*, 355, 1320-1325

Utzinger, J., Keiser, J., Xiao, S. H., Tanner, M. & Singer, B. H. (2003). Combination therapy of schistosomiasis in laboratory studies and clinical trials. *Antimicrobial Agents and Chemotherapy*, 47, 1487-1495.

Weiler, C. (1989). Efficiency of focal molluscicidal treatment against schistosomiasis re-infection in an irrigation scheme and in a small dams area in Mali. *Annals of Tropical Medicine and Parasitology*, 40, 234-236

Wilson, R. A. and Coulson, P. A. (2006). Schistosome vaccines: a critical appraisal. *Mem Inst Cruz Rio de Janeiro,10(Suppl.*10, 13-20.

World Health Organisation (1965). Molluscividing screening and evaluation. *Bulletin of the World Health Organisation* 33,567-81.

World Health Organisation (1985). The control of schistosomiasis. Report of the WHO Expert Committee. Geneva World Health Organisation (WHO Technical Report Series, No 728).

World Health Organisation (1990). Health education in the control of schistosomiasis. World Health Organisation, Geneva, 1-56

World Health Organisation (1992). The role of mollusciciding in schistosomiasis control. World Health Organisation, Geneva, WHO/SCHIST/92.107

World Health Organisation (1993). The control of schistosomiasis. Second Report of WHO Committee, WHO/TRS/830, 1-26.

World Health Organisation (1996). Report of the WHO Informal Consultation on the use of chemotherapy for the control of morbidity due to soil-transmitted nematodes in humans. World Health Organisation, Geneva. WHO/CTD/SIP/96.2

World Health Organisation (2000). Human health and Dams: the World Health Organisation's submission to the World Commission on Dams. Geneva. (Protection of the human Environment: Water, Sanitation and Health Series; document WHO/SDE/WSH/00.01)

World Health Organisation (2002). Prevention and control of schistosomiasis and soil-transmitted helmithiasis. Report of a WHO Expert Committee. Geneva, World Health Organisation (WHO Technical Report Series, No 912).

5

Directives for Schistosomiasis Control in Endemic Areas of Brazil

Tereza C. Favre et al.*
Laboratory of Eco-epidemiology and Control of Schistosomiasis and Soil-transmitted Helminthiases / Oswaldo Cruz Institute, Fiocruz
Brazil

1. Introduction

The World Health Organization (WHO, 2010) estimates that 7.1 million people are infected with *Schistsosoma mansoni* in the Americas, 95% of which in Brazil. Resolution CD49.R19 of the Pan American Health Organization (PAHO, 2009) urged Member States to commit themselves to eliminate or reduce neglected diseases and other infections related to poverty for which tools exist, to levels so that these diseases are no longer considered public health problems by year 2015. The resolution considered schistosomiasis as one of the diseases whose prevalence can be drastically reduced in the Americas with available cost-effective interventions, and approved goals and strategies to be adopted by the countries according to their health policies, epidemiological situation and health service structure.

The present chapter firstly compares similarities and differences in the main goals and primary strategies between the current recommendations of the Brazilian Schistomiasis Control Programme (PCE), Ministry of Health (MS), and those of CD49.R19, with particular emphasis on improving coverage of diagnosis and treatment. Secondly, it examines data from a representative endemic area to provide evidence that an approach including school-based diagnosis and treatment would enable short-term improved access to and coverage of the control actions targeted at the school-aged group. Thirdly, it applies spatial analysis to evaluate baseline and post-treatment prevalence data from an endemic locality to show the feasibility of mapping re-infection risk areas based on the identified "hot spots", thus contributing to improve preventive measures such as environmental sanitation and snail control. Finally, it will be argued that the current MS strategy can be further improved towards the goal of drastically reducing prevalence in the foreseeable future taking into account the epidemiological situation and health service structure without compromising the country's health policies.

---

*Carolina F. S. Coutinho[1], Kátia G. Costa[1], Aline F. Galvão[1], Ana Paula B. Pereira[1], Lilian Beck[1], Oswaldo G. Cruz[2] and Otavio S. Pieri[1]
[1]*Laboratory of Eco-epidemiology and Control of Schistosomiasis and Soil-transmitted Helminthiases / Oswaldo Cruz Institute, Fiocruz, Brazil*
[2]*Scientific Computation Programme, Fiocruz, Brazil*

2. Directives for schistosomiasis control

The MS (1998, 2008) current strategy for schistosomiasis control in endemic areas focus on periodical stool surveys of whole populations through active case detection followed by prompt treatment of the egg-positives at the municipal primary health care level, together with preventive measures such as environmental sanitation and health education. It is envisaged that early, regular detection and treatment of the positives would avoid increasing morbidity and transmission among all age-groups. The main goals are to prevent the occurrence of severe forms of the disease and to reduce prevalence to less than 25% at the community level. This strategy has contributed to decrease the country-wide percentage of egg-positives from 10.4% in 1997 (290,031 positives out of 2,791,831 examined) to 5.2% in 2009 (68,952 positives out of 1,329,585 examined), confirming a downward trend observed since the mid-1990s (Coura & Amaral, 2004; Amaral et al. , 2006); however, it has yielded unsatisfactory results in highly endemic areas mainly due to low population coverage (Favre et al., 2006a). Therefore, it has been advocated that control activities in such problematic areas should focus on high-risk groups like school-aged children rather than whole populations (Favre et al., 2009).

The PAHO Resolution CD49.R19 proposes that the main goal for drastically reducing schistosomiasis in the Americas is to decrease prevalence and parasite load in high transmission areas; the primary strategies are (i) regular administration of chemotherapy irrespective of infection status to at least 75% of school-aged children that live in at-risk areas, defined by a prevalence over 10% in school-aged children, (ii) improved excreta disposal systems and access to drinking water and (iii) health education. This strategy of preventive chemotherapy has been established in accordance with the WHO (2002) recommendations of targeting treatment to high risk groups without prior diagnosis in preference to the previously advocated community-wide approach.

The main differences in control strategy between PAHO/WHO and the MS are summarized in Table 1 and briefly discussed below.

2.1 Diagnosis

Kato-Katz (KK) thick smears remain the method of choice for diagnosing egg-positive individuals in schistosomiasis control actions aimed at whole populations and high-risk groups from endemic areas of Brazil (MS, 2008). At present, KK kits are provided by the Immunobiological Technology Institute (Bio-Manguinhos/Fiocruz) at a cost of U$ 0.41 per exam. A single KK slide (one exam) is recommended for active-search surveys due to its operational cost-effectiveness, as increasing the number of slides or stool samples significantly increases the diagnosis sensitivity only in cases of light-intensity infections (less than 100 eggs per gram of faeces, or epg) (Rabello, 1992).

2.2 Prevalence classes

The PCE/MS recommends a cut-off value of 5% for the lower prevalence class, instead of 10% as suggested by PAHO/WHO, to compensate for the low sensitivity of one single KK slide used in stool surveys. A study from a low prevalence area in Brazil showed that screening a population with one KK slide missed 61.1% of the egg-positive individuals compared with a gold standard, indicating a sensitivity of 38.9% (Enk et al., 2008). According to this estimation, a prevalence of 5% based on one KK slide would correspond to an actual prevalence of 12.8%, whereas 10% would correspond to 25.7%. As the majority of severe forms usually occur in areas with prevalence above 25% (Coura & Amaral, 2004), the cut-off value of 5% based on one KK slide is a more cautious approach than 10% for the low-prevalence class. Accordingly, the MS sets the cut-off value of 25% as a prevalence level from which the control measures should be intensified at the community level in order to prevent the occurrence of severe forms of the disease.

The cut-off value of 50% for the higher prevalence class based on a single KK slide implies that, in endemic localities with prevalence ≥ 50%, practically all individuals are egg-positive. Furthermore, as a significant, positive relationship between prevalence and intensity of infection is usually found in endemic areas, a prevalence of 50% or more may correspond to a geometric mean of 200 or more eggs per gram of faeces (epg) (Rabello et al., 2008). This is regarded as moderate-to-heavy intensity of infection (WHO, 2002), which requires urgent control actions.

Organ	Prevalence	Endemic localities
MS (1998, 2008)	≥ 50%	Annual screening and treatment of all population Health education and environmental sanitation
	From 25% to < 50%	Biennial screening of all population followed by treatment of the positives and their household cohabitants Health education and environmental sanitation
	From 5% to < 25%)	Biennial screening of all population followed by treatment of the positives Health education and environmental sanitation
	< 5%	Passive case detection and treatment Health education and environmental sanitation

Organ	Prevalence	School	Community
PAHO/WHO (2009)	High (> 50%)	Annual treatment of all school-aged children	Treatment of high-risk groups; passive case detection and treatment Improvements of excreta disposal systems and access to drinking water, education
	Moderate (From 10% to 50%)	Biennial treatment of all school-aged children	Passive case detection and treatment Improvements of excreta disposal systems and access to drinking water, education
	Low (< 10%)	Treatment of school-aged children on entry and on leaving primary schooling	Passive case detection and treatment Improvements of excreta disposal systems and access to drinking water, education

Table 1. Strategies for schistosomiasis control recommended by the Brazilian Ministry of Health (MS) and the Pan American Health Organization (PAHO/WHO) in endemic areas.

2.3 Stool surveys

The PCE/MS currently recommends regular household stool surveys of whole populations for actively searching for infection carriers in endemic areas. The suggested survey periodicity varies according to the local prevalence class: annual for high prevalence and biennial for moderate prevalence. Passive case detection is only recommended for the low prevalence class. However, as pointed out by Favre et al. (2006a), the municipal primary

health care services of endemic areas have already reached their maximum capacity due to the overload of duties and are unable to sustain community-wide stool surveys at a regular basis. As a result, the targets agreed upon by the municipalities to fulfil the MS recommendations in those areas are far from being accomplished (Favre et al 2009).
The PAHO/WHO strategy involves stool surveys only to collect baseline data of the community prevalence prior to intervention and to follow-up its impact. Samples of 200-250 school-aged children from each ecologically homogeneous area are used for parasitological monitoring just before treatment and at 2-3 years thereafter (Montresor et al., 2002).

2.4 Treatment

Praziquantel (PZQ) is the drug of choice for treating egg-positive individuals in the course of schistosomiasis control actions. At present, it is provided by the Medicines and Drugs Technology Institute (Far-Manguinhos/Fiocruz) as 600 mg tablets at a cost of U$ 0.15 per tablet. The PCE/MS recommends a single oral dose of 60mg/kg for children of 2-15 years and 50 mg/kg for older children and adults (MS, 2008). Following official advice by the Federal Council of Medicine (CFM), treatment without prior diagnosis is not currently recommended. The only exceptions are: (i) treatment of all population in areas of prevalence ≥ 50% assessed through annual screening, which is accepted by the CFM, and (ii) treatment of household cohabitants of egg-positive individuals in areas of prevalence between 25% and 50% assessed through biennial screening.
The PAHO/WHO strategy involves school-based and community-based treatment targeted at school-aged children and other high-risks groups without prior diagnosis, as well as treatment of egg-positives following passive-case detection. The periodicity of school-based treatment varies according to the prevalence class: annual for high prevalence, biennial for moderate prevalence and twice during elementary schooling (on entry and on leaving) for low prevalence. This strategy of targeted preventive chemotherapy is viewed by the MS as a step backward for the Americas, as studies conducted in Brazil had shown that mass chemotherapy had only a transitory effect on schistosomiasis indicators (Coura & Conceição, 2010); instead, the focus should be on strengthening capacity for diagnosis and treatment of infection carriers at the primary care level and on improving environmental sanitation (PAHO, 2009). As pointed out by Rabello & Enk (2006), targeted treatment irrespective of infection status has the following implications: (i) risk of increasing drug resistance; (ii) relative high cost and low sustainability as compared to individual treatment integrated into the primary health care system; (iii) ethical requirement of informing the patient about the risks and benefits of unnecessary treatment and the right to refuse it without positive diagnosis.
Table 2 shows parasitological data from a school-based stool survey followed by treatment of egg-positives in order to illustrate the issues involved in targeting preventive chemotherapy at school-aged children from a municipality with moderate prevalence in an endemic area of Brazil. Both stool survey and treatment were performed by the municipal primary health care team. A total of 2,625 school-aged children (6-15 years) were examined in 11 schools, and all 676 (25.8%) egg-positives were treated with 60 mg/kg PZQ. If all 2,625 children were given PZQ irrespective of infection status, 1,949 (73.9%) of them would take the drug unnecessarily. Moreover, in five schools more than 80% of the children would be treated with negative diagnosis.
It is noteworthy that, although the side effects of PZQ are considered to be mild and transient (Coura & Conceição, 2010), they are a major factor discouraging people from taking the drug (Fleming et al., 2009; Garba et al., 2009; Souza-Figueiredo et al., 2010). A

School	Number of			% of	
	Examined	Positives	Negatives	Positives	Negatives
A	126	1	125	0.8	99.2
B	192	2	190	1.0	99.0
C	490	55	435	11.2	88.8
D	252	36	216	14.3	85.7
E	61	12	49	19.7	80.3
F	327	84	243	25.7	74.3
G	126	43	83	34.1	65.9
H	103	37	66	35.9	64.1
I	340	136	204	40.0	60.0
J	580	256	324	44.1	55.9
K	28	14	14	50.0	50.0
Total	**2,625**	**676**	**1,949**	**25.8**	**74.2**

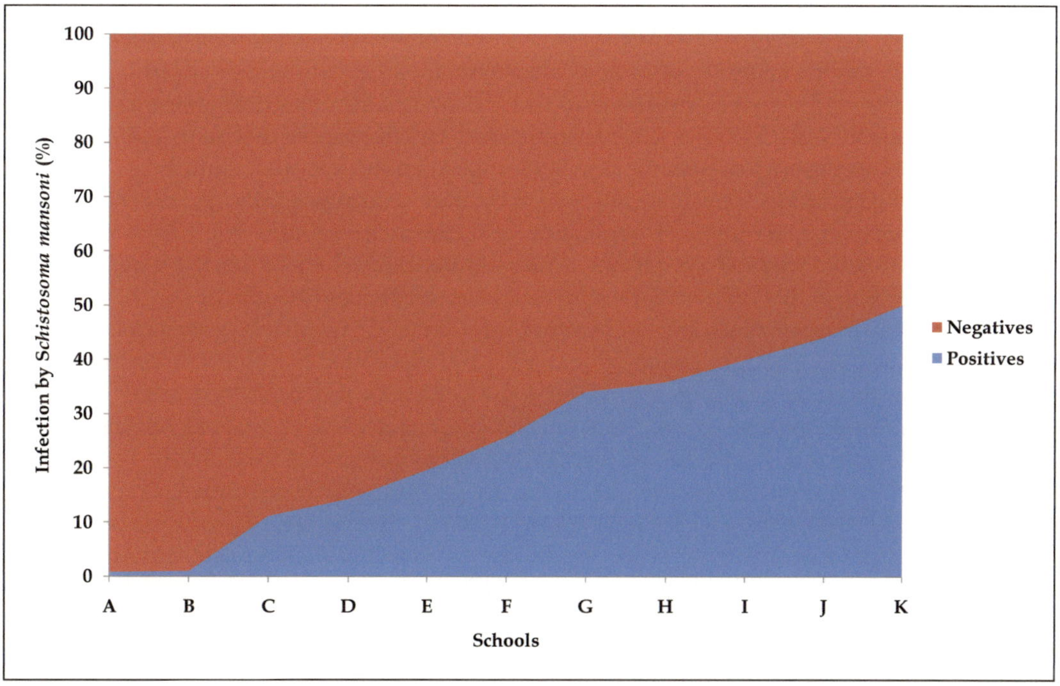

Table 2. Differences in treatment delivery to school-aged children between selective (positive only) and targeted (positive and negative) chemotherapy. The data are from school-based diagnosis followed by treatment of egg-positives carried out at the primary health care service from the municipality of Araçoiaba, North-east Brazil.

recent multi-country randomized controlled clinical trial on the efficacy and safety of single dose PZQ 40-60 mg/kg among adolescents (10-19 years) has shown that overall 78% of the patients reported adverse events up to four hours post-treatment; the most frequent were abdominal pain (40.4%), diarrhoea (17.5%), headache (10.7%), nausea (9.9%), vomiting (9.0) and dizziness (8.0%) (Olliaro et al., 2011). It is also worth mentioning that the bitter, disgusting taste of PZQ tablets is a major drawback for its administration among school-aged children (Meyer et al., 2009). Further evidence is needed to evaluate whether the bitter taste and side effects of PZQ can lower compliance, particularly in the absence of positive diagnosis.

2.5 Integrated measures

Some countries in sub-Saharan Africa have been successful in drastically reducing schistosomiasis infection using mass treatment with PZQ among school-aged children in high prevalence areas (Kabatereine et al., 2006; Kolaczinski et al., 2007; Touré et al., 2008; Tohon et al., 2008). However, to obtain sustained, satisfactory results mass treatment coverage should be kept around 90%, which has proven challenging over the years. In Brazil, selective treatment has reduced prevalence of infection in the short-term and morbidity in medium to long-term periods, but has not been sufficient to control disease transmission (Coura & Conceição, 2010). Studies from different endemic areas have shown that treatment strategies should be accompanied by auxiliary measures according to the epidemiological and geographical settings of each region (Guo et al., 2005; Wang et al., 2009; Sarvel et al., 2011). Accordingly, the MS advocates integrated measures combining selective treatment with environmental sanitation and health education incorporated into the primary health care system, as follows:

Recommended environmental sanitation measures include safe-water supply, adequate sewage collection and disposal, proper land use and occupation, soil drainage and control of intermediate snail hosts. Large-scale measures may be covenanted between the municipal and state level according to specific epidemiological requisites and complying with the environmental legislation. Local, small-scale measures to control intermediate host snails may include drainage, removal of vegetation and debris in habitats such as waste-water ditches and streams; methods aimed at direct elimination of snails such as molluscicide application are acceptable only under exceptional circumstances (MS, 2007)

Strategies of information, education, and communication (IEC) are also given special emphasis by the MS. A new approach to health education is recommended, involving interdisciplinary actions both in the school setting and in the community. As proposed by Massara & Schall (2004), the education process is seen not only as the acquisition of abilities but also as the building of affective and social relationships as well as environmental awareness.

As pointed out by Pieri & Favre (2007), an integrated approach aimed at improving coverage of both diagnosis and treatment and intensifying the use of auxiliary preventive measures is of paramount importance for scaling up the Brazilian schistosomiasis control programme within the Unified Health System (SUS). As the current directives of the MS and PAHO/WHO are not without drawbacks, an alternative strategy may be proposed to offset the issues raised.

3. An alternative strategy

An alternative strategy aiming to improve the MS current directives by further integrating the control actions into the primary health care system and involving diagnosis and selective treatment of school-aged children in the school setting is given in Table 3. It takes into account the operational difficulties faced by the most troubled municipalities without compromising the programme main goals. Thus, stool surveys are targeted at school-aged children as their prevalence is a suitable indicator of the community prevalence level (Guyatt et al 1999; Rodrigues et al 2000; Pereira et al 2010). Treatment is indicated in case of egg-positive diagnosis in conformity with prescribed indications and contraindications. Community-wide mass treatment is only considered if prevalence among school-aged children is more than 50%; treatment of cohabitants without prior diagnosis is not indicated.

Prevalence	Endemic localities
High (> 50%)	**Annual school-based screening of all school-aged children and treatment of all population** **Health education and environmental sanitation**
Moderate (From 5% to 50%)	**Biennial school-based screening of all school-aged children and treatment of the positives** **Health education and environmental sanitation**
Low (< 5%)	**Passive case detection and treatment** **Health education and environmental sanitation**

Table 3. An alternative strategy for schistosomiasis control in endemic areas of Brazil.

In endemic areas of Brazil for which there are reliable estimates of infection at the locality level, most prevalence levels are between 5% and 50% (Favre et al 2006b; Barbosa et al 2006). This situation is exemplified in Table 4 showing baseline parasitological data from stool surveys carried out in representative localities of an endemic area of Pernambuco, extracted from Pereira et al (2010). Those data may be used to compare the three strategies shown here as regards diagnosis and treatment.

According to the MS directives, in the locality of Paroés (prevalence 5%) only passive case detection should be carried out, as a part of the primary health care routine; in the eight localities with prevalence from 5% to 25%, all 4,934 residents should be screened and the 694 egg-positives, treated; in the five localities with prevalence from 25% to 50%, all 3,141 residents should be screened, and the 1,012 egg-positives and their 1,815 cohabitants (not in the table), treated; in the locality of Araújo (prevalence ≥50%), all 181 residents should be screened and treated. Overall 8,256 exams and 3,702 treatments should be performed.

In contrast, according to PAHO/WHO recommendations, all children aged 6-15 years should be screened except in Caricé and Sotave (where a representative sample of 250 children would be selected in each), totalling 1,447 exams and 2,088 treatments. It is of concern that this strategy would result in at 1,553 (74.4%) school-aged children being treated without positive diagnosis.

According to the proposed alternative strategy, in the locality of Paroés (prevalence 5%) only passive case detection should be carried out, as a part of the primary health care routine; in the 13 localities with prevalence from 5% to 50%, all 1,983 school-aged children should be screened and the 487 egg-positives, treated; in the locality of Araújo (prevalence ≥50%), all 68 school-aged children should be screened and all 181 residents, treated. On the whole, 2,051 exams and 668 treatments would be performed. It should be noted that none of the 1,553 school-aged children without positive diagnosis would receive treatment.

Locality	All ages				School-aged children (6-15 yrs)			
	Number residents	Number examined	Number positives	% positives	Number residents	Number examined	Number positives	% positives
Araújo	181	149	95	63.8	68	56	46	82.1
Poço Dantas	216	184	89	48.4	63	60	30	50.0
Sítio Bom Jesus	296	247	102	40.2	78	65	32	49.2
Caricé	1,882	1,532	609	39.8	409	349	170	48.7
Camorim	462	417	143	33.5	193	128	46	35.9
Covas	285	237	69	29.1	87	87	35	40.2
Sotave	3,330	2,271	562	24.7	731	527	138	26.2
Souto	127	103	17	16.5	23	19	5	26.3
Engenho Brasil	331	246	38	15.4	102	76	14	18.4
Palheta	109	109	15	13.8	35	35	2	5.7
Lagoinha	345	249	27	10.8	104	75	7	9.3
Anil	119	83	7	8.4	30	21	2	9.5
Engenho Bom Jesus	356	240	18	7.5	77	52	2	3.8
Chã de Aldeia	217	161	10	6.2	51	38	4	10.5
Paroés	143	96	4	4.1	36	24	1	4.2
All localities	8,399	6,324	1,805	28.5	2,088	1,612	534	33.1

Table 4. Parasitological data from whole populations and school-aged children in representative localities of an endemic area of schistosomiasis in Brazil. The data were extracted from Pereira et al (2010)

It must be borne in mind that population coverage of 75.3%, as observed in the given example, is rarely achieved by the health teams in the endemic areas. In fact, stool surveys of whole populations in the highly endemic Rainforest Zone of Pernambuco from 2003 to 2006 reached 19.7% of the population at risk (Favre et al, 2009); more recently, from 2007 to 2010, the coverage in the same zone was increased by only 4 percentage points to 23.7% (MS, 2011). This low coverage is due to the fact that the municipal authorities annually set covenanted quantitative targets for population diagnosis and treatment in line with the Priority Action Plan in Health Surveillance (PAP-VS) adjusted to the availability of personnel and financial resources. In the Rainforest Zone of Pernambuco the average target for 2006-2007 has been only 13.7% of the population at risk (Table 5).

It has been argued that the PAP-VS target for diagnosis and treatment set by the most troubled municipalities from endemic areas may be better accomplished if it is applied to school-aged children (Pieri & Favre, 2007). Firstly, school-aged children are particularly vulnerable to schistosomiasis and play an important role in maintaining transmission. Secondly, school-aged children are accessible and generally show good compliance. Thirdly, school-based actions involving teachers and children's families may help the health teams to scale up control actions as needed. Fourthly, detecting and treating infection in school-aged children prevent infection from increasing as they reach the pre-adult stage. Fifthly, the focus on school-aged children is a more realistic, feasible strategy to accomplish the PAP-VS target; as it can be seen in Table 5, the total target of 172,500 exams set for 2006-2007 would exceed in 3.6% the population in that age-group.

Municipalities	Prevalence (%)	Population (2006)		PAP-VS (2006-2007)	% PAP-VS	
		All ages	School-aged		All ages	School-aged
Água Preta	13.4	30,455	5,847	2,500	8.2	57.0
Aliança	20.6	36,992	6,550	8,000	21.6	162.8
Amaraji	13.4	22,279	4,230	3,000	13.5	94.6
Barreiros	11.2	38,082	7,215	3,000	7.9	55.4
Belém de Maria	13.3	9,460	1,951	2,100	22.2	143.5
Buenos Aires	9.8	11,671	2,074	5,000	42.8	321.4
Camutanga	1.5	8,107	1,411	3,000	37.0	283.5
Carpina	7.6	70,337	10,040	10,000	14.2	132.8
Catende	14.7	31,063	5,854	4,000	12.9	91.1
Chã de Alegria	11.8	11,252	2,165	5,000	44.4	307.9
Chã Grande	3.7	20,556	3,491	3,500	17.0	133.7
Condado	5.6	24,271	3,575	5,500	22.7	205.1
Cortês	18.7	12,823	2,607	2,000	15.6	102.3
Escada	33.1	58,450	10,279	6,000	10.3	77.8
Ferreiros	6.3	10,579	1,818	3,000	28.4	220.0
Gameleira	19.5	27,227	4,658	3,000	11.0	85.9
Glória do Goitá	9.4	28,105	5,547	8,000	28.5	192.3
Goiana	12.0	76,371	12,394	5,500	7.2	59.2
Itambé	10.0	35,523	6,488	6,000	16.9	123.3
Itaquitinga	18.0	15,632	2,765	4,000	25.6	192.9
Jaqueira	11.1	12,635	2,524	2,000	15.8	105.7
Joaquim Nabuco	5.2	16,090	3,263	1,600	9.9	65.4
Lagoa do Carro	17.7	14,599	2,252	2,500	17.1	148.0
Lagoa do Itaenga	5.6	22,880	3,921	3,000	13.1	102.0
Macaparana	4.7	23,706	4,274	3,500	14.8	109.2
Maraial	10.8	16,124	3,125	1,600	9.9	68.3
Nazaré da Mata	14.1	31,261	4,626	5,000	16.0	144.1
Palmares	4.6	54,355	10,286	6,000	11.0	77.8
Paudalho	10.5	49,225	8,093	5,000	10.2	82.4
Pombos	4.4	24,904	4,328	2,500	10.0	77.0
Primavera	16.5	11,937	2,195	2,000	16.8	121.5
Quipapá	7.3	22,894	5,151	3,000	13.1	77.7
Ribeirão	5.1	41,765	7,241	3,500	8.4	64.4
Rio Formoso	26.8	22,049	4,220	2,700	12.2	85.3
São Benedito do Sul	19.7	10,915	2,086	2,000	18.3	127.8
São Jose Coroa Grande	6.5	15,773	2,684	2,000	12.7	99.4
Sirinhaem	10.9	32,889	6,596	2,000	6.1	40.4
Tamandaré	19.8	19,110	3,471	2,500	13.1	96.0
Timbaúba	11.7	56,647	10,079	8,000	14.1	105.8
Tracunhaém	12.5	12,734	2,298	5,000	39.3	290.1
Vicência	20.1	29,413	5,620	7,000	23.8	166.1
Vitória de Santo Antão	9.8	125,563	19,989	6,000	4.8	40.0
Xexéu	12.8	15,752	2,721	2,000	12.7	98.0
TOTAL	**12.2**	**1,262,455**	**222,002**	**172,500**	**13.7**	**103.6**

(*) Source: Brazilian Institute of Geography and Statistics (IBGE)
(**)Source: State Health Secretariat of Pernambuco (SES-PE).

Table 5. Prevalence of schistosomiasis, population data* and number of stool exams targeted for 2006-2007 by the Priority Action Plan in Health Surveillance (PAP-VS)** for the municipalities of the Rainforest Zone of Pernambuco state. The percentages of 2006-2007 PAP-VS target for all ages and school-aged children (7-14 yrs) are also given.

It must be stressed that the proposed alternative of targeting diagnosis and treatment at school-aged children aims to assist the municipalities that do not have enough resources to follow the current MS recommendations of covering whole populations, as is the case of Araçoiaba (Table 6).

- Geographic coordinates : 07° 47' 24" S 35° 05' 27" W
- Area: 92 km ^{2}
- Main economic activity: cash-crop agriculture for the production of alcohol and sugar.
- Population (2009):
  - Total: 17,484
  - Municipal Human Development Index (IDH-M): 0.637;
  - Basic Education Index (IDEB): 2.8
- Schistosomiasis status
  - Covenanted target: (2005 – 2009): 7,346 exams (42% of the population)
  - Diagnosis coverage (2005 -2009): 6,070 exams (34.7% of the population)
  - Treatment compliance (2005 2009): 1,320 patients (75.9% of the positives)
  - Reasons for no treatment: absence (18.1%), contraindication (6.0%)
  - Prevalence: 40.9 % (2005), 32.2% (2006), 30.2% (2007), 19.8% (2009)
- School-aged children(6 -15 yrs):
  - Total: 3,418;
  - Enrolled: 3,273 (95.8%);
  - Drop-out: 13.6%
  - Elementary schools: 11

Table 6. Demographic and parasitological data of Araçoiaba, a municipality from the endemic area of North-east Brazil.

That municipality holds a relatively low index of human development (0.637) in the endemic area of schistosomiasis in Pernambuco. The covenanted target for schistosomiasis diagnosis between 2005 and 2009 was only 42% of the population at risk, but the actual cumulative coverage was even lower, 34.7%. Of the 6,070 exams carried out during that period, 1,739 (28.6%) were positive. It can be argued from the data on school-aged children that the elementary schools would provide a satisfactory setting for implementing control actions in the municipality. Thus, 95.8% of the school-aged children are enrolled at school and the drop-outs are negligible (13.6%) may be reached out from the school records.
According to the MS (2011), only two of the 99 endemic municipalities surveyed in Pernambuco between 2005 and 2009 had higher prevalence than Araçoiaba, namely, Escada (33.1%) and João Alfredo (47.3%). It is of note that treatment compliance was satisfactory (75.9%of the egg-positives), the main reason for non-treatment being absence (18.1%). As the contraindication cases were considerable (105 out of 1739), the importance of well-trained health staff during this phase cannot be underestimated.

4. Spatial analysis

Spatial analysis and Geographic Information Systems (GIS) are important tools that can be used for identifying environmental risk factors and delimiting risk areas of schistosomiasis, leading to optimization of resources and improvement of actions for the specific conditions

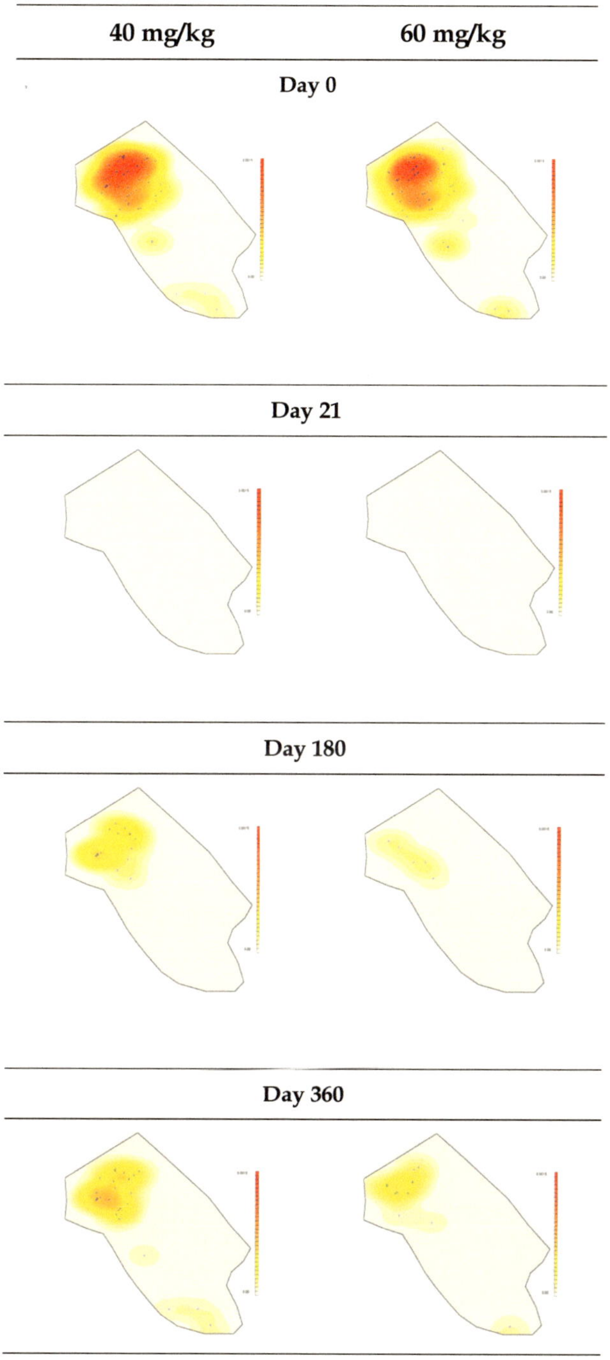

Fig. 1. Kernel intensity estimates of egg-positive subjects at baseline (Day 0), 21 days, 180 days and 360 days after treatment with PZQ 40 mg/kg or PZQ 60 mg/kg. The vertical bars indicate the kernel intensity scale. The original data are from Galvão et al., 2010.

of the disease (Bergquist, 2002). Thus, the MS recommends that data from stool surveys should include the geographic coordinates of the households obtained by a Global Positioning System (GPS) receptor for later insertion on a digitized map and a geo-referenced database. As egg-positive households tend to cluster within communities due to focal characteristics of risk factors and transmission, kernel density exploratory analysis has been of help to assess differences in their spatial distribution patterns and to relate them to potential sources of risk in endemic areas of schistosomiasis in Brazil (Gazzinelli et al., 2006; Araújo et al., 2007; Galvão et al., 2010; Cardin et al., 2011) and China (Zhang et al., 2009).

Figure 1 illustrates the use of kernel density estimator for visually identifying risk areas and comparing the magnitude of spatial clustering in individual infection before and up to one year after treatment with either 40mg/kg or 60mg/kg PZQ single dose. A bandwidth of 75 meters was used, and the colour pattern of the intensity scale varied from white (lowest intensity kernel) to red (highest intensity kernel). The data are from Galvão et al. (2010). Before treatment (D0) the clusters of egg-positives were similar with respect to intensity and extent, as the individuals were randomly assigned to each treatment group. The area-wide white seen at D21 reflects the fact that all individuals became egg-negative at 21 days after treatment. The highest kernel intensity and extent of clusters in the group of 40 mg/kg than in the 60 mg/kg, both at 180 and 360 days, indicate that reversion of individuals to egg-positive up to one year after treatment was higher in the lower-dose group. Figure 1 also indicates that infection tended to return to the pre-treatment level, although they might take longer among the patients who received the higher PZQ dose.

Based on this information, it can be recommended that primary health care teams should carry out snail surveys to identify potential transmission foci and implement local environmental sanitation and other preventive measures as appropriate.

5. Concluding remarks

It is clear from the above explanation that the current MS strategy for schistosomiasis control can be further improved without compromising the country's health policies, especially as regards the ethical requirement of delivering treatment only to egg-positive diagnosis. It is expected that the health authorities will incorporate sustained school-based actions for scaling up coverage and achieving rapid impact on schistosomiasis, particularly in the most troubled municipalities. However, the primary health care teams should include community-wide control actions as soon as the critical situation is overcome.

6. References

Amaral, R. S.; Tauil, P. L.; Lima, D. D. & Engels, D. (2006). An analysis of the impact of the schistosomiasis control programme in Brazil. *Mem Inst Oswaldo Cruz,*Vol. 101, Suppl. I, (October 2006), pp. 79-85, ISSN 0074-0276

Araújo, K. C.; Resendes, A. P. C.; Souza-Santos, R.; Silveira-Júnior, J. C. & Barbosa, C. S. (2007). Spatial analysis of *Biomphalaria glabrata* foci and human cases of mansoni schistosomiasis in Porto de Galinhas, Pernambuco State, Brazil, in the year 2000. *Cad Saúde Pública,* Vol. 23, No. 2, (February 2007), pp. 409-417, ISSN 0102-311X

Barbosa, C.S., Favre, T.C., Wadndeley, T.N., Callou, A.C., Pieri, O.S. (2006). Assessment of schistosomiasis through school surveys in the Forest zone of Pernambuco, Brazil. *Mem Inst Oswaldo Cruz,*Vol. 101, Suppl. I, (October 2006), pp. 55-62, ISSN 0074-0276

Bergquist, N.R. (2002). Schistosomiasis: from risk assessment to control. *Trends Parasitol*, Vol. 18, No. 7, (July 2002), pp. 309-314, ISSN 1471-4922

Cardim, L. L.; Ferraudo, A. S.; Pacheco, S. T. A.; Reis, R. B.; Silva, M. M. N.; Carneiro, D. D. M. T. & Bavia, M. E. (2011). Análises espaciais na identificação das áreas de risco para a esquistossomose mansônica no município de Lauro de Freitas, Bahia, Brasil. *Cad Saúde Pública*, Vol. 27, No.5, (May 2011), pp. 899-908, ISSN 0102-311X

Coura, J. R. & Amaral, R. S. (2004). Epidemiological and control aspects of schistosomiases in Brazilian endemic areas. *Mem Inst Oswaldo Cruz*, Vol. 99, Suppl. I, (August 2004), pp. 13-19, ISSN 0074-0276

Coura, J. R. & Conceição M. J. (2010). Specific schistosomiasis treatment as a strategy for disease control. *Mem Inst Oswaldo Cruz*, Vol. 105, No. 4, (July 2010), pp. 598-603, ISSN 0074-0276

Enk, M. J.; Lima, A. C. L.; Massara, C. L.; Coelho, P. M. Z. & Schall V. T. (2008). A combined strategy to improve the control of *Schistosoma mansoni* in areas of low prevalence in Brazil. Am J Trop Med Hyg, Vol. 78, No. 1, (January 2008), pp. 140-146, ISSN 0002-9637

Favre, T. C.; Ximenes, R. A. A.; Galvão, A. F.; Pereira, A. P. B.; Wanderley, T. N.; Barbosa, C. S. & Pieri, O. S. (2006a). Attaining the minimum target of resolution WHA 54.19 for schistosomiasis control in the Rainforest Zone of the state of Pernambuco, Northeastern Brazil. *Mem Inst Oswaldo Cruz*, Vol. 101, Suppl. I, (October 2006), pp. 125-132, ISSN 0074-0276

Favre, T.C.; Ximenes, R.A.A.; Galvão, A.F.; Pereira, A.P.; Wanderlei, T.N.; Barbosa, C.S. & Pieri, O.S. (2006b). Reliability of current estimates of schistosomiasis prevalence in the rainforest zone of the state of Pernambuco, Northeastern Brazil. *Mem Inst Oswaldo Cruz*,Vol. 101, Suppl. I, (October 2006), pp. 73-78, ISSN 0074-0276

Favre,T. C.; Pereira, A. P. B.; Galvão, A. F.; Zani, L. C.; Barbosa, C. S. & Pieri, O. S. (2009). A rationale for schistosomiasis control in elementary schools of the Rainforest Zone of Pernambuco, Brazil. *PloS Negl Trop Dis*, Vol. 3, No. 3, (March 2009), pp. e395, ISSN 1935-2735

Fleming, F.M.; Fenwick, A.; Tukahebwa, E. M.; Lubanga, R. G.; Namwangye, H.; Zaramba, S. & Kabatereine, N. B. (2009). Process evaluation of schistosomiasis control in Uganda, 2003 to 2006: perceptions, attitudes and constraints of a national programme. *Parasitology*, Vol. 136, No. 13, (November 2009), pp. 1759-1769, ISSN 0031-1820

Galvão, A. F.; Favre, T. C.; Guimarães, R. J. P. S.; Pereira, A. P. B.; Zani, L. C.; Felipe, K. T.; Domingues, A. L. C.; Carvalho, O. S.; Barbosa, C. S. & Pieri, O.S. (2010). Spatial distribution of Schistosoma mansoni infection before and after chemotherapy with two praziquantel doses in a community of Pernambuco, Brazil. *Mem Inst Oswaldo Cruz*, Vol. 105, No. 04, (July 2010), pp. 555-562, ISSN 0074-0276

Garba, A.; Touré, S.; Dembelé, R.; Boisier, P.; Tohon, Z.; Bosqué-Oliva, E.; Koukounari, A. & Fenwick, A. (2009). Present and future schistosomiasis control activities with support from the Schistosomiasis Control Initiative in West Africa. *Parasitology*, Vol. 136, (July 2009), pp. 1731-1737, ISSN 0031-1820

Gazzinelli, A.; Hightower, A.; LoVerde, P.T.; Haddad, J. P. A.; Pereira, W. R.; Bethony, J.; Correa-Oliveira, R. & Kloos, H. (2006). The spatial distribution of Schistosoma mansoni infection before and after chemotherapy in the Jequitinhonha Valley in

Brazil. *Mem Inst Oswaldo Cruz*, Vol. 101, Suppl. I, (September 2006), pp. 63-71, ISSN 0074-0276

Guo, J. G.; Cao, C. L.; Hu, G. H.; Lin, H.; Li, D.; Zhu, R. & Xu, J. (2005). The role of 'passive chemotherapy' plus health education for schistosomiasis control in China during maintenance and consolidation phase. *Acta Trop*, Vol. 96, No. 2-3, (November - December 2005), pp. 177-183, ISSN 0001-706X

Guyatt , H.L.; Brooker, S.& Donnely, C.A. (1999). Can prevalence of infection in school-aged children be used as an index for assessing community prevalence? *Parasitology*, Vol. 118, No. 3, (March 1999), pp.257-268, ISSN 0031-1820

Kabatereine, N. B.; Fleming, F. M.; Nyandindi, U.; Mwanza, J. C. L. & Blair. L. (2006). The control of schistosomiasis and soiltransmitted helminths in East Africa. *Trends Parasitol*, Vol. 22, No. 7, (July 2006), pp. 332-339, ISSN 1471-4922

Kolaczinski, J. H.; Kabatereine, N. B.; Onapa, A. W.; Ndyomugyenyi, R.; Kakembo A. S. L. & Brooker, S. (2007). Neglected tropical diseases in Uganda: the prospect and challenge of integrated control. *TRENDS in Parasitology*, Vol. 23, No. 10, (September 2007), pp. 485-493, ISSN 1471-4922

Massara, CL. & Schall, V.T. (2004). A pedagogical approach of schistosomiasis - an experience in health education in Minas Gerais, Brazil. *Mem Inst Oswaldo Cruz*, Vol. 99, Suppl. I, (August 2004), pp. 113-119, ISSN 0074-0276

Meyer, T.; Sekljic, H.; Fuchs, S.; Bothe, H.; Schollmeyer, D. & Miculka, C. (2009). Taste, a new incentive to switch to (R)-Praziquantel in schistosomiasis treatment. *PloS Negl Trop Dis*, Vol. 3, No. 1, (January 2009), pp. e357, ISSN 1935-2735

MS (1998). *Controle da Esquistossomose: Diretrizes Técnicas* (Second edition), Ministério da Saúde - Fundação Nacional de Saúde, ISBN 85-7346-028-8, Brasília

MS (2007). *Vigilância e Controle dos moluscos de Importância Epidemiológica: DiretrizesTécnicasdo Programa de Vigilância e Controle da Esquistossomose* (Second Edition), Ministério da Saúde - Secretaria de Vigilância em Saúde, ISBN 978-85-334-1438-9, Brasília, Retrieved from:
http://portal.saude.gov.br/portal/arquivos/pdf/manual_controle_moluscos.pdf

MS (2008). Esquistossomose, In: Vigilância em Saúde: *Esquistossomose, Hanseníase, Malária, Tracoma e Tuberculose* (Second Edition), Secretaria de Atenção Básica - Departamento de Atenção Básica, pp. 48-65, Ministério da Saúde, ISBN 978-85-334-1303-0, Brasília, Retrieved from:
http://portal.saude.gov.br/portal/arquivos/pdf/abcad21.pdf

MS (2011). Secretaria de Vigilância em Saúde. Programa de Controle da Esquistossomose. Departamento de Informática do Sistema Único de Saúde - DATASUS. (Assessed in 29/06/2011) http://tabnet.datasus.gov.br/cgi/tabcgi.exe?sinan/pce/cnv/pce.def

Montresor, A.; Gyorkos T.; Crompton D. W. T. & Savioli, L. (2002). *Helminth Control in School-Age Children*, World Health Organization, Retrived from:
http://www.who.int/wormcontrol/documents/helminth_control/en/

Olliaro, P. L.; Vaillant, M. T.; Belizario, V. J.; Lwambo, N. J. S.; Ouldabdallahi, M.; Pieri, O. S.; Amarillo, M. L.; Kaatano, G. M.; Diaw, M.; Domingues, A. L. C.; Favre, T. C.; Lapujade, O.; Alves, F. & Chitsulo, L. (2011). A multicentre randomized controlled trial of the efficacy and safety of single-dose praziquantel at 40 mg/kg vs. 60 mg/kg for treating intestinal schistosomiasis in the Philippines, Mauritania,

Tanzania and Brazil. *PloS Negl Trop Dis,* Vol. 5, No. 6, (June 2011), pp. e1165, ISSN 1935-2735

PAHO (October 2009). 49th Directing Council - Final Report, In: *61st Session of the Regional Committee,* 10.03.2011, Avaiable from: http://new.paho.org/hq/index.php?option=com_docman&task=doc_download&gid=3725&Itemid

Pereira, A. P. B.; Favre, T. C.; Galvão, A. F.; Beck, L.; Barbosa, C. S. & Pieri, O. S. (2010). The prevalence of schistosomiasis in school-aged children as an appropriate indicator of its prevalence in the community. *Mem Inst Oswaldo Cruz,* Vol. 105, No.4, (July 2010), pp. 563-569, ISSN 0074-0276

Pieri, O.S. & Favre, T.C. (2007). Incrementando o programa de controle da esquistossomose. *Cad Saúde Pública,* Vol. 23, No.7, (July 2007), pp. 1733-1734, ISSN 0102-311X

Rabello, A. L. T. (1992). Parasitological diagnosis of schistosomiasis mansoni : fecal examination and rectal biopsy. *Mem Inst Oswaldo Cruz,* Vol. 87, Suppl. IV, (1992), pp. 325-331, ISSN 0074-0276

Rabello, A. & Enk, M. (2006) Progress towards the detection of schistosomiasis. In *Report of the Scientific Working Group on Schistosomiasis 2005,* TDR/SWG/07 , pp. 67-71, WHO, Retrieved from: http://apps.who.int/tdr/publications/tdr-research-publications/swg-report-schistosomiasis/pdf/swg_schisto.pdf

Rabello, A.; Pontes, L. A.; Enk, M. J.; Montenegro, S. M. L. & Morais C. N. L. (2008). Diagnóstico Parasitológico, Imunológico e Molecular da Esquistossomose Mansoni, In: *Schistosoma mansoni & Esquistossomose uma visão multidisciplinar,* Omar dos Santos Carvalho, Paulo Marcos Zech Coelho & Henrique Leonel Lenzi, pp. 895-925, Fiocruz, ISBN 978-857541-150-6, Rio de Janeiro

Rodrigues, L.C.; Wheeler, J.G., Shier, R.; Guerra, H.L.; Pimenta, F. Jr. & Lima e Costa, M.F. (2000). Predicting the community prevalence of schistosomiasis mansoni from the prevalence among 7- to 14-year-olds. *Parasitology,* Vol 121, No. 5,pp. 507-512 (November 2000), ISSN 0031-1820

Sarvel, A. K.; Oliveira, A. A.; Silva, A. R.; Lima, A. C. L. & Katz, N. (2011). Evaluation of a 25-Year-Program for the Control of Schistosomiasis Mansoni in an Endemic Area in Brazil. *PloS Negl Trop Dis,* Vol. 5, No. 3, (March 2011), pp. e990, ISSN 1935-2735

Sousa-Figueiredo, J. C.; Pleasant, J.; Day M.; Betson M.; Rollinson, D.; Montresor, A.; Kazibwe, F.; Kabatereine, N. B. & Stothard R. (2010). Treatment of intestinal schistosomiasis in Ugandan preschool children: best diagnosis, treatment efficacy and side-effects, and an extended praziquantel dosing pole. *Int Health,*Vol. 2. No. 2, (June 2010), pp. 103-113, ISSN 1876-3413

Tohon, Z. B.; Mainassara, H. B.; Garba, A.; Mahamane, A. E.; Bosqué-Oliva, E.; Ibrahim, M. L.; Duchemin, J. B.; Chanteau, S. & Boisier P. (2008). *PloS Negl Trop Dis,* Vol. 2, No. 5, (May 2008), pp. e241, ISSN 1935-2735

Touré, S.; Zhang, Y.; Bosqué-Oliva, E.; Ky, C.; Ouedraogo, A.; Koukounari, A.; Gabrielli, A. F.; Sellin, B.; Webster, J. & Fenwick, A. (2008). Two-Year impact of single praziquantel treatment on infection in the national control programme on schistosomiasis in Burkina Faso. *Bulletin of the World Health Organization,* Vol. 86, No. 10, (October 2008), pp. 780-788, ISSN 0042-9686

Wang, L. D.; Guo, J. G.; Wu, X. H.; Chen, H. G.; Wang, T. P.; Zhu, S. P.; Zhang, Z. H.; Steinmann, P.; Yang, G. J.; Wang, S. P.; Wu, Z. D.; Wang, L. Y.; Hao, Y.; Bergquist,

R.; Utzinger, J. & Zhou, X. N. (2009). China's new strategy to block Schistosoma japonicum transmission: experiences and impact beyond schistosomiasis. *Trop Med Int Health*, Vol. 14, No. 12, (December 2009), pp. 1475-1483, ISSN 1360-2276

WHO (2002). *Prevention and control of Schistossomiasis and soil-transmitted helminthiasis*. Report of a WHO Expert Committee, ISBN : 92 4 1209127, Geneva

WHO (2010). Schistosomiasis. In : *Weekly Epidemiological Record*,Vol. 85, No. 18, (April 2010), pp. 158–164, ISSN 0049-8114

Zhang, Z.; Clark, A. B.; Bivand, R.; Chen, Y.; Carpenter, T. E.; Peng, W.; Zhou, Y.; Zhao, G. & Jiang, Q. (2009). Nonparametric spatial analysis to detect high-risk regions for schistosomiasis in Guichi, China. *Trans R Soc Trop Med Hyg*, Vol. 103, No. 10 (October 2009), pp. 1045-1052, ISSN 0035-9203

Schistosomiasis in Lake Malaŵi and the Potential Use of Indigenous Fish for Biological Control

Jay R. Stauffer, Jr.[1] and Henry Madsen[2]
[1]*School of Forest Resources, Penn State University, University Park, PA*
[2]*DBL Centre for Health Research and Development, Faculty of Life Sciences, University of Copenhagen, Frederiksberg*
[1]*USA*
[2]*Denmark*

1. Introduction

Schistosomiasis is a parasitic disease of major public health importance in many countries in Africa, Asia, and South America, with an estimated 200 million people infected worldwide (World Health Organization, 2002). The disease is caused by trematodes of the genus *Schistosoma* that require specific freshwater snail species to complete their life cycles (Fig. 1). People contract schistosomiasis when they come in contact with water containing the infective larval stage (cercariae) of the trematode.

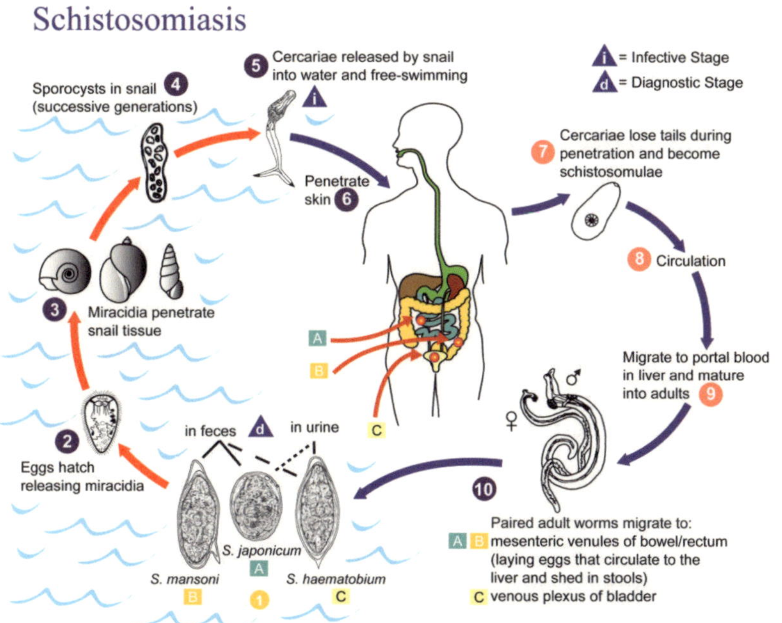

Fig. 1. Life cycle of schistosomes (Source: CDC/Alexander J. da Silva, PhD/Melanie Moser)

Schistosome transmission, *Schistosoma haematobium*, is a major public health concern in the Cape Maclear area of Lake Malaŵi (Fig. 2), because the disease poses a great problem for local people and reduces revenue from tourism. Until the mid-1980's, the open shores of Lake Malaŵi were considered free from human schistosomes (Evans, 1975; Stauffer et al., 1997); thus, only within relatively protected areas of the lake or tributaries would transmission take place. These areas were suitable habitat of intermediate host snail, *Bulinus globosus*. During mid-1980's, reports indicated that transmission also occurred along open shorelines. It is now evident that in the southern part of the lake, especially Cape Maclear on Nankumba Peninsula, transmission occurs along exposed shorelines with sandy sediment devoid of aquatic plants via another intermediate host, *Bulinus nyassanus* (Madsen et al., 2001, 2004). This species is endemic to Lake Malaŵi and is a diploid (2n=36) member of the *tropicus/truncatus* group of *Bulinus* where also the most important hosts of *S. haematobium* in North Africa belong, i.e., *B. truncatus* (4n=72). The changes in transmission pattern could be related in part to over-fishing which clearly has resulted in decline in density of several cichlid fish species (Stauffer et al., 1997), some of which are important predators of snails or a new strain of *Schistosoma haematobium* capable of exploiting *B. nyassanus* as host. Another diploid species of this group, *Bulinus succinoides* has not been shown to be a host. Stauffer et al. (1997) suggested that a lake-wide strategy for controlling schistosome intermediate hosts using fishes should be initiated to reduce the prevalence of this disease. Preliminary studies indicated that the facultative molluscivore and popular food fish, *Trematocranus placodon*, is effective at controlling schistosome intermediate host snails in fishponds (Chiotha et al., 1991a, b).
Although all types of fishing are prohibited within a 100-m zone along the shoreline within Lake Malaŵi National Park, this clearly is not respected. Seine-net fishing from the shoreline is often observed and gill-nets are often found within this sanctuary zone (pers. obs.). Beach seining, however, is the most damaging form of fishing, since nets are often very fine meshed (sometimes lined with mosquito nets) and since the near-shore zone of the lake is where juvenile fishes reside; thus, recruitment of fish populations is seriously affected. It is evident that densities of some cichlid species, including molluscivorous species, have declined markedly in shallow waters compared to densities during the early 1980s (Stauffer et al., 2006). Here we summarize the results of a six year study of the interactions among fish abundance, snail intermediate hosts for *Schistosoma haematobium*, and prevalence of human infections.

2. Study area

Lake Malaŵi (Fig. 2), the most southerly lake in the East African Rift Valley system, is over 600 km long (Beadle, 1974) and is 75 km wide at its widest point; its total surface area is approximately 29,600 km^2. As such, it is the third largest lake in the world by volume and the ninth largest by surface area. The lake is bordered by western Mozambique, eastern Malaŵi, and Tanzania. Its largest tributary is the Ruhuhu River and its outlet is the Shire River, a tributary of the Zambezi. The largest part of the lake is in Malaŵi, while about a quarter of the lake area is under the jurisdiction of Mozambique; this includes the area surrounding the Malaŵian islands of Likoma and Chizumulu, which are the lake's only two inhabited islands. It is bordered by Malaŵi, Mozambique, and Tanzania. It is also the second deepest lake in Africa. The lake harbors more fish species than any other lake on Earth.

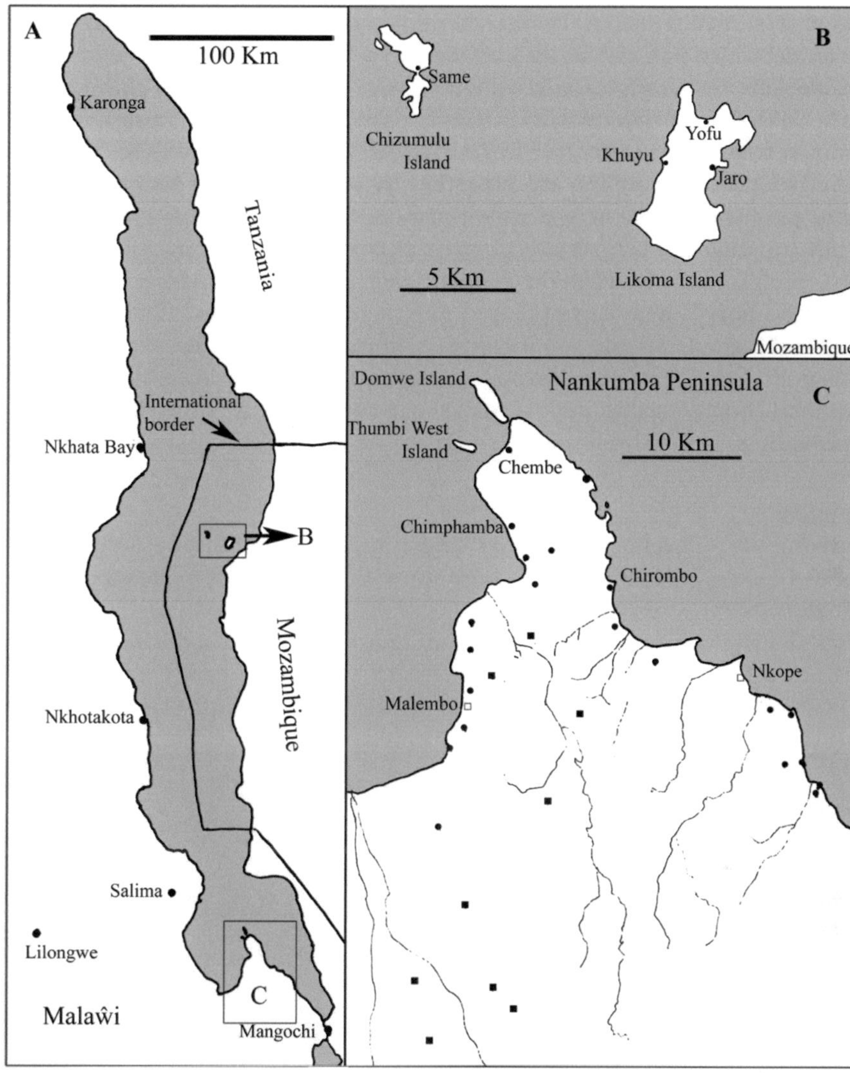

Fig. 2. Lake Malaŵi and some of our sampling sites (Source: Madsen et al. in press).

The climate is generally tropical with a rainy season from November to April. There is little to no rainfall throughout much of the country from May to October. It is hot and humid from September to April along the lake, with average daytime maxima of 27- 29°C. From June through August, the daytime maxima are around 23°C. During the cold months the prevailing wind is southerly.

Fishes from Lake Malaŵi are the major food source to the residents of Malaŵi. The Malaŵians prefer chambo, which consists of any one of four species of the cichlid genus *Oreochromis*, as well as the kampango, a large catfish (*Bagrus meridionalis*).

The water in Lake Malaŵi is typically alkaline with a pH of 7.7-8.6, a carbonate hardness of 107-142 mg l^{-1} and a conductivity of 210-285 µS cm-1. The lake water is generally warm, having a surface temperature that ranges from 24-29°C and a deep level temperature of 22°C.

Lake Malaŵi National Park, a World Heritage site since 1984 and the World's first freshwater underwater park, is located on and around the Nankumba Peninsula. The park includes some islands, the separate Mwenya Hills, Nkhudzi Hills and Nkhudzi Point at the eastern base of the peninsula, and an aquatic zone extending 100 m offshore of all these areas. Its aim is to protect portions of Lake Malaŵi's aquatic communities so the steep hills immediately behind the shoreline are protected to prevent eroded sediments polluting the lake. A managed fishing zone is designated just offshore incorporating some islands within the park, but trawling is prohibited. Other fishing methods such as gill netting, long line, and trapping are prohibited within the 100m aquatic zone of the reserve.

Much of the lakeshore is heavily populated. Five shoreline villages, Chembe, Chimphamba, Mvunguti, Zambo and Chidzale, are included within enclaves in the park. As the soil of the peninsula is poor and crops fail about 50% of the time, local people are dependent on fishing for a livelihood. Some 40,000 people make a living directly from the lake in offshore fisheries, providing most of the country's animal protein intake.

2.1 Study sites

In the following we will refer to specific villages and these are briefly described below. On Nankumba Peninsula, detailed studies were done in 4 villages, i.e. Chembe, Chimphamba, Mvunguti, and Chirombo Bay.

Chembe is a fishing village with a population of roughly 8,000-10,000. Chembe (Fig. 3) is located on an open bay on the northern part of the Monkey Bay peninsula. It is well protected from the strong winds which blow in the southern and eastern sections of Lake

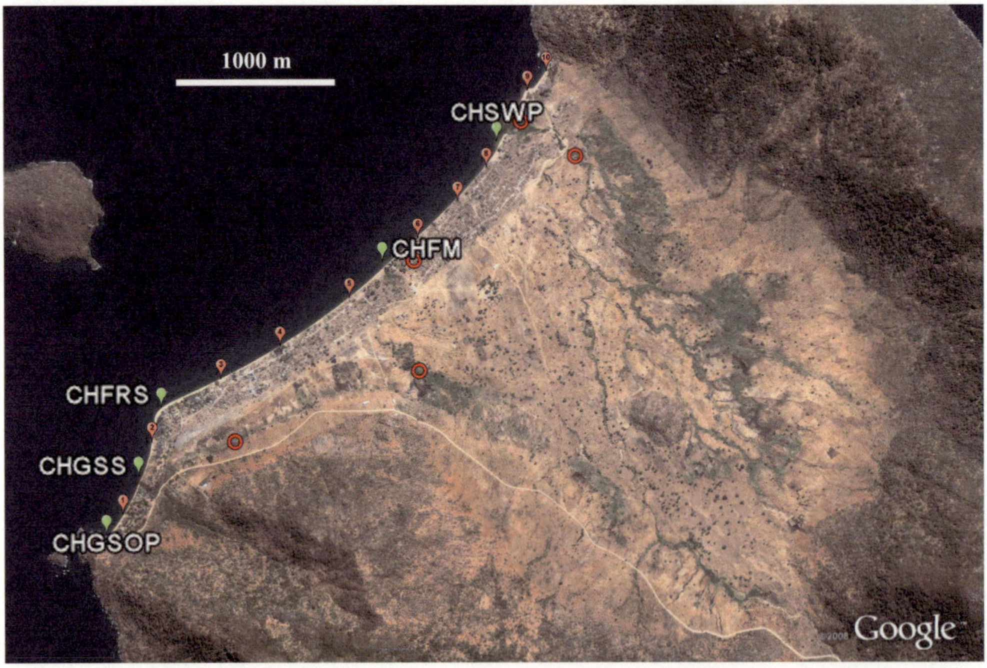

Fig. 3. Sampling sites in Chembe Village area. Green labeled symbols show transect sampling sites and red numbered symbols scooping sites. Red circles show inland sampling sites.

Malaŵi. People live primarily along an approximately 3000 m stretch of shoreline to a distance of about 250-300 m from the shore. The shoreline is facing northwest and the inland area is rather low and traversed by a number of streams and rivers, which are potential habitats for *Bulinus globosus*, an intermediate host for the urinary schistosome, *Schistosoma haematobium*. In the upland areas, some agricultural activities take place.

Chimphamba, with a population of about 2000 people, is located along an approximately 1.2 km shoreline facing southwest. The village area is surrounded by mountains and a few short streams cross the village area. To the south, there is a valley with one major in-flowing stream. The lake bottom outside the village is heavily polluted with various debris.

Mvunguti is located along an approximately 400 m sandy shoreline facing north and the village area extending up to about 300 m from the shore is surrounded by mountains. At each end of the village a small stream flows through the village area. Both streams are habitats for *B. globosus*. The lake bottom slopes steeply.

Chirombo Bay is located along an approximately 1700 m stretch of sandy shoreline facing east. Most people live along the southernmost 1000 m of this shoreline. The upland is flat and the lake bottom slopes gently, so the maximum depth sampled within 200 m from the shoreline was 4.5 m. Population density is not high. The upland areas contain a number of streams that can harbor *B. globosus*.

Kasankha is located along an approximately 1800 m stretch of sandy shoreline facing northwest. Houses are primarily found less than 400 m from the shoreline. The bottom slope is relatively gentle and the shoreline well protected. Close to the southern end of the beach, a river flows into the lake forming a swampy area, which is habitat for *B. globosus*. At the northern end of the beach, a small seasonal stream joins the lake. Crocodile and hippopotamuses are often seen in the bay and therefore this site was excluded from regular sampling. *Bulinus nyassanus* is abundant in the lake at this site.

Matola village is located along an open shoreline with gentle slope and the maximum depth that could be sampled within 200 m from shore was 4.5 m. *Bulinus nyassanus* was often found at high densities in relatively shallow water, but inland sites were not checked at this location. Also, *B. succinoides* was generally abundant in *Vallisneria* beds.

Finally, a number of sites were sampled along the Malaŵian shoreline in the northern part of the lake and most of these sites had relatively exposed sandy shorelines and generally density of *B. nyassanus* was low. Often inland sites, however, are important habitats for *B. globosus*. Some of these sites were close to the shore and kept flooded from wave action in the lake. Two sites were selected on the islands, i.e. Same Bay on Chizumulu Island and Yofu on Likoma Island. Same Bay is a protected bay with a stretch of sandy beach and a large area with very shallow water with stones and/or grass. Within this area, rice is cultivated and the area contains a dense population of *B. globosus*. The lake outside the sandy beach harbors *B. nyassanus* at relatively low density. Yofu is located along a sandy beach which is quite exposed to wave action.

Along the Tanzanian coast the lake bottom slopes very steeply at most sites and is therefore unsuitable for *Bulinus* snails. Only at Liuli did we find *B. nyassanus*. In one pool next to the lake, we found *Biomphalaria pfeifferi* infected with *Schistosoma mansoni*.

3. Schistosomiasis in people at Lake Malaŵi

Malaŵi is one of the countries where both urinary and intestinal schistosomiasis is endemic (Teesdale et al. 1986); around the lake, however, the urinary form caused by *S. haematobium* is dominant. Although schistosomiasis has been a major public health problem for many years in many lakeshore communities of Lake Malaŵi, there is evidence that transmission has increased in certain areas within the last 20 years (Stauffer et al. 2006). In addition to causing a major health problem for local people, the disease also affects an important source of income for the country, namely tourism. The area around Cape Maclear is a World Heritage Site and is visited by many tourists every year. Unfortunately, many visitors become infected with schistosomes and some health organizations such the United States Centers for Disease Control and Prevention (CDC) warn against visiting Lake Malaŵi (Centers for Disease Control, 2005).

On Nankumba Peninsula, in the southern part of the lake overall prevalence of *S. haematobium* infection in 1998/1999 ranged from 10.2% to 26.4% in inland villages and from 21.0% to 72.7% in lakeshore villages; for school children prevalence of infection ranged from 15.3% to 57.1% in inland schools and from 56.2% to 94.0% in lakeshore schools (see Madsen et al., in press). Inhabitants on the islands, Chizumulu and Likoma, also had lower prevalence of infection than those living in lakeshore villages on Nankumba Peninsula. This increased prevalence in lake shore villages is not necessarily linked to transmission taking place in the lake itself, but could also be due to the presence of more numerous typical transmission (back waters and inland sites such as streams, ponds) being close to the lake. Re-infection after treatment of school children in some villages, Chembe and Chimphamba) on Nankumba Peninsula is as high as 40% using parasitological examination, but using more sensitive serological tests reinfection rates are considerably higher (70%)(Madsen et al., in press).

3.1 Schistosome transmission

Two snail species are involved in transmission on the Nankumba Peninsula, i.e. *B. globosus* and *B. nyassanus*. *Bulinus globosus* (Morelet, 1866) is found in most of the sub-Saharan Africa in various freshwater habitats including streams, rivers, seasonal pools, and lakes (Brown, 1994; Mandahl-Barth, 1972; Cantrell, 1981; Madsen et al., 1987; Ndifon & Ukoli, 1989). *Bulinus nyassanus* (Smith, 1877) is a member of the *B. truncatus/tropicus* group and is endemic to Lake Malaŵi; it is found on open sandy areas and has a preference for habitats devoid of vegetation and with substratum consisting of coarse and, to a smaller extent, fine sand, where it is normally found in the upper 2-3 cm of the substratum (Wright et al., 1967; Phiri et al., 2001; Madsen et al., 2004). Its status as intermediate host was not recognized prior to these studies (Madsen et al., 2001) and an alternative explanation for the changed transmission pattern was that another strain of *S. haematobium,* capable of using *B. nyassanus* as host, had been introduced on Nankumba Peninsula. Molecular data, however, do not suggest existence of two *S. haematobium* strains and *S. haematobium* from Likoma Island can infect *B. nyassanus* from Nankumba (Stauffer et al., 2008).

Transmission in the lake takes place both in back waters and in the lake proper and also in further inland habitats. Transmission in inland sites and back waters is through *B. globosus* and starts towards the end of the rainy season or early dry season in March/April and continues until sites dry; which could be as early as June/ July or 1-2 months later (Madsen et al., in press). A few sites may, however, persist for longer but *B. globosus* populations often disappear before sites dry. Usually several of such sites exist in village areas at the lake shore and these clearly contribute to the higher infection levels in lake shore communities. Many of these inland water bodies (Fig. 4) are actually streams that after rains become isolated from the lake (Madsen et al., 2004). Inland transmission can be found throughout the lake's upland. Especially, in the northern part of the lake such sites may be kept under water due to wave action. Some of the inland sites may support *Biomphalaria pfeifferi* and *S. mansoni* transmission (Fig. 5).

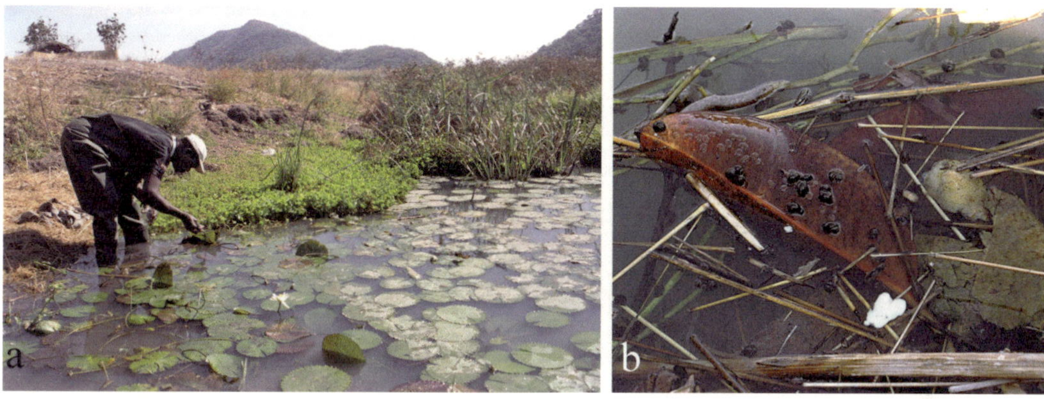

Fig. 4. Typical inland transmission site (a) with high density of *Bulinus globosus* (b).

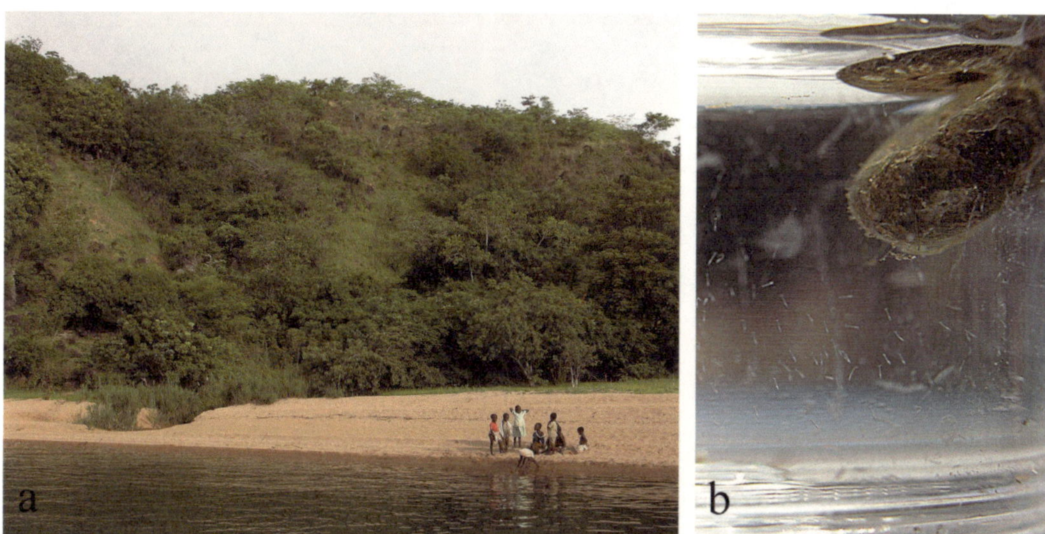

Fig. 5. A "stream" site (a) along the foothill harbouring *Biomphalaria pfeifferi* that shed cercariae of *Schistosoma mansoni* (b).

Transmission in the lake can be either by *B. globosus* along protected shorelines often with aquatic vegetation or presence of boulders in the water (Fig. 6) and/or through *B. nyassanus* along open sandy shorelines (Fig. 7) on the Nankumba peninsula (Madsen et al., 2004). Transmission by *B. globosus* within the lake or backwaters may commence towards the end of the rainy season or shortly after and may continue through October/November which is much longer than transmission in sites further inland (Madsen et al., in press). Transmission through *B. nyassanus* will start May/July when populations increase in shallow water and persist into November/December depending on weather conditions, i.e. storms coming

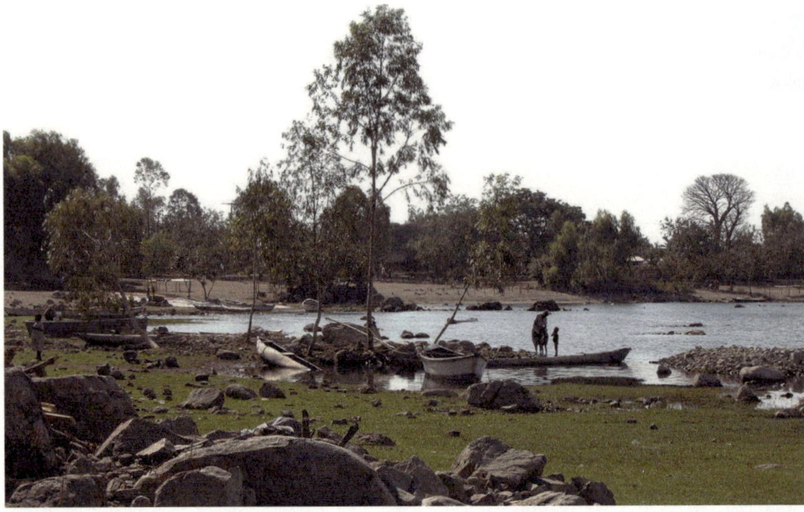

Fig. 6. Protected harbour site at Same Bay with transmission through *Bulinus globosus*.

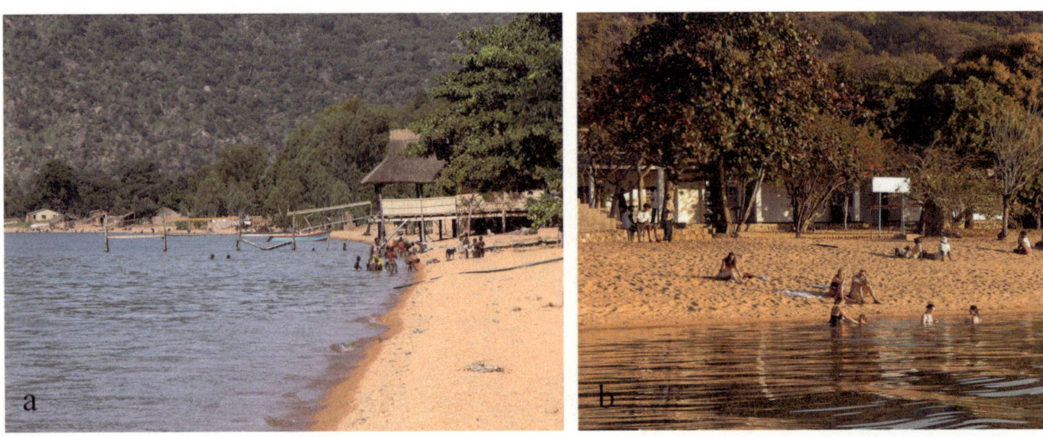

Fig. 7. Open beach at Chembe (a) where transmission of *Schistosoma haematobium* occurs with *Bulinus nyassanus* as intermediate host. This is the shoreline where many tourists (b) get infected.

from a northerly direction which can cause high mortality in *B. nyassanus* populations (Madsen et al., in press). *Schistosoma haematobium* transmission through *B. nyassanus* is limited to sites where snail occurs in shallow water close to shore. Infected *B. nyassanus* have been found only on Nankumba Peninsula. Density of *B. nyassanus* is generally higher in the southern part, especially in shallow water, of the Lake (Nankumba and Matola) than in the northern part. Density of *B. nyassanus* is partly governed by sediment composition (Genner & Michel, 2003; Madsen & Stauffer, in press) and further there is a negative association between density of *B. nyassanus* and density of *T. placodon* (Madsen & Stauffer, in press).

4. Snail fauna

Lake Malaŵi has an impressive snail fauna (Fig. 8), though the snail fauna is less diverse than Lake Tanganyika's (Brown, 1994). For many years, the molluscs of Lake Malaŵi continued to be known almost entirely from empty shells (Crowley et al., 1964). Later, collections of living specimens allowed substantial revision (Mandahl-Barth, 1972, Wright et al., 1967). A total of 28 gastropod species is recognized to live within the lake and on the swampy parts of its shores (Brown, 1994) of which 16 are endemic. Amongst these are the medically important species.

The prosobranch gastropods are dominated by *Melanoides* spp. (Oliver, 1804). Their shell is medium to large (max shell height 27 mm), slender and dextral. It is the most abundant snail genus in Lake Malaŵi and distinction between species is an ongoing debate (Eldblom & Kristensen, 2003; Sørensen et al., 2005). *Gabbiella stanleyi* (Smith, 1877) is a small (max size: 5.3 mm) snail with a thick-walled dextral shell and is endemic to Lake Malaŵi (Brown, 1994). Four species of *Lanistes* (Montfort, 1810) are found in Lake Malaŵi; they have a sinistral shell with a max height of 75 mm. *Lanistes nyassanus* (Dohrn, 1865) and *L. solidus* (Smith, 1877) are both endemic to Lake Malaŵi and found in shallow water and most common on sand among weedbeds (Louda et al., 1984; Brown, 1994). Several species *Bellamya* are known from Lake Malaŵi.

4.1 *Bulinus globosus*

Bulinus globosus (Morelet, 1866) belongs to the *Bulinus africanus* group and reaches a maximum of 22.5 mm in shell height (Brown, 1994). The globose shell has a blunted spire. *Bulinus globosus* is found in sub-Saharan Africa in various freshwater habitats including streams, rivers, seasonal pools, and lakes (Mandahl-Barth, 1972; Cantrell, 1981, Madsen et al., 1987, Ndifon & Ukoli, 1989). The snail lives in shallow water, where it may occur on bare substrata, but is more common among aquatic plants (Thomas & Tait, 1984). *Bulinus globosus* may be flushed into Lake Malaŵi during the rainy season, when lagoons and ponds adjacent to the lake overflow or are captured by the rising lake (Phiri et al., 2001). *Bulinus globosus* has been reported at several sites in Lake Malaŵi, especially in sheltered corners and near inflowing streams (Fryer, 1959; Madsen et al., 2004).

Bulinus globosus is the most widespread and probably the most important intermediate host for *Schistosoma haematobium* in Tropical Africa (Brown, 1994) and was until recently the only confirmed intermediate host for *Schistosoma haematobium* in Malaŵi (Teesdale et al., 1986, Brown, 1994, Msukwa & Ribbink, 1997). Stauffer et al. (1997) and Msukwa & Ribbink (1997) suggested that other *Bulinus* species, apart from *Bulinus globosus*, may also act as intermediate host for *S. haematobium*.

4.2 *Bulinus nyassanus*

Bulinus nyassanus (Smith, 1877) is a member of the *B. truncatus/tropicus* group and has a more thick-walled shell with a more pointed apex (barely projecting above the last whorl) compared to *B. globosus*. The maximum shell height of *B. nyassanus* is 13.6 mm (Brown, 1994). *Bulinus nyassanus* is endemic to Lake Malaŵi and is found on open sandy areas and has a preference for habitats devoid of vegetation and with substratum consisting of coarse and, to a smaller extent, fine sand, where it is normally found in the upper 2-3 cm of the substratum (Wright et al., 1967; Louda et al., 1983; Phiri et al., 2001; Madsen et al., 2004). *Bulinus succinoides* (Smith, 1877) is in the same group as *B. nyassanus* but smaller (maximum size: 6 mm), more slender, and with a thinner shell living upon *Vallisneria* plants (Wright et al., 1967; Brown 1994).

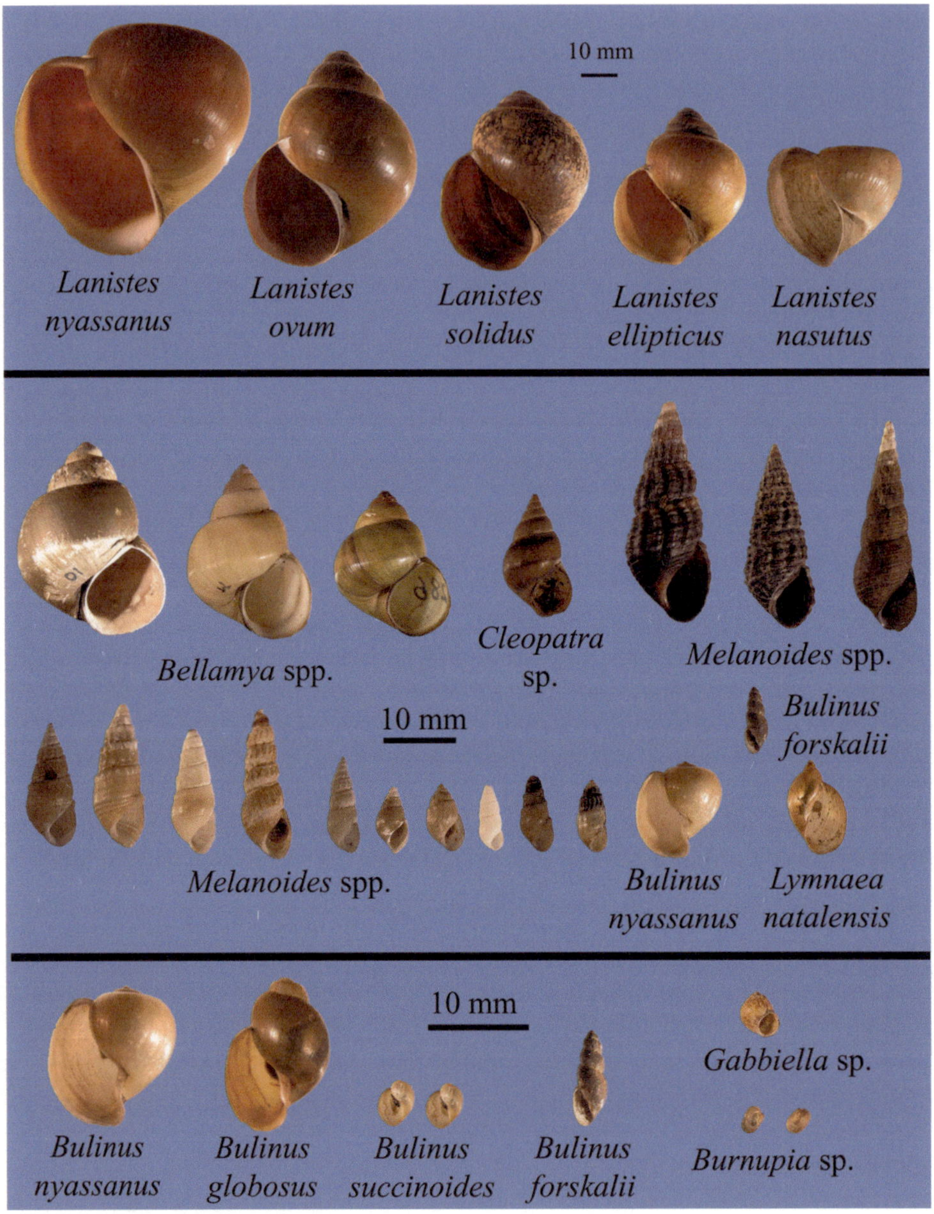

Fig. 8. Snail shells from Lake Malaŵi.

4.3 *Biomphalaria pfeifferi*

This genus comprises most of the larger planorbid snails in Africa and with a few exceptions these are of medical importance as intermediate hosts of *Schistosoma mansoni* (Danish Bilharziasis Laboratory, 1977). Eleven species are known from Africa and four of these are found in South-east Africa. The shell is discoid of medium size up 12-15 mm in diameter. Both in size and shell shape *Biomphalaria pfeifferi* (Fig. 9) is very variable and many local forms have been described as distinct species, but it is impossible to regard them even as subspecies. It is common throughout tropical Africa and the most important intermediate host of *S. mansoni*. In South-east Africa it is widely distributed, but rare or absent in the coastal area and in the great lakes.

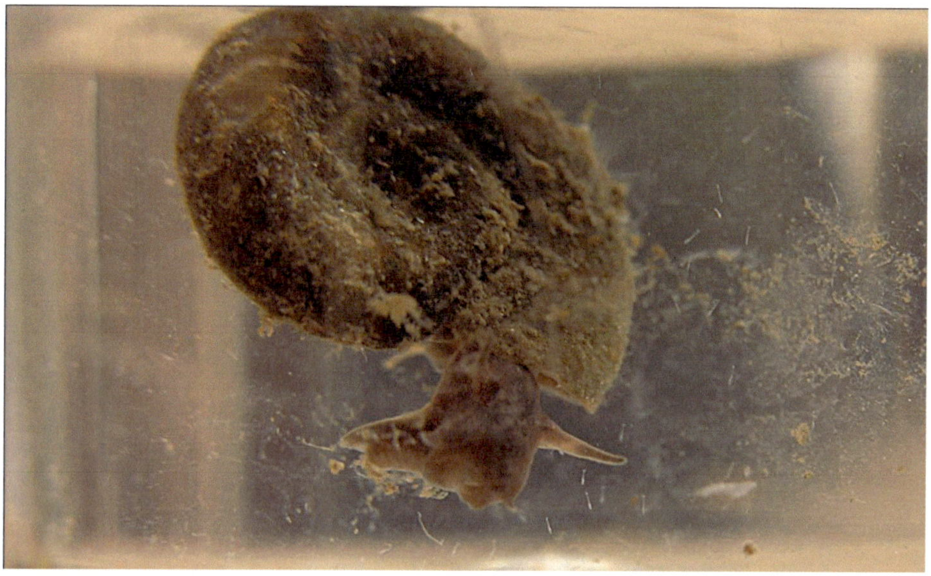

Fig. 9. *Biompalaria pfeifferi*

5. Fish and fishing in Lake Malaŵi

Lake Malaŵi harbors the most diverse ichthyofauna of any freshwater lake in the world, with as many as 850 species occurring (Konings, 2001). Lake Malaŵi cichlids exhibit spectacular diversity in trophic morphology, including specialist algal scrapers, planktivores, insectivores, piscivores, paedophages, snail crushers, and fin biters (Stauffer et al., 1995).

The rich fauna of this lake is primarily attributable to the explosive adaptive radiation and speciation of the haplochromine cichlids (Regan, 1922; Trewavas, 1935; Greenwood, 1979). As early as 1893, the diversity of the fishes inhabiting Lake Malaŵi was recognized by Günther (Eccles &Trewavas, 1989). Regan's (1922) revision of the fishes of Lake Malaŵi encouraged several collecting expeditions, which provided the material for Trewavas' (1935) classic synopsis of the fauna. The cichlids of Lake Malaŵi are characterized, in part, by both their inter- and intra-lake endemicity. The status of many of the groups described as genera, however, remain questionable as precise locality information is lacking for 32 of the 38 type species used to define these genera. In some cases, the validity of the type species of the genus is questioned. For example, the type species of *Ctenopharynx* is *Ctenopharynx intermedius* (Günther), and the type collection of *C. intermedius* consists only of the holotype, which is a relaxed skin with broken fins (Eccles & Trewavas, 1989). Surveys have been undertaken of the cichlids in Lake Malaŵi (Ribbink et al., 1983; Lewis et al., 1986; Konings, 1990; Turner 1996), and, although these surveys resulted in new facts and speculation of the different forms, they did not result in comprehensive and formal descriptions of new taxa. The rapid speciation within these fishes has resulted in a paucity of characters needed to distinguish among taxa. This dearth of information about unique characters is at odds with the need to be able to delimit species for the conservation and utilization of these fishes for food, tourism, disease control, and scientific investigations. Certainly, there is an inherent obligation for all the species in a World Heritage Site, such as Lake Malaŵi, to be documented and recognized.

5.1 Diversity of Lake Malaŵi cichlids

Cichlids are one of the most speciose families of vertebrates, with conservative estimates quoting more than 2000 extant species. Although native to tropical areas of the world, with the exception of Australia, some 70-80% of cichlids are found in Africa, with the greatest diversity found in the Great Lakes (lakes Victoria, Tanganyika, and Malaŵi). Their highly integrated pharyngeal jaw apparatus permits cichlids to transport and process food; thus enabling the mandibular jaws to develop specializations for acquiring a variety of food items. This distinct feature has allowed cichlids to achieve great trophic diversity, which in turn has lead to great species diversity.

By far, the greatest radiation of cichlids is found in the Great Lakes of Africa, with Lake Malaŵi alone having as many as 850 species. The phylogenetic diversity ranges from the single invasion of Lake Malaŵi, which resulted in the endemism of all but a few species, to multiple invasions in Lake Tanganyika, which resulted in the presence of 12 different tribes. The rich fauna of these lakes is primarily attributable to the explosive adaptive radiation and speciation of the pseudocrenilabrine cichlids. The driving mechanism for these speciation events is unknown. The two most widely proposed methods are allopatric speciation and intrinsic isolating mechanisms. Furthermore, biologists generally agree that female mate choice can act as a strong driving force in runaway speciation where the average female preference for a specific male trait differs between two allopatric populations. Thus, behavioral traits are important tools for the diagnosis of these African cichlids, primarily because behavioral traits played a very important role in and facilitated the rapid radiation of these fishes, which may not always be accompanied by discernable morphological changes. The importance of behavioral traits in delimiting the many species of Lake Malaŵi cichlids necessitates the use of SCUBA gear to document and record unique behaviors of the species being studied. In many cases, unique species can only be discerned by recording their different behaviors.

The driving mechanisms for the speciation events that led to the explosive radiation of the haplochromine cichlids in Lake Malaŵi is undiscovered; the two most widely proposed methods are allopatric speciation (Fryer & Iles, 1972) and intrinsic isolating mechanisms. Several authors (Lande, 1981, West-Eberhard, 1983) proposed that rapid divergence of mate recognition via sexual selection could promote behavioral isolation and facilitate speciation. Runaway sexual selection has been proposed to partially explain rapid radiation of these fishes and Deutsch (1997) provided evidence that sexual selection may be associated with the color diversification of the Lake Malaŵi rock-dwelling cichlids.

5.2 Fisheries in Lake Malaŵi

The traditional fishing methods on Lake Malaŵi consisted of traps and beach seines operated from dugout canoes and small plank boats (Cohen et al., 1996). Fishing was originally artisanal using small craft, open water seines (chirimila), and gillnets. The fisheries consisted of *Oreochromis* spp. (chambo), the catfishes especially *Bagrus meridionalis*, the small pelagic cyprinid *Engraulicypris sardella* and small zooplanktivorous cichlid species (utaka). *Labeo mesops* was the most important riverine fishery and was originally second only to the chambo fishery. Ringnets were introduced in 1943, initially for catching *Oreochromis* species, and later to catch small pelagic species such as *E. sardella* (usipa) and small, zooplanktivorous haplochromine cichlids (utaka) (Ogutu-Ohwayo et al., 1997). The cyprinid *L. mesops* which was the most important riverine species was, as in the case of the Lake Victoria *L. victorianus* (Ogutu-Ohwayo, 1990), depleted due to intensive gillnetting of gravid individuals on breeding migrations (Cohen et al., 1996).

The first fishery survey of Lake Malaŵi showed that the main commercial fisheries were supported by cichlid tilapia caught in shore seines and open water ringnets. Since then however, tilapia abundances have declined and the species of endemic tilapia are now so scarce that the main commercial fishery (Maldeco, which works in association for the Malaŵi fisheries department) has resorted to breeding tilapia in fish farm ponds to stock large enclosures fixed in open waters in the south east arm of the lake (Lowe-McConnell, 2009). Here they rear endemic tilapia *Oreochromis shiranus* (Lowe-McConnell, 2009).

Research into environmental conditions affecting fish production in Lake Malaŵi has included, for example, the work by Duponchelle et al. (2005) on food partitioning within the species-rich benthic fish community. Using a combination of stable isotopes and stomach analysis, they found that, although benthic algal production contributed to the energy requirement of offshore fishes living in water 10-30 m deep, the larvae of the abundant lake fly *Chaoborus edulis* were the most important food source for demersal fishes; thus supporting the hypothesis that demersal fish production in Lake Malaŵi is sustained mainly through the pelagic food chain, rather than from benthic detritus.

Systematic overfishing of fresh waters is largely unrecognized because of weak reporting and because fishery declines take place within a complex of other pressures (Allan et al., 2005). Indeed, one of the symptoms of intense fishing in inland waters is the collapse of particular stocks even as overall fish production rises--a biodiversity crisis more than a fisheries crisis (Allan et al., 2005).

The annual trawl catch for the entire lake has fluctuated between 1000 and 3000 tonnes over the last 40 years. The small-scale fisheries exploit an estimated 110 species, with 25 species comprising 80% of the total catch by weight (FAO, 1993; Turner, 1995; Turner et al., 1995; Weyl et al., 2005). There is, however cause for caution as surveys in southern Lake Malaŵi have shown considerable overlap between artisanal and trawl fisheries (Weyl et al., 2005) and there is evidence that the artisanal gill net fishery is now operating at depths greater than 50 m (Weyl et al., 2005).

In addition, degradation of the spawning grounds due to excessive siltation following deforestation and de-vegetation of the catchment area may have affected *L. mesops* (Cohen et al., 1996). An industrial trawl fishery which was introduced on Lake Malaŵi during the 1970's to harvest small cichlids (Turner, 1977), accelerated the decline in stocks of certain species in the lake. The size and the number of cichlid species caught was reduced by 20% in some parts of the lake.

5.3 Molluscivores

Several molluscivorous fish species exist in Lake Malaŵi and of these, *Trematocranus placodon* (Regan, 1922) is the most abundant and widely distributed (Fig. 10) and it has been considered the potentially most active biological control agent for schistosomiasis (Chiota et

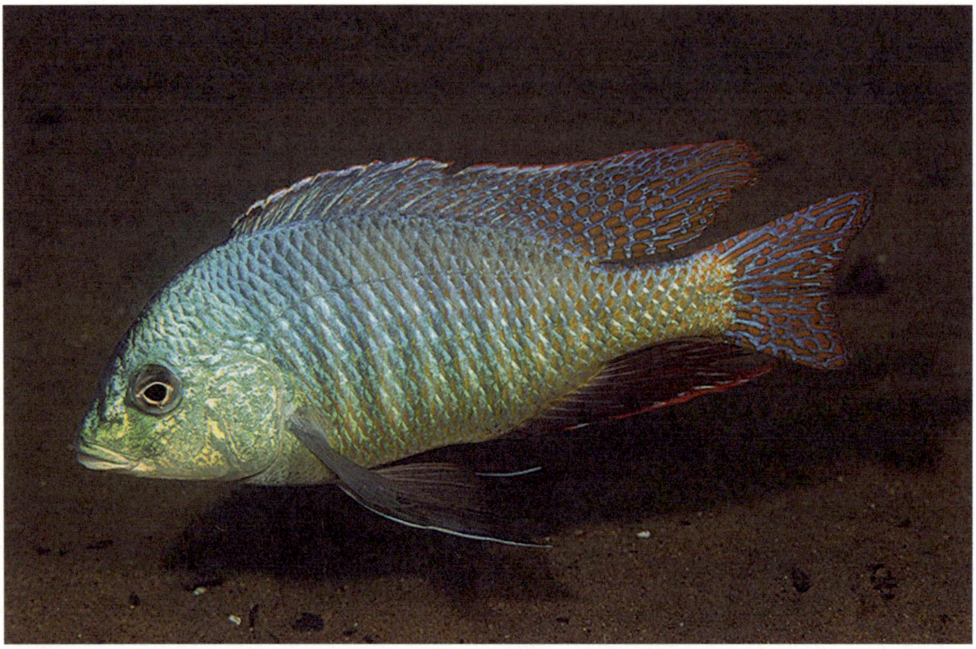

Fig. 10. *Trematocranus placodon* (Photo by Dr. Adrianus Konings).

al., 1991a,b; Msukwa & Ribbink, 1997). Since then, experiments have been conducted to understand its foraging behavior and impact on snail distribution in natural and semi-natural environments (Chiota et al., 1991a; Msukwa & Ribbink, 1997). *Trematocranus placodon* has earlier been described as *Haplochromis placodon*, *Cyrtocara placodon* and *Lethrinops placodon* (Regan, 1922;Fryer & Iles, 1972; Axelrod & Burgess 1979; Slootweg, 1994). *Trematocranus placodon* is placed in the endemic "Hap" species flock, compared to the endemic Malaŵian rock fishes or the "mbuna" flock (Fryer & Iles, 1972). The cichlid is widespread throughout the lake (Axelrod & Burgess, 1979) and it has three black spots on a silvery body and reaches a maximum total length of 23 cm (Konings, 2001). It is common in shallow waters on sandy bottoms where it forages mainly on gastropods. It exhibits sexual dimorphism during the breeding season from July to September, where the ripe male assumes a blue color, probably caused by hormones causing the chromatophores to expand (Fryer & Iles, 1972; Konings, 2001). *Trematocranus placodon* has a very well developed pharyngeal jaw apparatus including upper and lower pharyngeal bones and ingested snails are moved to the pharynx where they are crushed (Fryer & Iles, 1972). During the breeding season, the males are territorial, constructing bowers, which function as spawning sites. The females are mouth brooding (Konings, 2001). *Trematocranus placodon* possibly forage in groups, relying on group members to locate food (Chiota et al., 1991a); it feeds on benthic insects, detritus and fish scales before reaching maturity (at about 10 cm) where it almost exclusively feed on bivalves and gastropods (Msukwa & Ribbink, 1997). *Trematocranus placodon* locates snails in the sediment by their movements. When *T. placodon* detects a movement in the sediment via its enlarged pores on its chin, it attacks.

The molluscivorus fishes are particularly vulnerable to the artesian fishing gear when they are spawning or in shallow areas. We attribute the observed decrease in density of *Trematocranus placodon*, which is one of the most widespread snail-eating fish species, from

1980 to 2003 to overfishing and the increased use of fine-meshed beach seines that collect juvenile fishes. During the 1970s and early 1980s most fishing activity took place in offshore waters. As these fishing stocks became depleted, fishermen moved inshore with illegal fine-meshed nets. As these fishing pressures built, people started using beach seines and the fish in water less than 7 m were removed. The peak abundance of *T. placodon* then shifted to deeper waters where they were not susceptible to beach seines. We therefore concluded that we must encourage people from Chembe Village to consider a fish ban during certain times of the year in an effort to restore *T. placodon* to it former population levels in the shallow waters of Lake Malaŵi.

Trematocranus placodon feeds in preference on *B. nyassanus* although *Melanoides* species dominate in its stomach content. The proportion of large (>4 mm) *B. nyassanus* of all *B. nyassanus* consumed increased with fish size (Evers *et al.* 2006). *Bulinus nyassanus* seems to constitute a more profitable prey than *Melanoides* when evaluated on the basis of organic material gained relative to effort invested in shell crushing (Evers *et al.*, 2011).

Our data suggest a negative relationship between density of *T. placodon* and density of *B. nyassanus*, and of *Melanoides* spp., while there is a positive relationship between densities of the two snail species (Madsen & Stauffer, in press). Both snail species are the major elements in the diet of *T. placodon* and *B. nyassanus* appears to be the preferred species (Evers et al., 2006) especially during times of this snail's highest abundance in the field (Madsen et al., 2010).

6. Controlling *B. nyassanus* through protection of fishes at village areas

From the data, it is likely that prior to the mid 1980's, density of *B nyassanus* was kept low due to predation by *T. placodon*, i.e. biological control at work. Whether the changed distribution pattern of *T. placodon* is entirely the result of overfishing should be evaluated by following changes in fish and snail distribution after implementation of a fish-ban. Changes in fish populations may occur rapidly; when fish population density is high, beach-seining is attractive to the local people but after a period of intense beach seining fish population density will drop to levels where beach seining is no longer attractive. Subsequently, when beach seining is reduced fish populations will recover.

Because of the observed trend, we are optimistic about reversing the situation through an effective fish ban in village areas. Whether this would be sufficient to also reduce schistosome transmission remains to be seen. The intermediate host, *B. nyassanus*, undergoes marked seasonal variation in density in the very shallow water (i.e. water depth less than about 1.5 m) close to the shore. Each year in December-January, *B. nyassanus* is virtually eliminated from these depths at Chembe Village and possibly other shore lines with a northerly exposure owing to wave action. During this period, *B. nyassanus* populations, however, persist in deeper water, where the density fluctuations are much less pronounced than in the shallows. Populations of *B. nyassanus* in the shallow water will then increase again close to the shore as the prevailing wind direction shifts from a northerly to a southerly direction. At present, snails in the very shallow water close to the shore appear not to be vulnerable to predation from *T. placodon*, but if *T. placodon* could return to forage in shallow water through implementation of a fish ban, as in 1978 (Stauffer et al., 1997), the annual increase of *B. nyassanus* in shallow water might be prevented, because it must be recruited from snails living in slightly deeper waters. Certainly, this was the situation in the late 1970s, when the open waters of Lake Malaŵi were regarded as schistosome free.

It is interesting that also for *Melanoides* density there is a significant inverse relationship with density of *T. placodon*. Evers et al. (2006) showed that although *T. placodon* preferentially feeds on *B. nyassanus*, the major component in its stomach content is actually *Melanoides* due to its dominance in the snail fauna (94%-96% as opposed to the 3-5% for *B. nyassanus*). Evers et al. (2006) also showed that the maximum size (shell height) of *Melanoides* consumed by *T. placodon* of up to 230 mm (standard length) was about 15 mm. Larger *T. placodon* probably would be able to handle slightly larger snails, but it is likely that the largest *Melanoides* specimens are not susceptible to predation by *T. placodon*. Another interesting observation is that density of *B. nyassanus* is positively related to density of *Melanoides*, contrary to the prediction of Genner et al. (2004).

The only realistic possibility for reducing density of *B. nyassanus* and thereby hopefully *S. haematobium* transmission is to protect populations of *T. placodon* in the near-shore areas of the lake. Although the use of fish for biological control of freshwater snails has failed in some areas (Slootweg et al. 1994, Slootweg 1995), this should not happen in the case of *T. placodon* in Lake Malaŵi, because nothing really changes i.e. the food availability for the fishes does not change and due to interactions with other fish species that are also protected we would expect its feeding repertoire to remain unaltered. Attempts should be made through government extension workers to introduce a community enforced shallow water fishing ban. We assisted in forming a committee at Chembe that should be promoting such a fish-ban by educating community members on the need for practicing sustainable use of fish resources. The committee engaged local leaders, villagers as well as fishermen on the need for implementing a community enforced fish ban in the period during which fish should be allowed to breed. Initially the committee worked well but at the end of the project, there was evidence that it was no longer effective. Thus, there has been no estimation of fish population density after implementation of the fish ban.

7. Controlling *B. globosus* in back waters and inland sites

Even if *T. placodon* can control *B. nyassanus* and transmission along open shorelines, *S. haematobium* transmission will persist in inland habitats and other measures will have to be implemented in those areas. Many villages have several inland sites where *B. globosus* can exist – e.g., often streams that during the dry season turn into a series of ponds. Several of the inland sites may contain water through the dry season almost until the following rainy season, while many others just contain water for a few months into the dry season. Beach seining probably constitutes an important source of protein for local people and, if banned, many people may not afford to purchase fish from fishermen who catch outside the fish ban zone. We therefore think that, possibilities of utilizing these inland sites for aquaculture should be explored. Although aquaculture have well documented positive effects (e.g., improved nutrition, better food security, better job opportunities and financial benefits), there are also concerns that such activities may lead to increased transmission of various water related diseases because installations (canals and ponds) often function as excellent habitats for intermediate hosts of trematodes (notably schistosomes and liver flukes). Furthermore, cultured species should be from the local watershed due to the high risk of escape to the lake. Fish ponds would probably be organically loaded and this might favor proliferation of the intermediate host snails, i.e. *Bulinus globosus* and possibly *Biomphalaria pfeifferi*. Aquaculture using polyculture including molluscivore species might not control the intermediate host snails although Chiotha et al. (1991a, b) have demonstrated that a mix culture that included *T. placodon* significantly reduced intermediate hosts. Experience from Cameroon and elsewhere was not promising because soft food items might be abundant in inland waters and molluscivores might shift to such food items and this can lead to reduction in the crushing mill reduing their ability to crush snails. Slootweg et al. (1993) even warns against aquaculture in schistosomiasis endemic areas. It may be necessary to control access to the fish ponds such that they do not become transmission sites even if they sustain dense populations of intermediate host snails.

8. Conclusion

Fishes from Lake Malaŵi comprise most of the animal protein consumed by Malaŵians, thus fishing pressure on inshore fishes is intense. We attribute the observed decrease in density of *T. placodon* from 1980 to 2003 in the shallow waters to overfishing and the increased use of seine-meshed beach seines. It is obvious that the peak abundance of *T. placodon* has shifted to deeper waters when compared to observations in earlier years (Stauffer et al., 1997; Stauffer et al., 2006). Furthermore, as density of snail-eating fishes decreased the density of the intermediate host, *B. nyassanus*, increased.

There is no doubt, that *B. nyassanus* is a major player in the transmission of urinary schistosomes in Lake Malaŵi. In those areas where both *B. globosus* and *B. nyassanus* are intermediate hosts, the prevalence of infection in school-aged children is 2-3 times higher than where only *B. globosus* is a host (Stauffer et al., 2006; Stauffer et al. 2008). Relative to *B. nyassanus*, we found: (1) *Schistosoma haematobium* transmission through *B. nyassanus* is limited to sites where it occurs in shallow water close to shore; (2) Infected *B. nyassanus* have been found only on Nankumba Peninsula; (3) Density of *B. nyassanus* is generally higher in the southern part of the Lake (Nankumba and Matola) than in the northern part; and (4) Density of *B. nyassanus* is partly governed by sediment composition, i.e. particularly a high content of the clay fraction is a negative predictor.

Based on the above, we initially postulated that a different strain of *S. haematobium* was introduced into Lake Malaŵi that was preadapted to infect *B. nyassanus. Bulinus nyassanus* is a diploid member of the *Bulinus truncatus/tropicus* group. Most members of this group that are intermediate hosts are tetraploid, thus it was surprising that *B. nyassanus* was a player in transmission of urinary schistosomes in Lake Malaŵi. Stauffer et al. (2008) reported that the schistosomes found in *B. globosus* and *B. nyassanus* could not be genetically differentiated. Furthermore, they demonstrated that miracidia shed from children that originated from *B. globosus* could infect *B. nyassanus*. Thus, Stauffer et al. (2008) suggested that *S. haematobium* in Lake Malaŵi always had the potential to infect both *B. globosus* and *B. nyassanus*.

Finally, we concluded that if reductions in prevalence of schistosome infections in people are achieved through chemotherapy campaigns, we will need to protect native fish populations in near shore areas of the lake. The question is whether an effective prevention of fishing within a 100 m zone from the shore will restore fish populations and will this lead to reduced density of *B. nyassanus*, especially in the shallow waters. We have shown that a fish ban can be established and implemented, but it will require continued support from extension workers in the village. In order to reduce fishing pressure in the lake, we should consider creating alternative sources of fish protein and thereby reduce dependence on the natural fish populations.

9. Acknowledgment

We thank the government of Malaŵi for giving us permission to work in Lake Malaŵi and the University of Malaŵi for providing us with the proper permits to collect fishes and snails. For the parasitological studies on people, we would like to express our gratitude to the National Health Sciences Research Committee of the Ministry of Health for ethical clearance of the studies. We also thank the District Health Officers in the Mangochi and Likoma districts for their involvement and assistance in the implementation of the research. The work was conducted in collaboration with Malaŵi Fisheries Department and Malaŵi Parks and Wildlife Department. We are grateful for the help provided by Dr. Adrianus Konings and all our staff. Funding was provided by the NSF/NIH joint program in ecology of infectious diseases (DEB-0224958).

10. References

Allan, J. D.; Abell, R.; Hogan, Z.; Revenga, C.; Taylor, B. W.; Welcomme, R.L. & Winemiller, K. (2005). Overfishing of inland waters. *BioScience*, 55, 1041-1051

Axelrod, H.R. &Burgess, W.R. (1979). *African Cichlids of Lakes Malaŵi and Tanganyika.* 8th Edition. Tropical Fish Hobbyist Publications. Neptune, New Jersey

Beadle, L.C. (1974). *The inland waters of Tropical Africa. An introduction to tropical limnology.* Logham Group Ltd. 365 pp.

Brown, D.S. (1994). *Freshwater Snails of Africa and Their Medical Importance.* 2nd Edition. Taylor and Francis, London.

Cantrell, M. A. (1981). Bilharzia snails and water level fluctuations in a tropical swamp. *Oikos*, 36, 226-232

Centers for Disease Control. (2005). Health information for travelers to East Africa. Available: www.cdc.gov/travel/eafrica.gtm [accessed 12 May, 2005]

Chiotha, S.S.; McKaye, K.R. & Stauffer, J.R. (1991a). Prey handling in *Trematocranus placodon*, a snail-eating cichlid fish from Malaŵi. *Ichthyological Exploration of Freshwater*, 2, 203-208

Chiotha, S.S.; McKaye, K.R. & Stauffer, J.R. (1991b). Use of indigenous fishes to control schistosome snail vectors in Malaŵi, Africa. *Biological Control*, 1, 316-319

Cohen, A., Kaufman, L., & Oguto-Ohwayo, R. (1996). Anthropogenic threats, impacts, and conservation stragegies in the African Great Lakes - A review. In: *The Limnology, Climatology, and Paleoclimatology of the East African Lakes* (Editors: Johnson, T. & Odada, E.) Gordon & Breach Publishers, Newark, New Jersey, 575-624

Crowley, T. E., Pain, T. & Woodward, F.R. (1964). A monographic review of the Mollusca of Lake Nyasa. *Annales de la Musée royal de l'Afrique Centrale: Sciences Zoologiques*, 131, 1-58

Danish Bilharziasis Laboratory (1977). *A field guide to identification of African freshwater snails. 4: South East African species.* Danish Bilharziasis Laboratory

Deutsch, J.C. (1997). Colour diversification in Malaŵi cichlids: evidence for adaptation, reinforcement, or sexual selection? Biological Journal of the Linnean Society, 62,1-14

Duponchelle, F.; Ribbink, A. J.; Msukwa, A.; Mafuka, J.; Madere, D. & Bootsma, H. (2005). Food partitioning within the species-rich benthic fish community of Lake Malaŵi, East Africa. *Canadian Journal of Fisheries and Aquatic Sciences*, 62, 1651-1664

Eccles, D.H. & Trewavas, E. (1989). *Malaŵian cichlid fishes: The classification of some haplochromine genera.* Lake Fish Movies, Herten, West Germany

Eldblom, C. & Kristensen, T.K. (2003). A revision of the genus *Melanoides* (Gastropoda: Thiaridae) in Lake Malaŵi. *African Zoology*, 38, 357-369

Evans, A.C. (1975). *Report on visit to Malaŵi, 19th-31st May 1975: Investigations into schistosomiasis potential in and around lake-shore resorts and other tourist sites, with suggestions and recommendations*. Report to Ministry of Trade, Industry, and Tourism

Evers, B.N. ; Madsen, H.; McKaye, K.R. & Stauffer, J.R., Jr. (2006). The schistosome intermediate host, *Bulinus nyassanus*, is a preferred food for the cichlid fish, *Trematocranus placodon*, at Cape Maclear, Lake Malaŵi. *Annals of Tropical Medicine*, 100, 75-85

Evers, B.N.; Madsen, H. & Stauffer, J.R., Jr. (2011). Crush-resistance of soft-sediment gastropods of Lake Malaŵi: Implications for prey selection by molluscivorous fishes. *Journal of Freshwater Ecology*, 26, 85–90

Food and Agriculture Organization. (1993). Fisheries management in south-east Lake Malaŵi, the Upper Shire River and Lake Malombe. CIFA Technical Paper 17. 106 pp. FAO, Rome

Fryer, G. (1959). The trophic interrelationships and ecology of some littoral communities of Lake Nyasa with especial reference to the fishes, and a discussion of the evolution of a group of rock-frequenting Cichlidae. *Proceedings of the Zoological Society of London*, 132, 153–281

Fryer, G. & Iles, T. D. (1972). *The Cichlid Fishes of the Great Lakes of Africa*. Tropical Fish Hobbyist Publications. Neptune, New Jersey

Genner, M.J. & Michel, E. (2003). Fine-scale habitat associations of soft-sediment gastropods at Cape Maclear, Lake Malaŵi. *Journal of Molluscan Studies*, 69, 325–328

Genner, M.J.; Michel, E.; Erpenbeck, D.; De Voogd, N.; Witte, F. & Pointier, J.-P. (2004). Camouflaged invasion of Lake Malaŵi by an Oriental gastropod. *Molecular Ecology*, 13, 2135–2141

Greenwood, P.H. (1979). Towards a phyletic classification of the 'genus' Haplochromis (Pisces: Cichlidae) and related taxa. Part 1. *Bulletin of the British Museum (Natural History) Zoology*, 35, 265-322

Konings A. F. (1990). *Book of Cichlids and All Other Fishes of Lake Malaŵi*. Tropical Fish Hobbyists Publications. Neptune, New Jersey

Konings, A. F. (2001). *Malaŵi cichlids in their natural habitat*. (3rd edition). Cichlid Press. El Paso. USA.

Lande, R. (1981). Models of speciation by sexual selection on polygenic traits. *Proceedings of the National Academy of Sciences*, 78, 3721-3725

Lewis, D.; Reinthal, P. & Tremdall, J. (1986). *A Guide to the Fishes of Lake Malaŵi National Park*. World Conservations Centre. Gland, Switzerland

Louda, S.M.; Gray, W.N.; McKaye, K.R. & Mhone, O.J. (1983). Distribution of gastropod genera over a vertical depth gradient at Cape Maclear, Lake Malaŵi. *The Veliger*, 25, 387-392.

Louda, S.M.; McKaye, K.R.; Kocher, T.D. & Stackhouse, C.J. (1984). Activity, density and size of *Lanistes nyassanus* and *L. solidus* (Gastropoda, Ampullaridae) over the depth gradient at Cape Maclear, Lake Malaŵi, Africa. *The Veliger*, 25, 145-152

Lowe-McConnell, R. (2009). Fisheries and Cichlid Evolution in the African Great Lakes: Progress and Problems. *Freshwater Reviews*, 2, 131-151

Madsen, H.; Bloch, P.; Kristensen, T.K. & Furu. P. (2001). *Bulinus nyassanus* is intermediate host for *Schistosoma haematobium* in Lake Malaŵi. *Annals of Tropical Medicine and Hygiene*, 95, 353-360

Madsen, H.; Bloch, P.; Makaula, P.; Phiri, H.; Furu, P. & Stauffer, J.R. Jr. (in press). Schistosomiasis in Lake Malaŵi villages. *EcoHealth*

Madsen, H.; Coulibaly, G. & Furu, P. (1987). Distribution of freshwater snails in the river Niger basin in Mali with special reference to the intermediate hosts of schistosomes. *Hydrobiologia*, 146, 77-88

Madsen, H. & Stauffer, J.R. Jr. (in press). Density of *Trematocranus placodon* (Pisces: Cichlidae): A predictor of density of the schistosome intermediate host, *Bulinus nyassanus* (Gastropoda: Planorbidae), in Lake Malaŵi. EcoHealth

Madsen, H.; Stauffer, J.R., Jr.; Bloch, P.; Konings, A.; McKaye, K.R. & Likongwe, J.S. (2004). Schistosomiasis transmission in Lake Malaŵi. *African Journal of Aquatic Science*, 29, 117-119

Madsen, H., Kamanga, K.C.J., Stauffer, J.R. Jr. & Likongwe, J. (2010). Biology of the molluscivorous fish *Trematocranus placodon* (Pisces: Cichlidae) from Lake Malaŵi. *Joumal of Freshwater Ecology*, 25, 449-454

Mandahl-Barth, G. (1972). The freshwater mollusca of Lake Malaŵi. *Revue de zoologie et de botanique Africaines*, 86, 257-289

Msukwa, A.V. & Ribbink, A.J. (1997). The potential role of sanctuary areas for biological control of schistosomiasis in Lake Malaŵi national park. In: Proceedings of "Workshop on Medical Malacology in Africa", Harare, Zimbabwe, Sep. 22- 26 (Eds. Madsen, H., Appleton C.C. & Chimbari, M.) p.305- 317

Ndifon, G.T. & Ukoli, F.M.A. (1989). Ecology of freshwater snails in south-western Nigeria. I: Distribution and habitat preferences. *Hydrobiologia*, 171, 231-253

Ogutu- Ohwayo, R. (1990). The decline of the native fishes of Lakes Victoria and Kyhoga (East Africa) and the impact of introduced species, especially the Nile perch, *Lates niloticus* and Nile tilapia, *Oreochromis niloticus*. *Environmental Biology of Fishes*, 27, 81-96

Ogutu- Ohwayo, R.; Hecky, R.E.; Cohen, A.S. & Kaufman, L. (1997). Human impacts of the African Great Lakes. *Environmental Biology of Fishes*, 50, 117-131

Phiri, H., Bloch, P. Madsen, H. & Dudley, C. (2001). Distribution and population dynamics of *Bulinus globosus* and *B. nyassanus* on Nankumba Peninsula, Mangochi District, Malaŵi. Preliminary findings. In: Proceedings of "Workshop on Medical and Veterinary Malacology in Africa", Harare, Zimbabwe, Nov. 8-12, (Eds. Madsen, H., Appleton C.C. & Chimbari, M.) p. 273-286.

Regan, C.T. (1922). The cichlid fishes of Lake Nyassa. *Proceedings of the Zoological Society of London*, 1921, 675–727.

Ribbink, A.J.; Marsh, B.A.; Marsh, A.C.; Ribbink, A.C. & Sharp, B.J. (1983). A preliminary survey of the cichlid fishes of rocky habitats in Lake Malaŵi. *South African Journal of Zoology*, 18, 149-310.

Slootweg, R. (1994). *A multidisciplinary approach to schistosomiasis control in Northern Cameroon with special reference to the role of fish in snail control.* ICG Printing Dortrech. DSc thesis. University of Leiden. The Netherlands

Slootweg, R. (1995). Snail control by fish: an explanation for its failure. *NAGA, The ICLARM Quarterly*, 16-19.

Slootweg, R.; Malek, E.A. & McCullough, F.S. (1994). The biological control of snail intermediate hosts of schistosomiasis by fish. *Reviews in Fish Biology and Fisheries*, 4, 67-90

Slootweg, R.; Vroeg, P. & Wiersma, S. (1993). The effects of molluscivorous fish, water quality and pond management on the development of schistosomiasis vector snails in aquaculture ponds in North Cameroon. *Aquaculture and Fisheries Management*, 24, 123-128

Stauffer, J.R.; Arnegard, M.E.; Cetron, M.; Sullivan, J.J.; Chtsulo, L.A.; Turner, G.F.; Chiotha, S. & McKaye, K.R. (1997). Controlling Vectors and hosts of parasitic diseases using fishes. A case history of schistosomiasis in Lake Malaŵi. *BioScience*, 47, 41-49

Stauffer, J. R., Jr.; Bowers, N.J.; McKaye, K.R. & Kocher, T.D. (1995). Evolutionarily significant units among cichlid fishes: The role of behavioral studies. *American Fisheries Society Symposium*, 17, 227-244

Stauffer, J.R. Jr.; Madsen, H.; McKaye, K.; Konings, A.; Bloch, P.; Ferreri, C.P.; Likongwe, J. & Makaula, P. (2006). Molluscivorous Fishes - Potential for Biological Control of Schistosomiasis. *EcoHealth*, 3, 22-27

Stauffer, J. R., Jr.; Madsen, H.; Konings, A.; Bloch, P.; Ferreri, C.P.; Likongwe, J.; Black, K. & McKaye, K.R. (2007). Taxonomy: A precursor to understanding ecological interactions among schistosomes, snail hosts, and snail-eating fishes. *Transactions of the American Fisheries Society*, 136, 1136-1145

Stauffer, J. R., Jr.; Madsen, H.; Webster, B.; Black, K.; Rollinson, D. &Konings A. (2008). *Schistosoma haematobium*in Lake Malaŵi: snail hosts (*Bulinus globosus, Bulinus nyassanus*) susceptibility and molecular diversity. *Journal of Helminthology*,82, 377-382

Sørensen, L. V.G., Jorgensen, A. & Kristensen, T. K. 2005. Molecular diversity and phylogenetic relationships of the gastropod genus *Melanoides* in Lake Malaŵi. *African Zoology*, 40, 179-191

Teesdale, C.H.; Choudhry, A.W.; Pugh, R.N.; Ellison, R.N. & Alford, D.P. (1986). *Bilharzia – A manual for health workers in Malaŵi National Bilharzia Control Programme*. Ministry of Health, Malaŵi

Thomas, J.D. & Tait, A.I. (1984). Control of the snail hosts of schistosomiasis by environmental manipulation: a field and laboratory appraisal in the Ibadan area, Nigeria. *Philosophical Transactions of the Royal Society, London*, B, 305, 201-254

Turner, G. F. (1995). Management, conservation and species changes of exploited fish stocks in Lake Malaŵi. In: *The Impact of Species Changes in African Lakes*. (Editors: Pitcher, T. J. & Hart, P. J. B.) 365-397

Turner G.W.; Tweddle, D. & Makwinja, R. D. (1995). Changes in demersal cichlid communities as a result of trawling in southern Lake Malaŵi. In: *The Impact of Species Changes in AFrican Lakes* (Editors: Pitcher, T. J. & Hart, P. J. B.) 339-412

Turner, G.R. (1996). *Offshore Cichlieds of Lake Malaŵi*. Cichlid Press, El Paso, Texas.

Turner, J.L. (1977). Some effects of demersal traŵling in Lake Malaŵi (Lake Nyasa) from 1968 to 1974. *Journal of Fish Biology*, 10, 261-271

Trewavas, E. (1935). A synopsis of the cichlid fishes of Lake Nyassa. *Annals and Magazine of Natural History, ser. 10,* Vol.16, 65–118

West-Eberhard, M.J. (1983). Sexual selection, social competition, and speciation. *Quarterly Review of Biology*, 58, 155-183

Weyl, O.L.F.; Nyasula, T., & Rusuwa, B. 2005). Assessment of catch, effort, and species changes in the pair trawl fishery of southern Lake Malaŵi, Malaŵi, Africa. *Fisheries Management and Ecology*, 12, 395-402

World Health Organization (2002). Prevention and control of schistosomiasis and soil transmitted helminthiasis: Report of a WHO expert committee. World Health Organization, Technical Report Series 912

Wright, C.A., Klein, J. & Eccles, D.H. (1967). Endemic species of *Bulinus* in Lake Malaŵi. *Journal of Zoology, London*, 151, 199-209

Part 4

Clinical Manifestations

7

Schistosomasis and Bladder Cancer

Saad S. Eissa, M. Nabil El-Bolkainy and Mohab S. Eissa
Department of pathology, National Cancer Institute, Cairo University
Egypt

1. Introduction

Schistosomiasis also known as *Bilharziasis,* is a parasitic disease that dates back to antiquity. The ancient Egyptians, through settling and cultivating the Nile valley, were among the first to contract the disease. Thus, the main symptom hematuria was mentioned in Egyptian papyri (1500-1800 B.C.), and schistosome eggs were identified in Egyptian mummies through paleopathologic studies. In 1852, Theodor Bilharz, a German pathologist working in Cairo, discovered the worms in the portal circulation and was the first to describe the Pathology of the disease. Ferguson in 1911 was the first to report on the high frequency of bladder cancer in Egypt and to suggest an etiologic relation with urinary *Schistosomiasis,* a fact which is now generally accepted (Bolkainy & Chu 1981a). The aim of this article is to review the pathobiology of *Schistosoma* associated bladder cancer (SACB), describe the relationship between *Schistiosomiasis* and bladder cancer with respect to the mechanisms of carcinogenesis with emphasis on special features of SABC and recent methods of early detection.

2. Incidence and risk factors

An estimated 386,300 new cases and 150,200 deaths from bladder cancer occurred in 2008 worldwide (Jemal et al.,2011). The majority of bladder cancer occurs in males and there is a 14-fold variation in incidence internationally. The highest incidence rates are found in the countries of Europe, North America, and Northern Africa. Egyptian males have the highest mortality rates (16.3 per 100,000), which is twice as high as the highest rates in Europe (8.3 in Spain and 8.0 in Poland) and over 4 times higher than that in the United States (Ferlay et al., 2010) Smoking and occupational exposures are the major risk factors in Western countries, whereas chronic infection with *Schistosoma hematobium* in developing countries, particularly in Africa and the Middle East, accounts for about 50% of the total burden.(Parkin,2006) A majority of bladder cancers associated with *schistosomiasis* are squamous cell carcinoma, (SCC) while those associated with smoking are transitional cell carcinoma (TCC) (Sliverman et al.,2006).In the United States, mortality rates have stabilized in males and decreased in females from 1997 through 2006, (Edwards et al.2010) and in Europe declines have been observed in most countries since the 1990s, (Karim-Kos et al.,2008) due in part to reductions in smoking prevalence and reductions in occupational exposures known to cause bladder cancer. Bladder cancer continues to be the most common cancer among males in Egypt (Ferlay et al.2010), despite the large decreases in schistosomiasis.This is likely the result of a reduction in *schistosoma*-related bladder cancers being offset by an increase in tobacco-related bladder cancers.(Althuis et al., 2005). The association with *Schistosomiasis* determines a distinct clinico-pathologic entity quite different from that experienced in the Western world. It is commonly a well-differentiated SCC (80 %) with a limited tendency to lymphatic and blood stream metastasis despite the locally advanced stage of tumors in the majority of patients. Compared with Western series the tumors are multiple in 22% of cases and are frequently associated with atypical epithelial changes in the rest of the urothelium. SABC was encountered at an earlier age in patients with schistosome eggs in the specimens. About 95% of cases are muscle invasive at the time of presentation and, in absence of effective systemic therapy, these cases are often fatal. In fact, until recently, SABC has been the most common cause of death among men age 20- 44 years (Freedman et al.,2006). *Schistosomiasis,* is now a widespread endemic disease currently found in 75 countries. In the Nile Delta area, mixed infection with S. haematobium and *S. mansoni* is endemic, while *S. haematobium* is more prevalent in Upper Egypt due to the greater abundance of the specific intermediate host snails in that area. In *schistosomiasis* due to *S. haematobium*, the intensity of infection is correlated with morbidity, the degree of hematuria and proteinuria, and the pathological changes observed in the urinary bladder and ureters and malignancies of the bladder. The evidence associating *S. haematobium* infection with the development of bladder cancer is, however, far greater than that for any other parasitic infection; it has been supported by several major studies in countries in Africa and the Middle East (Moustafa et al.,1999). Cigarette smoking is now recognized as a major cause of bladder cancer in developed countries, increasing the risk two to three fold in North America and Europe and accounting for 50% of these cancers in males and 25% in females. Although much less information is available from developing countries, a recent study in Egypt indicated that smoking was strongly associated with bladder cancer in males and could account, at least in part, for 75% of these cancers (Freedman et al.,2006). Other risk factors includes certain organic chemicals - particularly aromatic (aryl)-amines such as naphthalene, benzidine, aniline dyes, and 4-aminobiphenyl - are known bladder carcinogens and have helped identify high-risk occupations, including petroleum chemical/rubber workers, hairdressers, painters, textile workers, truck drivers, and aluminum electroplaters. Bladder cancer may also result from pelvic radiotherapy, phenacetin use, and cyclophosphamide exposure, resulting in a four- to five-fold relative risk increase, particularly when exposure is in a chronic low-dose form (Ibrahim & Khaled,2006).

3. Evidence supporting the relationship between schistosomiasis and bladder cancer

3.1 Epidemiological evidence

The association of bladder cancer with *schistosomiasis* seems to be related to the endemicity of the parasite. Urinary *Schistosomiasis* is endemic throughout most of Africa, the Middle East, Madagascar, Reunion, Mauritius and India. In Africa, a high frequency is reported in countries along river Nile such as Egypt and Sudan, as well as, countries around lake Victoria as Kenya and Uganda. The disease is also prevalent in the west of the continent (Gold Coast and Senegal) and the eastern side of the continent below the Equator (Mozambique, Zambia and New Guinea) (Moustafa,et al.,1999). In the Middle East, it occurs in Iraq, Iran, Syria, Saudi Arabia and Yemen (Al-Saleem et al.,1990, Al-Shukri et al.,1987, Elem, & Purohit,1983).The consensus of available information strongly implicates an association between *S. haematobium* infection and the induction of bladder cancer. In Egypt, bladder cancer has been the most common cancer during the past 50 years. In 2002, Egypt's World-standardized bladder cancer incidence was 37/ 100,000, representing approximately 30,000 new cases each year(Parkin et al.,2005). Interestingly, the most common histopathological type of bladder cancer in Egypt has been SCC, constituting from 59% to 81% of reported bladder cancers between 1960 and 1980 (El-Mawla et al.,2001). Contrary to the leading etiology of smoking and occupational exposures in Western countries, chronic bladder infection with *Schistosoma haematobium,* the nematode causing urinary schistosomiasis, has been the most important risk factor for bladder cancer in Egypt (Moustafa et al.1999) This neoplasm accounts for 30.8% of the total cancer incidence and is ranked first among all types of cancer recorded in Egyptian males and second only to breast cancer in females (Mokhar et al.,2007). Changes in exposures linked to bladder cancer have occurred recently in Egypt. Prior to the 1964 completion of the Aswan High Dam, approximately 60%of people in North and South Egypt were infected with S. haematobium; a similar proportion was infected with *S. mansoni* (causing intestinal disease) in North Egypt, but rarely seen in southern parts of the country(El-Khoby et al.,2000). The dam appears to be responsible for a gradual replacement of *S. haematobium* by *S. mansoni* in North Egypt, and *S. mansoni* has expanded into southern regions (Felix et al.,2008). Another change in bladder cancer risk involves rising cigarette smoking in Egypt, which is now 32% among males (but only 7% among females) (WHO, 2000). In other countries, such as Iraq, Malawi, Zambia and Kuwait, where the endemicity of *schistosomiasis* due to either mixed or *S. haematobium* infestations is high, bladder cancer was also reported to be the leading cancer (Felix et al.,2008). In contrast, in *schistosome*-free countries bladder carcinoma ranks from the 5th to the 7th most common cancer in men and from the 7th to the 14th in women (Moustafa et al. 1999). With the reduction in *schistosomiasis* due to control efforts over the past 30–40 years, the epidemiology of bladder cancer in Egypt has shifted dramatically. This is exemplified by a recent study from Gouda et al (2007) in which they reviewed 9843 patients treated for bladder cancer by Egypt's National Cancer Institute (NCI) in Cairo between 1970 and 2007. The authors identified a dramatic decline in the proportion of patients with bladder cancer who had *schistosoma* ova on pathological evaluation (82.4% vs 55.3%) and in the proportion of patients treated for bladder cancer (from 27.6% of patients treated for cancer to 11.7%). They also describe an increase in the median age at presentation (from 47.4 years to 60.5 years), a decrease in the male to female ratio (from 5.4 to 3.3) and a decrease in the proportion of patients with SCC histology (from 75.9% to 33.0%). A similarly designed study from the Egyptian NCI in Cairo showed that patients treated for bladder cancer in 2005 had a six-fold increased risk of TCC of the bladder (vs SCC) compared with patients treated in 1980 (Felix et al.,2008) They also evaluated the incidence of SABC at several other institutions in Egypt during this period and showed no rise in incidence at other institutions as the incidence decreased at the NCI. Furthermore, these epidemiological trends have also been documented in the Egyptian nation-wide tumor registries (Salem et al., 2000, Freedman et al., 2006). The increase in frequency of TCC and decrease in frequency of SCC relative to previous reports indicate a transition phase from the SABC to the Western type of bladder cancer related to smoking, exposure to occupational and agricultural related chemicals. (Ibrahim & Khaled, 2006)

3.2 Experimentally induced schistiosomiasis

Several attempts were made to evaluate the carcinogenic potential of experimentally induced schistosomiasis. It has been suggested that chronic tissue injury could provide a promoting factor which acts to increase the rate of cell turnover via the induction of restorative hyperplasia and squamous metaplasia. Most of this focal hyperplasia is subsequently reversible However, in some situations, hyperplasia and dysplasia may become irreversible, particularly during concomitant exposure to low (sub-carcinogenic) doses of carcinogens e.g., N-nitroso compounds (Hicks,.et al., 1980).

3.2.1 Inflammatory cells

Schistosomiasis induces chronic irritation and inflammation in the urinary bladder, and this could facilitate changes in at least two stages of the development of the disease: first, initiation of premalignant lesions, and second, action as a promoting agent to increase the likelihood of the conversion of these lesions to the malignant state. At the stage of initiation, activated macrophages induced at the sites of inflammation are implicated in the generation of carcinogenic N-nitrosamines (NNA)and reactive oxygen radicals (Moustafa et al., 1994) that lead to DNA damage and subsequently to events such as mutations, DNA strand breaks, and sister chromatid exchanges. Inflammatory cells have also been shown to participate in the activation of other bladder carcinogens such as the aromatic amines (Badawi et al., 1992, 1995a).

3.2.2 Bacterial infections

Various species of bacteria including nitrate –reducing bacteria have been found in greater numbers in the urine of patients with *schistosomiasis* than in the urine of uninfected patients (Mostafa et al.1994). These higher levels of infection probably result from the tissue damage caused in various parts of the urinary tract by the egg-laying activities of the worms (Lehman et al.,1973, Falagas et al.2010). Injury to the urothelium from the passing eggs and/or bacterial infection might decrease the effectiveness of the mucosal barrier to reabsorb carcinogens in urine. Several of these bacterial species can mediate the N-nitrosation of amines, thereby providing a source of carcinogenic NNA in addition to those from exogenous sources (EL-Merzabani et al.,1979, Moustafa 1999).

3.2.3 N-Nitrosamines

Attention has focused on nitrite and N-nitroso compounds (NNCs).(Badawi et al.1995a) NNCs can be formed endogenously following the secondary infection by nitrate-reducing bacteria that invariably accompany schistosomal cystitis. NNCs, including nitrosamines and the direct-acting nitrosamides, are carcinogenic, inducing tumorigenic alkylation of specific bases and DNA sequences(O'Brien et al., 1988, Badawi et al.,1993,1994). Evidence of the interaction of carcinogens, with the genetic material of the bladder has been obtained by analyzing bladder mucosal DNA for the presence of mutations (Marletta,1988,Badawi et al.,1995b). Mutations have been observed in oncogenes, tumor suppressor genes, and genes associated with cell cycle control. In particular, mutations in the tumor suppressor gene p53 have been observed more frequently in patients with SABC than in patients with non-SABC(Badawi 1996). Changes in these and other genes and in microsatellite DNA, presumably arising as a result of carcinogenic insults, may lead to greater genetic instability and hence to the malignant transformation (Yamamoto, et al., 1997). Genomic DNA hypomethylation has been recently suggested as biomarker for to identify individuals who are more susceptible to the development of bladder cancer (Theodorescu 2003) Moreover, Inflammatory cells also participate in the activation of procarcinogens, such as aromatic amines and polycyclic aromatic hydrocarbons, to their ultimate carcinogenic metabolites (i.e., the final reactive form of the carcinogen) (Badawi et al.,1993). Since the aromatic amines are an important group of bladder carcinogens, an increased number of inflammatory cells in the urinary bladder of *schistosomal* patients may enhance the carcinogenic potential of these agents by increasing their rate of activation (Moustafa et al., 1994).

3.2.4 Cigarette smoking

Tobacco use is a well-documented risk factor for developing bladder cancer, but specific carcinogen(s) and molecular pathway(s) have not been elucidated. Much interest has focused on aromatic amines such as 4-aminobiphenyl (ABP) because they are found not only in cigarette smoke but also in several industrial chemicals. One potential mechanism by which amines cause carcinogenesis is by forming DNA adducts that result in transitional mutations(Kadlubar & Badawi 1995, Kaderlik, & Kadlubar 1995,). Habuchi et al., 1993 suggested that cigarette smoking might have a significant impact on the mutations of the p53 gene in urothelial cancers. Urothelial carcinogenesis in the presence of schistosomiasis seems to proceed along pathways different from those linked to smoking, since cigarette smoking appears to have a significant impact on the mutation of the p53 gene with A:T to G:C transitions which are not observed in SABC (Habuchi et al., 1993). The association of human papilloma virus (HPV) and non-schistosomal bladder squamous cell cancers has been reported in isolated cases in the USA (Maloney et al., 1994). An Egyptian study has also demonstrated HPV DNA in six of 16 (38%) SABC (Zekri et al.,1995). While SABC in South Africa showed no associated HPV (Cooper et al.,1997).

3.2.5 Occupational exposure

Exposure to chemicals used in dye, rubber, and textile manufacturing have been estimated to be responsible for up to 20% of bladder cancer cases (Cole et al.,1972). Most of these chemicals are aromatic amines that take several years to accumulate and thus account for the long latent periods before the development of bladder cancer. Aromatic amines from occupational exposures are activated and detoxified through the same reactions that aromatic amines in cigarette smoke are activated and detoxified. Hence, bladder cancer susceptibility depends on the cumulative expression profiles of these activating and detoxifying enzymes. It also means that exposures to occupational agents and cigarette smoke may be additive (Jung & Messing, 2000).

3.3 Genetic changes

The major differences in the clinico-pathologic features observed between the Western type of bladder cancer and SABC probably reflect underlying alternate tumor biology and carcinogenic pathways. Several studies attempted to characterize the chromosomal aberrations of SABC, including both SCC and TCC subtypes. Data were compared with those of the Western world.

3.3.1 Chromosomal studies

Over representation of 5p,6p,7p,8q,11q,17q and 22q of chromosomal material has been detected by Cytogenetic and molecular analysis. Aberrations of chromosomes 7, 9, and 17 showed reciprocal patterns in TCC and SCC, whether associated with Schistiosomiasis or not (Pycha et al. 1998). Few sporadic SCC cases examined by comparative genomic hybridization (CGH) have shown gains at 1q, 8qa, and 20q, as well as loses of 3p,9p, and 13q (El-Rifai et al.2000). Changes were observed at similar frequencies in SCC and TCC, irrespective to schistosomal status suggesting that these changes may be involved in a common pathway for bladder cancer development and progression independent of schistosomal status or histological subtype (Badawi,1996).

3.3.2 Cancer genes

Currently, it would appear that chromosome 9 and P53 changes may occur relatively early in the genesis of bladder cancer (Simoneau et al., 1996 , Reznikoff et al., 1996). The retinoblastoma (Rb) gene on chromosome 13 (13q) and the p53 gene on chromosome 17 (17p) play an important role in the progression of bladder cancer and possibly its development (Esrig et al., 1994). Rb gene mutations are seen in approximately 30% of bladder cancer (Cordon cardo et al.,1992). Inability to detect pRb immunohistochemically is associated with increased tumor grade and stage, especially muscle invasion (Xu et. al.,1993, Grossman et al.,1993) Some Studies revealed that Allelic losses in chromosome 17p, where the p53 gene resides, were less frequent in SCC (38%) than TCC (60%) Gonzalez-Zulueta,1995 while in South Africa, p53 mutations were recorded in 57% of SABC. (Badawi et al. 1999). It was also demonstrated that the histopathological subtype rather than the schistosomal impact itself determines the pattern of chromosomal changes for SABC. The pattern of point mutations in p53 appears to reflect the site of tumor origin, with most of the transitions occur in mutational hot spots at CpG dinucleotides (Hollstein et al., 1991). TP53 mutations in SABC included more base transition at CpG dinucleotids than seen in urothelial TCC. p53 inactivation ranged from 0 to 38% at the early stage of the disease, as opposed to 33% to 86% in the advanced tumor stage (Weintraub et al.1995, Badawi et al. 1996,) Excess mutations might be due to high levels of urinary nitrates in Schistoma infected patients producing nitric oxide by inflammatory cells. In these cases, there is usually an overexpression of MDM2 as well (Osman et al.1997). Elevated levels of DNA alkylation damage have been detected in *schistosome*-infected bladders and are accompanied by an inefficient capacity of DNA repair mechanisms. Whereas the p53 mutation frequency in SCC was similar to that reported for invasive TCC, there were differences in the type and position of these mutations between the two tumor types (Gonzalez-Zulueta et al., 1995). The ras oncogene does not seem to be strongly implicated in the differential process of carcinogenesis in SABC, judging from studies in different countries (Czerniak et al., 1990, Ibrahim & Khaled,2006). Deletions on chromosome 9 not only appear to occur in > 60% of bladder cancer across all grades and stages, but also are likely an initiating event (Jung & messing 2000). The p21 region of chromosome 9 (9p21) has been found to be mutated in a variety of malignancies suggesting the presence of a common tumor suppressor gene.(Theodorescu, 2003). Tamimi et al.(1996) found that a $p16^{INK4}$ deletion was present in 23 of 47 samples from SABC patients and that mutations were present in another 2 patients (i.e; 53% of tumors exhibited $p16^{INK4}$ gene alterations). They concluded that $p16^{INK4}$ alterations are more frequent in SABC than in other bladder tumors and may thus be associated with a specific etiology.

3.3.3 Microsatellite Instability

Microsatellite abnormalities found in cancer bladder appear to be early changes (Linnenbach et al., 1994; Orlow et al., 1994, Gonzalez-Zulueta et al., 1995), they may be reflecting severe deregulation of cellular DNA which if left unchecked may lead to unrepaired mutations in key regulatory genes such as p53. Importantly, microsatellite alterations are common in bladder cancer and analysis of genomic instabilities in urine samples has been recently evaluated as a method for bladder cancer screening with promising results in terms of sensitivity, specificity compared to classical techniques (Seripa et al., 2001; Zhang et al., 2001; Berger et al., 2002; Utting et al., 2002).

3.3.4 Oncogenes

Oncogenes may contribute to transformation and progression by being either overexpressed or mutated to produce an oncoprotein. One of the more important mechanisms by which oncogenes are overexpressed in bladder Cancer is through gene amplification (increased copies of the gene). In small series of SABC HER-2/ neu was overexpressed in all the studied TCC and none of SCC studied by Immunohistochemistry (Coombs et al., 1991, Cote et al.,1998, Wishahi,.et al.2000).

3.4 Cancer progression

Bladder Cancer cells require the acquisition of certain properties prior to being able to grow rapidly, invades, and metastasizes. These properties include uncontrolled growth and cellular mobility, mediated at least in part via EGF and EGFRs, expression or loss of expression of specific cell adhesion molecules, and overproduction of angiogenic factors. These factors may be produced by the tumor cells or released by the surrounding extracellular matrix or tumor associated stromal cells, or they may be products of inflammatory cells that infiltrate tumors. Folkman et al., (1987) using immunohistochemistry, increased microvascular density as a surrogate for angiogenesis has been found to be associated with tumor progression and decreased overall survival in Bladder Cancer patients.(Bochner et al.1995). The association of the apoptosis related proteins Bcl-2, Bcl-x, Bax and Bak, p53, E-cadherin, epidermal growth factor receptor and c-erbB-2, OCNA and Ki-67 were correlated with the clinical outcome of SACB in Cystectomy specimens from 109 patients with organ confined, muscle invasive stage, pT2pN0M0 were studied by Haitel and coworkers (2001) Immunohistochemical results were correlated with tumor progression. On multivariate analysis p53 emerged as a significant prognostic factor Additional independent prognostic factors were proliferating cell nuclear antigen for squamous cell carcinoma, and MIB-1, Bcl-x and Bax for transitional cell carcinoma.

4. Age and gender ratios

In *schistosome*-free countries throughout the world, the peak incidence of bladder cancer is in the sixth or seventh decade of life (La Vecchia et al., 1991) and is maximal between the ages of 65 and 75 years). Only 12% of bladder cancer cases occur in people younger than 50 years(Burnham, 1989). By contrast, in Egypt, Sudan, Iraq, Zambia, Malawi, and Zimbabwe, the mean age of the highest incidence of SABC is between 40 and 49 years (Moustafa et al., 1999), which clearly contrasts with the findings for *non-schistosoma* areas. The ratio of bladder cancer incidence (males to females) in countries with endemic infection was reported to be 5:1 but may vary within the range of 4:1 to 5.9:1 (Ibrahim,1986). The relatively higher gender ratio in the countries with endemic infection has been suggested to be because in rural areas the main route for infection is through contact with infected waters during agricultural activities, which are normally done by men rather than women. The predominantly male development of SABC has been explained by the high frequency of loss of chromosome Y using the FISH technique. Khaled et al.,(2000) demonstrated that 41% of cases of SABC showed loss of chromosome Y.

5. Pathobiology of schistosoma associated bladder cancer

SABC is histopathologically distinct from *non-S. haematobium* associated bladder cancer that occurs in North America and Europe. The former cancer is usually, sparing the bladder's trigone. Although the majority of bladder tumors formed due to *Schistosoma* infection are squamous cell carcinomas (SCC), adenocarcinomas and transitional cell carcinomas (TCC) or undifferentiated carcinomas can develop (Johansson & Cohen, 1997) Furthermore, it appears that there is a proportional increase of TCC due to schistosomal infections over time (Koraitim et al.,1995). Some researchers believe that TCC need more time to progress than SCC and are closely related with a less devastating inflammatory infiltrate (Michaud et al., 2007).

5.1 Gross features

The tumors commonly appeared as large nodular masses (Figure. 1) whereas papillary types are rare (2%). The carcinoma usually arises from the upper vesical hemisphere, at the posterior wall or vault. The trigone is rarely the site of the tumor origin (2%) (Khafagy et al.,1972) in contradistinction to the *non-shistosoma* associated cancer bladder where it involved in 21% (Mostofi,1975).

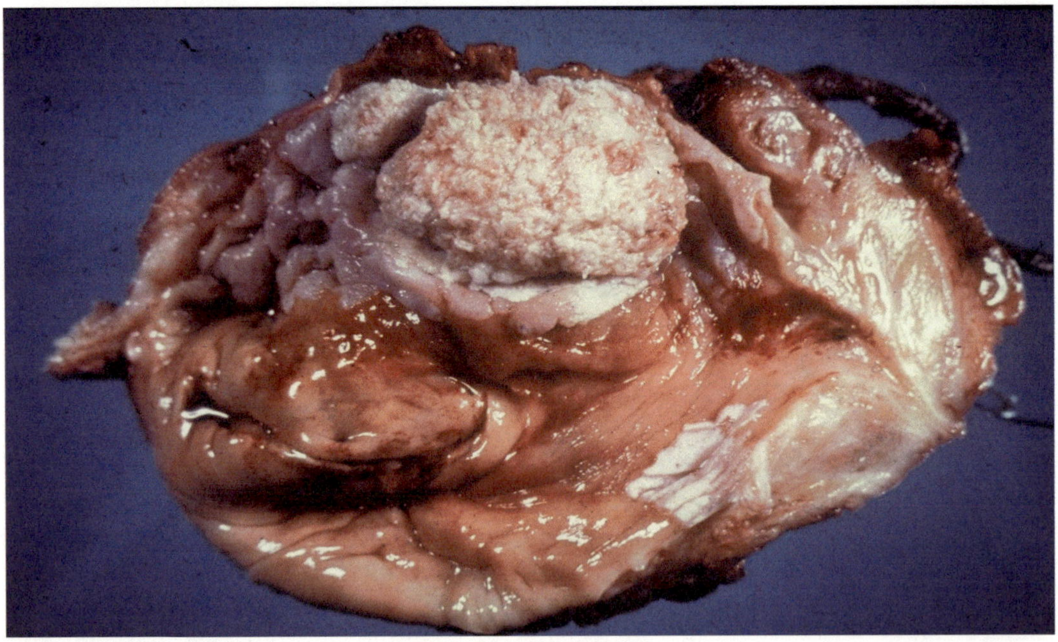

Fig. 1. SABC nodular type associated with leucoplakia

5.2 Precursor lesions

In the *Schistosoma* infested urinary bladder, the urothelium usually undergoes various metaplastic, proliferative and atypical changes (Khafagy et al., 1972). Metaplasia refers to a change in cell type, and this explains the histogenesis of non-transitional tumors in the bladder. Thus SCC and adenocarcinoma arise on top of squamous metaplasia and columnar metaplasia respectively. It is important to distinguish simple hyperplasia of the urothelium from atypical lesions (dysplasia and carcinoma insitu). The former is a simple reversible change, but the latter are associated with an increased risk of neoplastic development. Dysplasia, or low grade intraurothelial neoplasia, referred to pre-neoplastic atypical epithelial changes short of frank malignancy. Conversely, carcinoma insitu (CIS), or high grade intraurothelial neoplasia, is a preneoplastic atypical lesion which is cytologically

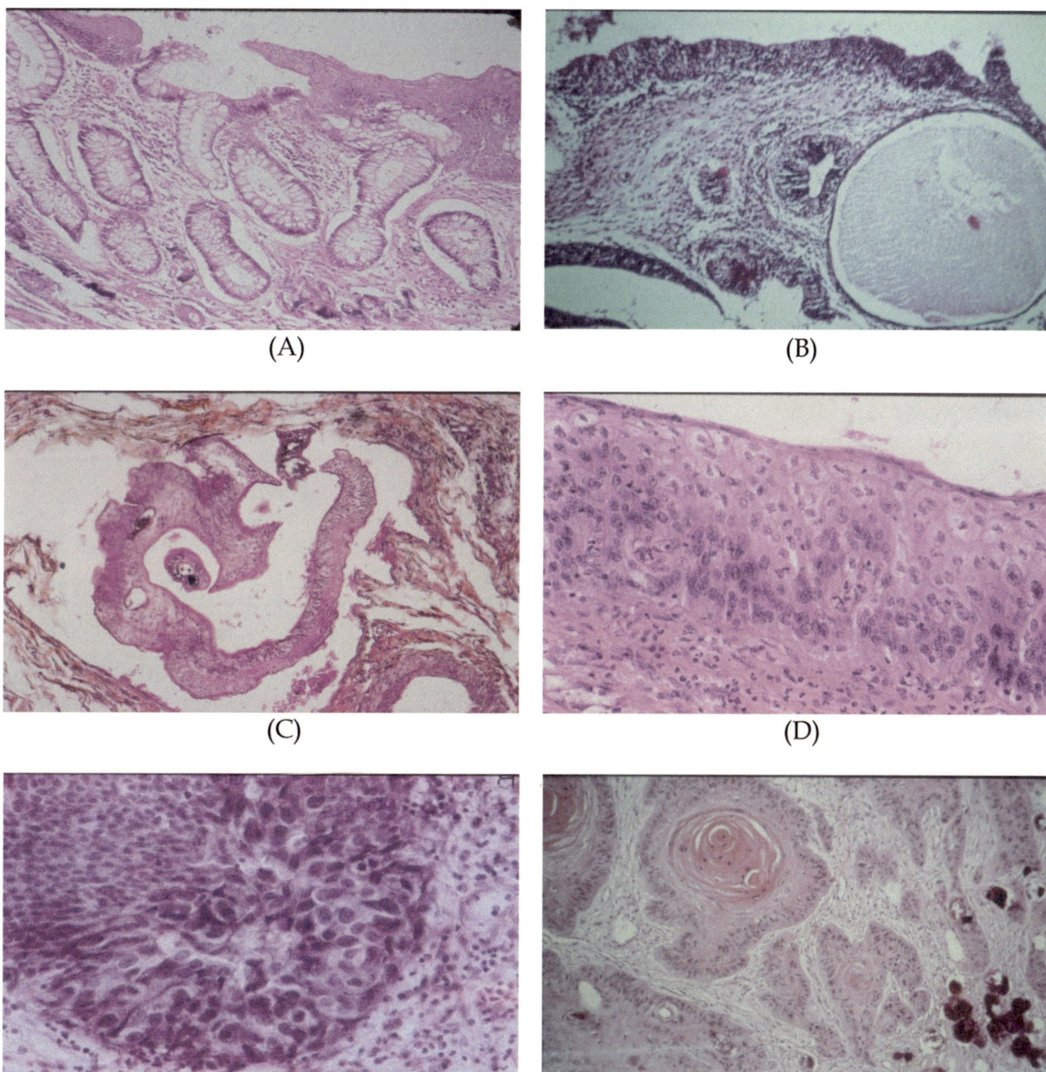

(A) (B) (C) (D) (E) (F)

Fig. 2. A) Simple Squamous metaplasia. B) Cystitis glandularis & cystica. C) Schistosoma worm in a vein. D) Squamous dysplasia. E) CIS in Brunn's nest F) SAB- Squamous cell carcinoma grade I.

indistinguishable from invasive cancer, but without invasion of the basement membrane. The rate of progression to invasive cancer is 15 % in cases of dysplasia (Cheng et al., 2000) and 35 % in CIS (Cheng et al., 1999). The SABC is frequently associated with a variety of pathologic changes in the bladder mucosa including: leucoplakia, cystitis cystica, carcinoma in situ and different *schistosoma* lesions (Zahran et al., 1976). In a series of Khafagy et al., (1972) of SABC 26 % of cases showed squamous metaplasia, 53 % of these lesions were non-keratinizing and 29 % showed surface keratinization and 18 % showed basal cell hyperplasia and atypia (Figure. 2).
Columnar metaplasia in the form of Brunn's nests, cystitis glandularis and cystica was observed in 52%-63 % (Khafagy,et al., 1972 & Zahran et al., 1976) of cystectomy specimens. Cystitis glandularis with atypia has been described by El-Bolkainy & Chu (1981a) at the tumor margin of adenocarcinoma. The natural history of these proliferative lesions has not been adequately studied due to lack of prospective follow up evaluation. Some of these changes such as simple hyperplasia and non- keratinizing squamous metaplasia without atypia are probably benign, however there is considerable evidence that atypical forms especially keratinizing squamous metaplasia (leucoplakia) may in fact have a premalignant potential. Similar evolutions may be expected in simple and atypical lesions of transitional epithelium. (Weiner et al., 1997).

5.3 Tumor histologic types

The urothelium is a multipotential unstable epithelium hence the multiple tumor types which may arise from it.

5.3.1 Transitional cell Carcinoma

In the SABC, transitional cell carcinoma contributed about 25 % of cases in large series collected over several years (Ghoneim et al., 1997), but there has been an increase in its relative frequency in recent years (Table 1). Three histologic subtypes and 10 rare variants are recognized.

Years No. of patients	(1976-1978) 1059	(1991-1993) 1256	(2000-2002) 923
Squamous carcinoma	78%	53%	40%
Transitional carcinoma	16%	36%	49%
Adenocarcinoma	4%	6%	5%
Undifferentiated	2%	5%	6%
Schistosoma ova	82%	59%	52%

Table 1. Time trend analysis of histologic types of bladder carcinomas in cystectomy specimens (Zaghloul et al., 2008).

5.3.2 Papillary transitional neoplasm of low malignant potential

This type is a papillary noninvasive tumor (Ta) which resembles a papilloma but with epithelial thickening exceeding the normal 6 layers. It contributes about 20% of all papillary tumors. Histologically, it shows preserved normal cell polarity with intact umbrella cells and intact basement membrane, no cellular atypia, and infrequent mitosis restricted to basal cell layer. Rarely may it show a prominent endophytic or inverted pattern. Such tumors were previously classified as grade I TCC. However, long term follow up studies have confirmed its rather benign nature. Thus, whereas 52 % of cases recurred, only 2% progressed to muscle invasive, and hence are considered favorable tumors of borderline malignancy or very low malignant potential.

5.3.3 Papillary transitional carcinoma

This refers to papillary tumors, which are composed partially, or entirely of malignant transitional epithelium. This type may be invasive or noninvasive. It is usually exophytic in pattern, rarely endophytic. Histologically, it shows both architectural disorder, as well as, cellular atypia of variable degree. They are graded either on a scale of three or a scale of two (low and high grades).

5.3.4 Invasive transitional carcinoma

This describes a non-papillary urothelial carcinoma (Figure.3) that invades the bladder wall; hence an aggressive behavior is expected. Such invasive property may complicate a papillary tumor, or may arise de novo. Also, these tumors are graded either on a scale of 3, or a scale of 2 (low and high grades). For therapeutic and prognostic implications, it is important to describe the pattern of invasion at tumor margin, namely: expansile with broad-front or tentacular growth, as well as, the depth of invasion, namely: infiltration of lamina propria(focal or extensive) or muscularis propria. In SABC the majority of tumors are invasive and 86% are high grade (Ghoneim et al., 2008).

5.3.5 Squamous Cell Carcinoma

The high frequency of SCC is one of the main distinctive features of carcinoma in the SABC and has been noted for a long time in different reports from Egypt, A relative frequency of 59% was recently reported (Ghoneim et al., 1997, 2008). This contrasts sharply with the relative infrequency of true squamous cell carcinoma in the Western world, which varied between 3% and 7% (El-Bolkainy et al., 1981b). The predominance of SCC in SACB series is probably related to squamous metaplasia and dysplasia which are relatively common in chronic Schistosomal cystitis that are frequently associated (65%) with this type of carcinoma (Khafagy et al.,1972). Fibrosis of the bladder wall of schistosomal origin has long been suspected as a limiting factor against tumor spread. Tissue reactions to schistosome eggs in the bladder wall, pelvic lymphatics, and regional lymph nodes were proposed as limiting factors against neoplastic spread. However the limited tendency of lymphatic spread of advanced tumors in schistosomal patients was explained by others as caused by predominance of low grade tumors in these patients (El-Bolkainy et al., 1981b). Histologically, SCC is composed of one cell type exhibiting squamous differentiation throughout the tumor. Malignant squamous cells may exhibit one or more of the following features according to their grade: eosinophilic cytoplasm, sharp cell borders, intercellular bridges, and concentric cellular formations of cell nests (squamous pearls). In bilharzial series, one half of cases are grade 1 or low grade with numerous cell nests and only slight nuclear anaplasia

5.3.6 Verrucous carcinoma

This rare variant of SCC, which has only been reported to occur in the *schistosomal* bladder, (Figure 4) is characterized by a low-grade malignancy and absence of lymph node or distant spread. It contributing 4.6% of SCC or 3.4% of all types of SABC (El-sebai, 1978)).

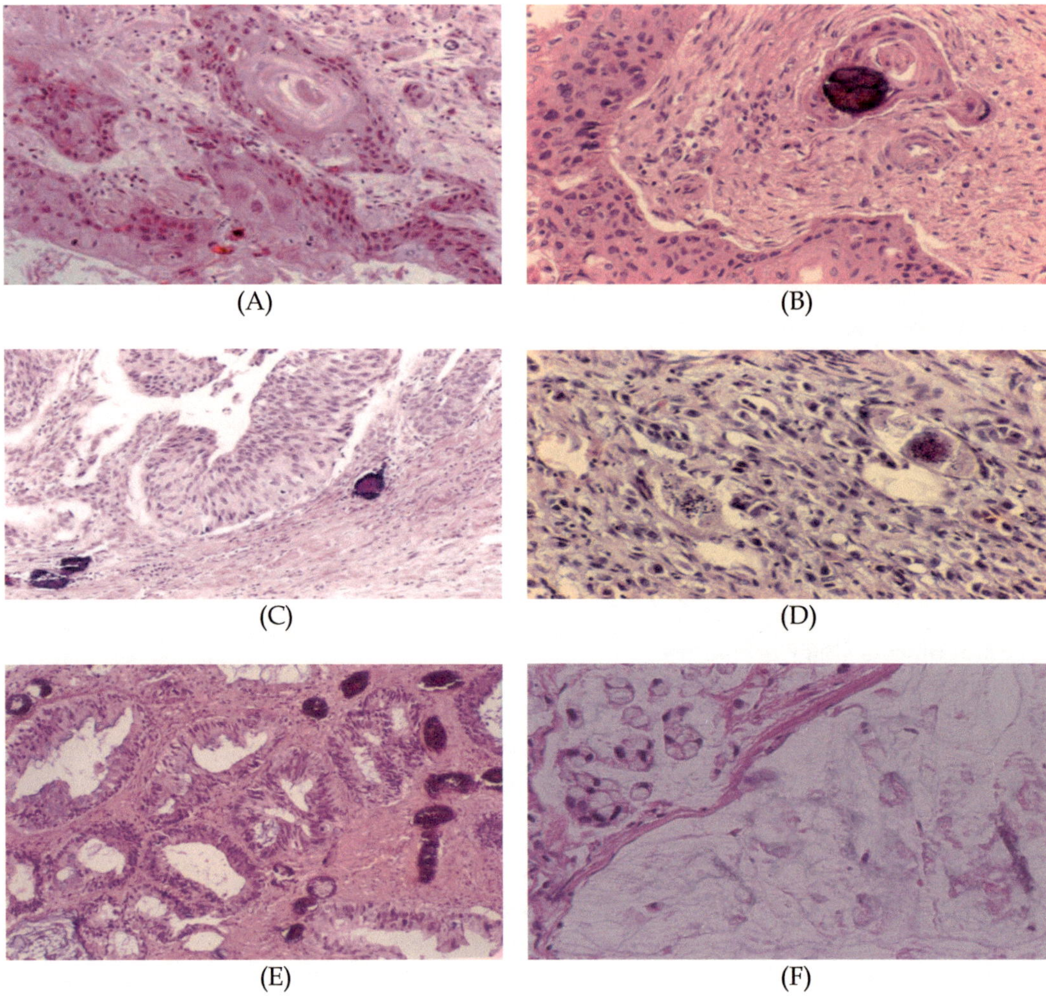

Fig. 3. A) Squamous cell carcinoma. B) Squamous cell carcinoma, urinary bladder. Notice the Schistosoma ova. C) Transitional cell carcinoma. D) Transitional cell carcinoma, Notice the vaible Schistosoma ova. E) Adenocarcinoma intestinal type. F) Mucinous adenocarcinoma

Verrucous carcinomas are divided into pure form which is exceptionally rare, and verrucous carcinoma associated with an invasive component (verrucoid carcinoma) which is more common. The former is a tumor of low malignant potential, but the latter will rather behave as conventional squamous cell carcinoma. Histologically, the tumor is a well differentiated, hyperkeratotic squamous cell carcinoma with elongated surface projections and down growths of club-shaped finger-like processes. The deeply advancing margin has a pushing rather than infiltrating border, where the cells are arranged in large bulbous masses of cohesive squamous cells.

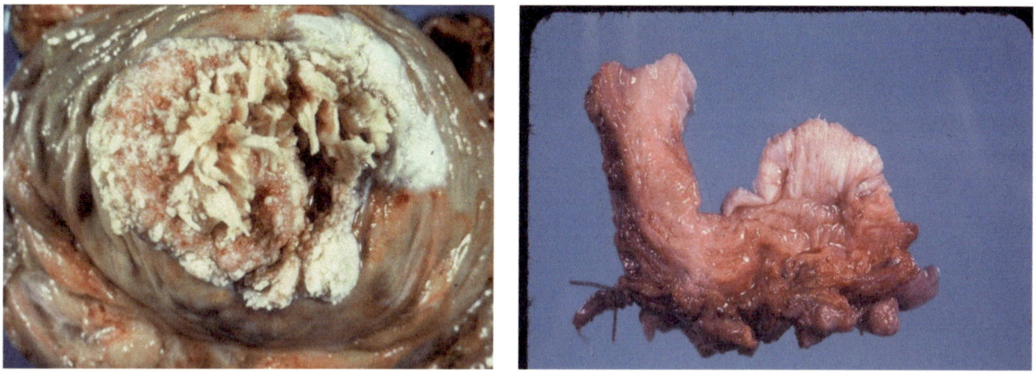

Fig. 4. SABC verrucous carcinoma cystectomy & cut section. Courtesy El-Bolkainy

5.3.7 Rare variants

The decline in the prevalence of *Schistosomiasis* in Egypt during the past two decades was associated with significant changes in the pathology of bladder carcinoma. This was confirmed by a time trend analysis study which demonstrated a significant decrease in Schistosoma eggs in tissues, a decline in the relative frequency of squamous carcinoma and an increase of transitional carcinoma (Zaghloul et al., 2008). Ten unusual variants of urothelial carcinomas are recognized (Mostofi et al.,1975), namely: urothelial carcinoma with squamous or glandular metaplasia, urothelial carcinoma with lymphocytic infiltrate (lymphoepithelioma), urothelial carcinoma clear cell type, urothelial carcinoma with ectopic placental glycoprotein production, plasmacytoid variant, lipid cell variant, micropapillary variant nested or deceptively benign variant, microcystic variant and osteoclastic variant.

5.3.8 Adenocarcinoma

Primary adenocarcinoma arises on top of cystitis glandularis, and is a rare tumor in western literature with a reported incidence of about 2%. This tumor type is more frequently encountered in areas where Schistosomiasis is endemic with a reported frequency variable between 6% (El-Bolkainy et al., 1981a) and 11% (Ghoneim et al.,1997). In a series of 185 patients of Schistosoma -associated primary adenocarcinoma, (El-Mekresh et al.,1998) 32% were non-mucin producing enteric type (Figure 3), 54% with interstitial mucin production, 10% with intraluminal mucin and 4% with intracellular mucin or signet ring type.

5.3.9 Undifferentiated tumors

About 2% of bladder carcinomas are too undifferentiated to be included in any of the above-mentioned histologic types. This heterogeneous group is generally highly aggressive and associated with very poor prognosis. It includes: small cell carcinoma, spindle and giant cell carcinoma and carcinosarcoma.

6. Early detection

Current methods of investigation of bladder cancer involve cystoscopy, ultrasound scanning and contrast urography, with additional information provided by cytology. These methods, although having a high detection rate, are expensive, time-consuming, invasive and uncomfortable.

6.1 Urine cytology

Cytology of voided urine or bladder washes is the most established noninvasive method in the work-up of haematuria (the most common presentation of bladder cancer) and follow-up in patients with a history of bladder cancer and is used as an adjunct to cystoscopy. This involves microscopic identification of exfoliated tumor cells based on cytological criteria (Figure 5). El-Bolkainy and Chu (1981a) used urine cytology for selective screening of rural high -risk population from 15 villages in Nile delta in Egypt for early detection of SABC. The high-risk group included farmers aged 20 years and above, and they contributed 19% of the total rural population. The tumor yield was 2 per 1000 high-risk screened and the majority of the detected tumors were at an early stage. The method has a high specificity but relatively low sensitivity, particularly in well-differentiated bladder tumors (Carmack & Soloway 2006). A meta-analysis that included data on 18 published series with 1,255 patients reported a sensitivity of 34% and specificity of 99% respectively (Lotan et al., 2003). Several factors contribute to this poor ability of urine cytology to detect cancer cells: only a small sample of urine can be processed and only a fraction of the sample can be used for final analysis which reduces the chance of capturing tumor cells. Background cells such as erythrocytes and leukocytes also confound the cytologic technique. Furthermore, cytological criteria that differentiate between low grade tumors and reactive cells can be ambiguous. (Wiener et al., 1993)

6.2 Urinary tumor markers of the bladder

The low sensitivity of urine cytology limits its use as a detection tool. Interest has been reported in identifying tumor markers in voided urine that would provide a more sensitive and objective test for tumor recurrence. Detection of bladder cancer using morphologic molecular tests could improve patient management in two ways. It would allow diagnosing tumors of the aggressive phenotype earlier and thus improve the prognosis of patients. In cases of less aggressive tumors, it could identify early disease onset and recurrences, thereby potentially reducing the need for expensive cystoscopic monitoring and surveillance procedures (Mitra et al., 2009). The following table 2 reflects the sensitivities and specificities of urine tumor markers in bladder cancer as reported in various publications

Commercially available marker	**Sensitivity (%) mean/ range**	**Specificity (%) mean/ range**
Cytology	48/ 16-89	96/ 81-100
Hematuria dipstick	68/ 40-93	68/ 51-97
BTA STAT	68/ 53-89	74/ 54-93
BTA TRAK	61/ 17-78	71/ 51-89
NMP22	75/ 32-92	75/ 51-94
NMP22 BLADDER CHEK	55.7	85.7
IMMUNOCYT	74/ 39-100	80/ 73-84
UROVYSION	77/ 73-81	98/ 96-100

Table 2. The sensitivities and specificities of selected urine tumor markers in bladder cancer (Urinary Tumor Markers for Bladder Cancer Corporate Medical Policy available at (www.bcbsnc.com)

There are several potential applications of urine tumor marker tests in patient surveillance, including: a) serial testing to detect recurrent disease earlier, b) as an adjunct to urine cytology in order to improve the detection of disease recurrence, c) providing a less expensive and more objective alternative to urine cytology, and d) directing the frequency of cystoscopy evaluation in the follow-up of patients with bladder cancer (Mitra, 2010). Currently available bladder cancer tumor markers and some of those in development are listed in Table 3,4, with an assessment of each marker and the level of evidence (LOE) for its clinical use. The LOE grading system is based on that of Hayes et al., (1996)

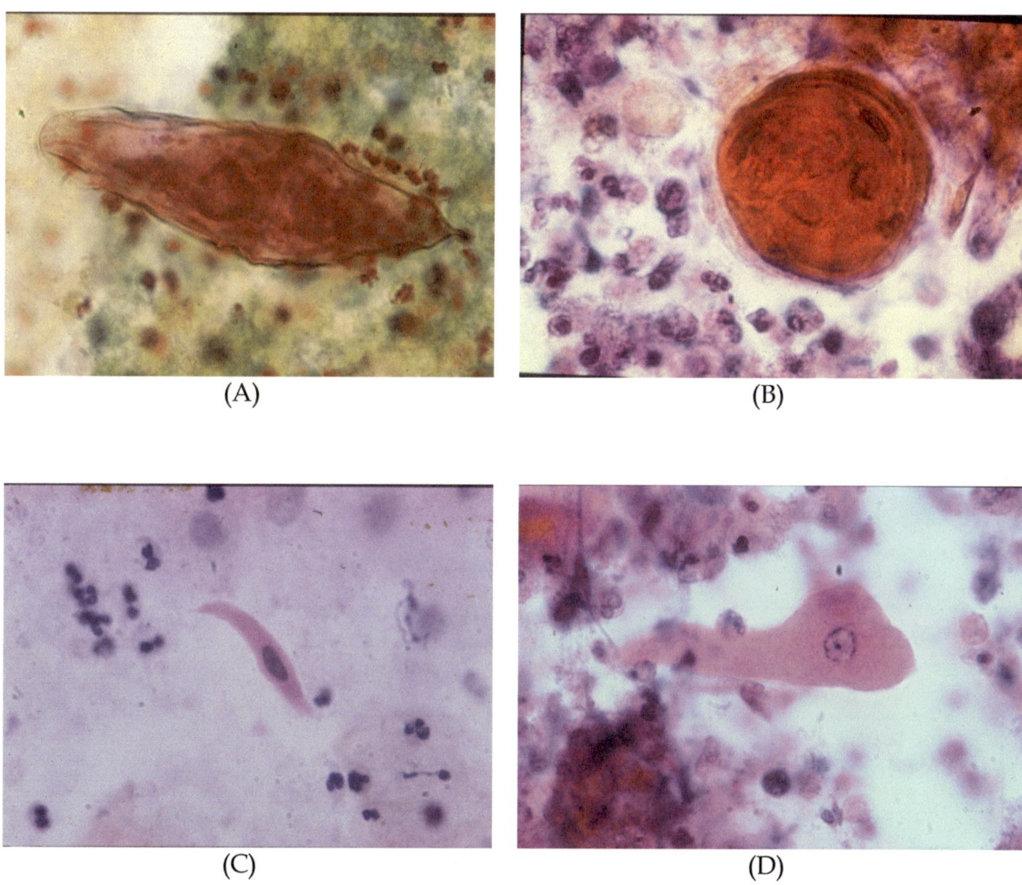

Fig. 5. A) Schistosoma ova terminal spine in urine. B) Squamous cell carcinoma, urine cytology. C) Squamous cell carcinoma spindle cell urine cytology. D) Squamous cell carcinoma tadpole, urine cytology.

Level	Type of evidence
I	Evidence from a single high-powered prospective controlled study specifically designed to test the marker, or evidence from a meta-analysis, pooled analysis or overview of level II or III studies.
II	Evidence from a study in which marker data are determined in relationship to a prospective therapeutic trial that is performed to test a therapeutic hypothesis but not specifically designed to test marker utility.
III	Evidence from large prospective studies.
IV	Evidence from small retrospective studies.
V	Evidence from small pilot studies.

Table 3. Levels of evidence (LOE) for grading clinical utility of tumor markers

Cancer Marker	LOE
BTA Stat	II
BTA Trak	II
NMP 22	II
Bladder Chek	II
Immunocyt	II
UroVysion	II
Cytokeratins 8, 18, 19	III
Telomerase - TRAP, hTert, hTR	III
BLCA-4	II
Survivin - protein and mRNA	II
Microsatellite markers	III
Hyaluronic acid / hyaluronidase	III
DD23 monoclonal antibody	II
Fibronectin	III
HCG - protein and mRNA	IV
DNA promotor regions of hypermethylated tumor suppressor and apoptosis genes	IV
Proteomic profiles (Mass spectrometry)	V

HCG, human chorionic gonadotropin; HTR, human telomerase; hTERT, human telomerase reverse transcriptase; TRAP, telomeric repeat amplification protocol; LOE, Levels of evidence(Fritsche. et al.2010)

Table 4. Currently available urine markers for bladder cancer.

6.2.1 Commercially available bladder tumor biomarkers in urine

BTA (bladder tumor antigen) stat® test, is a qualitative, point-of-care test with an immediate result that identifies a human complement factor H-related protein that was shown to be produced by several human bladder cell lines but not by other epithelial cell lines. The BTA *stat* test is an in vitro immunoassay intended for the qualitative detection of bladder tumor associated antigen in urine of persons diagnosed with bladder cancer The BTA stat test is an in vitro immunoassay intended for the qualitative detection of bladder tumor associated antigen in urine of persons diagnosed with bladder cancer. This test is indicated for use as an aid in the diagnosis and monitoring of bladder cancer patients in conjunction with cystoscopy. **The BTA TRAK® test** provides a quantitative determination of the same protein. Both tests have sensitivities comparable to that of cytology for high-grade tumors and better than cytology for low-grade tumors. **Nuclear matrix protein 22 (NMP-22)** is a protein associated with the nuclear mitotic apparatus. It is thought that this protein is released from the nuclei of tumor cells during apoptosis. Normally, only very low levels of NMP-22 can be detected in the urine, but elevated levels may be associated with bladder cancer. NMP-22 may be detected in the urine using an immunoassay. for use in the initial diagnosis and surveillance of bladder cancer. Testing for BTA or NMP-22 has been proposed as an adjunct or alternative to urinary cytology as a technique for bladder cancer surveillance. In addition, both tests have been investigated as initial tests in patients with signs and symptoms suggestive of bladder cancer (Bas et al.,2009).

Fluorescence in situ hybridization (FISH) DNA probe technology has also been used to detect chromosomal abnormalities in voided urine to assist not only in bladder cancer surveillance but also in the initial identification of bladder cancer. fluorescence in situ hybridization (FISH) DNA probe technology is a technique to visualize nucleic acid sequences within cells by creating short sequences of fluorescently labeled, single-strand DNA, called probes, which match target sequences. The probes bind to complementary strands of DNA, allowing for identification of the location of the chromosomes targeted. The UroVysion Bladder Cancer Kit designed to detect aneuploidy for chromosomes 3, 7, 17, and loss of the 9p21 locus via in urine specimens (Figure 6). It is used as an aid for initial diagnosis of bladder cancer in patients suspicion of disease, and in conjunction with cystoscopy to monitor bladder cancer recurrence. Better performance has been reported in identification of carcinoma in situ and high grade tumors (lokeshwar et al.,2005). Another potential advantage is apparent from a study of 69 cases of bladder wash where 3 cases showed no visible mass on cystoscopy, urine cytology was negative but was positive by FISH (Badawi, 2011).

The ability of the test in detecting occult tumors that are not initially visible on cystoscopy is apparent from finding of chromosomal. (Chromosomal abnormalities detected in exfoliated cells in urine of patients under surveillance have preceded cystoscopically identifiable bladder tumors by 0.25 to 1 year in 41%-89% patients (Mitra et al., 2009). The ImmunoCyt™ testuses fluorescence immunohistochemistry with antibodies to a mucin glycoprotein and a carcinoembryonic antigen (CEA). These antigens are found on bladder tumor cells. It used mainly for monitoring bladder cancer recurrence in conjunction with cytology and cystoscopy.

6.2.2 Other urinary markers

A number of other urinary tumor markers not currently commercially available are under investigation (Steiner et al.,1997, Stein et al.,1998).The availability of many new markers for bladder cancer raises the possibility of improving the rate of cancer detection by combined use of selected markers, measured either simultaneously or sequentially (Sanchez-Carbayo et al.,2001). The objective of such panel testing should be to improve both the sensitivity and the specificity for bladder cancer detection.

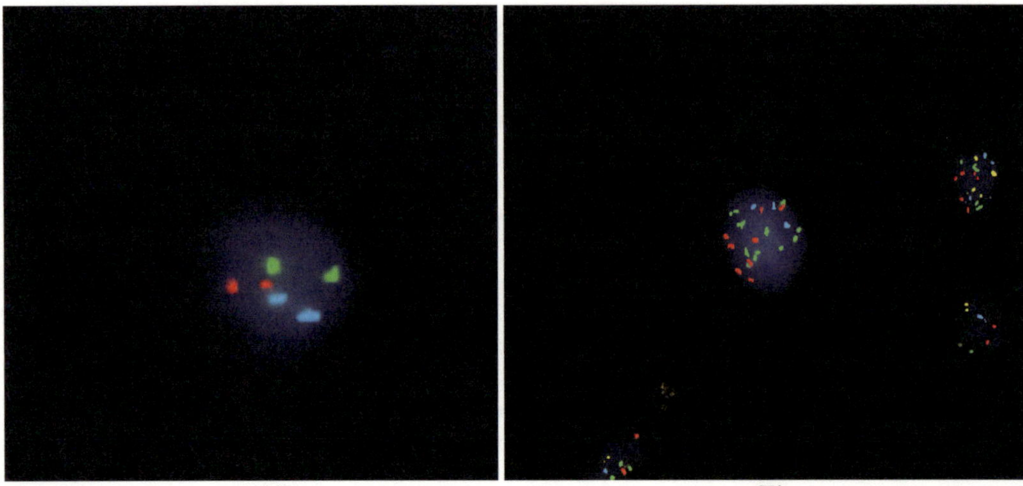

(A) (B)

Fig. 6. (A) Multicolor FISH Notice absence of yellow signals denoting 9p21 deletion X1250. (B) polysomy of chromosomes 3(red signals), 7 (green signals), and 17 (aqua signals) & deletion of chromosome 9p21 (absence of yellow signals X 1000). The background shows inflammatory cells with 2 copies of each of the studied chromosomes (normal pattern). Courtesy Omnia Badawi.

7. Prognostic factors

The major challenges confronting the urologist after treatment of bladder cancer are tumor recurrence and progression. In this regard, some pathologic parameters may serve as predictors of the biologic behavior of bladder tumors. Such prognostic factors are most valuable to stratify patients and to select high-risk patients for adjuvant treatment. Transurethral resection is commonly practiced for superficial bladder carcinoma in the west, but very rarely in the SABC. In the latter, most of the patients (95.3%) present with muscle invasive carcinoma, hence radical cystectomy is the treatment of choice. (El-Sebai,1978).For this reason, we will limit our discussion here for prognostic factors for invasive tumors after radical cystectomy, of Schistosoma associated series.

7.1 Prognosis in SABC

Ghoneim and associates (2008) analyzed a large series of 2720 cases of bladder cancer in a single institution of these 2090 were men and 630 women. The average age was 43 years, which is considerably lower than in European and American series. The Median follow up was 5.5 years. *Schistosoma* eggs were found in 85% of the cystectomy specimens. Of particular interest is the histology of the tumors removed. Squamous bladder tumors were encountered in 59%, transitional cell carcinoma in 22% and adenocarcinomas (non-urachal) were seen in 11% of the cases. About 7% of the tumors were mixed or unclassified. Nodal involvement has been universally associated to a poor outcome. Regional lymph nodes were involved in 20.4%. Bilateral lymph node involvement was reported in 39.6%.There is a sentinel region which is the endopelvic region. There is no skipped metastasis. Negative nodes in the endopelvic region indicate that more proximal dissection is not necessary and bilateral endopelvic dissection is required. Lymph node positivity is a significant and independent prognostic factor. The relative risk for the development of treatment failure among node positive patients was computed to be 1.8%. The investigators used univariate and multivariate analysis to test the following prognostic factors on disease free survival: sex, histology, stage, grade, lymph node status and presence or absence of *Schistosoma* ova. Noteworthy is that they found the same results as Bassi et al.(1999) In the multivariate analysis only tumor stage and grade as well as lymph node status had a significant impact on survival. The 5-year survival rate was 48%, also comparable to other published series (El-Mawla et al., 2001). The problem of correct clinical staging was also addressed by the authors. Clinical staging was not correct in 32% of the cases with the tendency to under stage the extent of the disease. The 5-year survival was 55% for lymph node negative patients and only 18% for patients with positive lymph nodes. Survival was strongly correlated to the stage of the disease. Stage pT3a patients 5-year survival was 43%, for pT3b it was 31% and for pT4 tumors only 8% survived 5 years and 2.6% died postoperatively These data are in concordance with data published on cystectomy series comprising transitional cell cancers (Stein et al 2001). Extended radical lymphadenectomy in treatment of SACB assures the removal of many nodal cancer deposits increases the accuracy of staging, is likely to result in improved postoperative survival (Ghoneim et al.,1979), (Leissner et al., 2004) Postoperative mortality was 2.6%. They concluded that contemporary cystectomy with continent diversion for muscle invasive disease provide minimal morbidity, offers good locoregional disease and results in acceptable quality of life (Abol-enein et al., 2004) The results published by others are remarkably similar (Stein et al., 2001, Herr et al., 2002).

7.2 Newer prognostic factors

A more sophisticated procedure may be used to evaluate the likelihood of recurrence or progression by DNA ploidy measurement, immunohistochemical staining of the basement membrane components, evaluation of cell adherence molecules, growth factors, proteases, cell surface antigens and blood group antigens, as well as by the determination of cell-cycle related proteins in bladder carcinoma (Stein et al.,1998; Grossman 1998; Zlotta & Schulman 2000,). All of these are experimental and none have reached clinical significance or become part of clinical routine. (lokeshwar et al.,2005).

8. Future prospects

SABC is theoretically a good example of a preventable malignant disease, if the parasite could be eliminated on a nationwide scale. This is far from being an easy problem. The current strategy adopted in Egypt involves a combination of snail control and mass therapy of the exposed population. Since screening projects are usually of limited nature, both in time and place, they only succeed in lowering the prevalence rate of the disease. There is still much to be learned about *Schistosomiasis* and its control. Other possibilities for bladder cancer prevention lie in smoking cessation, reduction of the occupational exposure (mainly to aromatic amines) by appropriate regulations and education activities, reduction of infection by *Schistosoma haematobium* (in endemic areas), and promotion of consumption of fruits and vegetables.

9. References

Aboul-Enein H., El-Baz M., Abdelhameed M., Abdel Latif & Ghoneim M., et al. (2004). Lymph node involvement in patients with bladder cancer treated with radical cystectomy: A path anatomic study -A single center experience. *J Urol* 172, 5, Part 1, 1818-1821.

Al-Saleem T., Alsh N & Tawfikh L. E. (1990). Bladder cancer in Iraq: The histological subtypes and their relationship to schistosomiasis. *Ann. Saudi Med.* 10:161–164.

Al-Shukri, S. M, Alwan, H., Nayef, M. & Rahman, A. (1987). Bilharsiasis in malignant tumors of the urinary bladder. *Br. J. Urol.,* 59:59–62.

Althuis MD, Dozier JD, Anderson WF, Devesa SS & Brinton LA.(2005). Global trends in breast cancer incidence and mortality 1973- 1997. *Int J Epidemiol.;* 34:405-412.

Badawi O. (2011).Evaluation of FISH for diagnosis and detection of recurrence of bladder TCC. MD thesis, PP 82-95NCI, Cairo Egypt.

Badawi A. F., Mostafa M. H.; Aboul-Asm, T. Haboubi, N. Y.; O'Connor, P. J. & D. P. Cooper. (1992). Promutagenic methylation damage in bladder DNA from patients with bladder cancer associated with schistosomiasis and from normal individuals. *Carcinogenesis* 13:877–881.

Badawi, A. F., Cooper D. P., M. H. Mostafa., M. H. Doenhoff, A. Probert, P. Fallon, R. Cooper, & P. J. O'Connor.(1993). Promutagenic methylation damage in liver DNA of mice infected with *Schistosoma* mansoni.*Carcinogenesis* 14:653–657.

Badawi, A. F., D. P. Cooper, M. H. Mostafa, T. Aboul-Asm, R. Barnard, G. P. Margison & P. J. O'Connor. (1994). *O*6-Alkylguanine-DNA-alkyltransferaseactivity in schistosomiasis associated human bladder cancer. *Eur. J. Cancer* 30:1314–1319.

Badawi, A. F.; Hirvonen, A.; Bell, D. A.; Lang, N. P. & Kadluba, F. F. (1995a). Role of aromatic amine acetyltransferases NAT1 and NAT2 in increasing carcinogen-DNA adduct formation in the human urinary bladder.*Cancer Res.* 55:5230–5237.

Badawi, A. F.; Mostafa, M. H.; Probert, A. & O'Connor, P. J.(1995b). Role of schistosomiasis in human bladder-cancer—evidence of association, etiologic factors, and basic mechanisms of carcinogenesis. *Eur. J. Cancer* Prev.4:45–49.

Badawi, AF.(1996).Molecular and genetic events in schistosomiasis associated human bladder cancer: role of oncogenes and tumor suppressor genes. *Cancer Lett.;* 105:123-138.

Bas, W.G. van Rhijn Henk G. van der Poel Theo & H. van der Kwast (2009). Cytology and Urinary Markers for the Diagnosis of Bladder *Cancer. European urology supplements* 8 536–541.

Bassi P.F. Drago Ferrantc G & Piazza N. (1999). Prognostic factors of outcome after radical cystectomy for bladder cancer: a retrospective study of a homogeneous patient cohort. *J Urol* 161.1494-1497.

Berger, A.P. Parson, W. Stenzl, A., Steiner, H., Bartsch, G. & Klocker, H. (2002). Microsatellite alterations in human bladder cancer: detection of tumor cells in urine sediment and tumor tissue. *Eur.Urol.* 41, 532-553.

Bochner, BH., Cote, RJ., Weidner, N., et al.(1995) Angiogenesis in bladder cancer: relationship between microvessel density and tumor prognosis. *J Natl Cancer Inst.;* 87:1603-1612.

Carmack, AJ & Soloway, MS.(2006).The diagnosis and staging of bladder cancer: From RBCs to TURs. *Urology;* 67(3 Suppl 1):3-8.

Cheng 1., Chenille, I.C., Neumann, R.M. & Bostwick, D.G.(2000). Flat intraepithelial llesions of the urinary bladder cancer, 88:625-631.

Cheng 1. Cheville, lC., Neumann, R.M. & Bostwick, D.G., (1999).Natural history of urothelial dysplasia of Bladder. *Am. J. Surg. Pathol* 23:443.
Cole P, Hoover R, Friedell GH. (1972). Occupation and cancer of thelower urinary tract. *Cancer*. 29:1250-1260.
Cooper, Z Haffajee & L Taylor (1997). Human papillomavirus and schistosomiasis associated bladder cancer I Clin Pathol: *Mol Pathol;* 50:145-148.
Cote, R.J.; Dunn, M. D & Chatterjee S. J, et al. (1998). Elevated and absent pRb expression is associated with bladder cancer progression and has cooperative effects with p53. *Cancer Res.;* 58:1090-1094.
Cordon-Cardo, C.; Wartinger, D & Petrylak, D. et al.(1992) Altered expression of the retinoblastoma gene product: prognostic indicator in bladder cancer. *J Natl Cancer Inst.;* 84:1251-1256.
Coombs, LM, Piggott, DA , Sweeney, E, et al.(1991) Amplification and over-expression of c-erbB-2 in transitional cell carcinoma of the urinary bladder. *Br J Cancer.;* 63:601-608.
Czerniak, B, Deitch, D & Simmons, H, et al. (1990) Ha-ras gene codon 12 mutation and DNA ploidy in urinary bladder carcinoma. *Br J Cancer.;* 62:762-763.
Edwards BK, Ward E, Kohler BA, et al.(2010). Annual report to the nation on the status of cancer, 1975-2006, featuring colorectal cancer trends and impact of interventions (risk factors, screening, and treatment) to reduce future rates. *Cancer*. 116:544-573.
El Bolkainy, M.N. & Chu, E.W. (1981a).Organization of a screening project for the detection of bladder cancer, in El Bolkainy MN, Chu EW (eds): *Detection of Bladder Cancer Associated with Schistosomiasis.*Cairo, Egypt, AI-AhramPress, pp 19-28.
EI-Bolkainy, M.N., Mokhtar, N.M., Ghoneim, M.A. & Hussein, M.H.(1981b). The impact of schistosomiasis on the pathology of bladder carcinoma.*Cancer*, 48:2643-2648.
Elem, B. & Purohit, R. (1983). Carcinoma of urinary bladder in Zambia: aquantitative estimate of Schistosoma haematobium infection. *Br. J. Urol.*55:275–278.
El-Khoby T, Galal N, Fenwick A, Barakat RA, El-Hawey A & Nooman A et al (2000) The epidemiology of schistosomiasis in Egypt: summary findings in nine governorates. *Am J Trop Med Hyg* 62:88–99.
El- Merzabani, M: El-Aaser A. & Zakhary N. (1979). A study on the etiological factors of Bilharzial bladder cancer in Egypt - 1. Nitrosamines and their precursors in urine, *Europ. J. Cancer.*15: 287-291.
El-Sebai, I. (1978). Cancer of the Bilharzia bladder. *Urol. Res.* 6:233–236.
Esrig D, Elmanjian D & Groshen S, et al. (1994) Accumulation of nuclear p53 and tumorprogression in bladder cancer. *N Engl J Med.;* 331:1259-1264.
EI-Mekresh, M.M., EI-Baz., Abol-Enein, H., & Ghoneim, M.A.(1998). Primary adenocarcinoma of the urinary bladder: a report of 185 cases. *Brit. J Urol.*, 82:206-212.
El-Mawla N.G, El-Bolkainy M.N & Khaled H. M. (2001). Bladder cancer in Africa: update. *Semin Oncol;* 28:174-178.
El-Rifai, W. Kamel, D. Larramendy, ML, Shoman, S., Gad, Y., Baithun, S., El Awady, M, Eissa, S & Khaled, et al. (2000). DNA copy number changes in Schistosoma associated and non-Schistosoma-associated bladder cancer. *Am J Pathol.;* 156(3):871-878.

Falagas M.; Vassilis S; Rafailidis, P; Eleni G. Mourtzoukou, Peppas G., & Matthew E. (2010). Chronic bacterial and parasitic infections and cancer: a review *J Infect Dev Ctries;* 4(5):267-281.

Felix AS, Soliman AS & Khaled H et al. (2008) The changing patterns of bladder cancer in Egypt over the past 26 years. *Cancer Causes Control*; 19: 421–429.

Ferlay J, Shin HR, Bray F, Forman D, Mathers CD & Parkin D. (2010.) GLOBOCAN (2008) Cancer Incidence and Mortality Worldwide: *IARC Cancer Base* No. 10. Lyon, France: International Agency for Research on Cancer; Year. Available at: http://globocan.iarc.fr.

Folkman, J & Klagsbrun, M.(1987) Angiogenic factors. *Science.*; 235:442-447.

Freedman LS, Edwards BK, Ries LA & Young JL eds.(2006). Cancer Incidence inFour Member Countries (Cyprus, Egypt, Israel, and Jordan) of the Middle East Cancer Consortium(MECC) Compared with US SEER. Bethesda, MD: National Cancer Institute, : NIH Available at: http://seer.cancer. gov/publications/mecc.

Fritsche H., Grossman B., Seth P & Lerner S Ihor SawczukNACB I (2010). Practice Guidelines And Recommendations For Use Of Tumor Markers In The Clinic Bladder Cancer National Academy of Clinical Biochemistry Guidelines for the Use of Tumor Markers in Bladder Cancer 1-17 available at hfritsche@mdanderson.org.

Ghoneim, M..A., EL-Mekresh. M..M., El-Baz, M.a., El-Attar, LA. & Ashamallah, A. (1997).Radical cystectomy for carcinoma of the bladder: critical l evaluation of the results of 1, 026 cases. *J Urol.*, 158:399.

Ghoneim, M., Abdel Latif, M., El-Mekresh, M. & Abol-Enein, H. (2008). Radical cystectomy for carcinoma of the bladder: 2, 720 consecutive cases 5 years later. *J. of urology* 180:121-127.

Grossman, H.B.; Liebert, M & Antelo M, et al.(1998); p53 and RB expression predict progression in T1 bladder cancer. *Clin Cancer Res.* 4:829-834.

Gonzalez-Zulueta M, Shibata A, Ohneseit PF, Spruck CH, III, Busch C, Shamaa M, et al. (1995).High frequency of chromosome 9p allelic loss and CDKN2 tumor suppressor gene alterations in squamous cell carcinoma of the bladder.*J Natl Cancer Inst;* 87:1383-93.

Gouda I, Mokhtar N, Bilal D, El-Bolkainy T & El-Bolkainy NM.(2007). Bilharziasis and bladder cancer: a time trend analysis of 9843 patients. *J Egypt Natl Canc Inst;* 19:158–62.

Habuchi, T., Takahashi, R., Yamada, H., Ogawa, O., Kakehi, Y., Ogura, K., Yamasaki, S., Toguchida , J., Shitake, K & Fujita, J. (1993). Influence of cigarette smoking and schistosomiasis on p53 gene mutation in urothelial cancer. *Cancer Res.* 53, 3795-3799.

Hayes, D. F., Bast, R., Desch, C. E., Fritsche, H., Kemeny, .NE & Jessup J, et al. (1996).A tumor marker utility grading system (TMUGS): A framework to evaluate clinical utility of tumor markers. *J Natl Cancer Inst;* 88:1456-1466.

Haitel A, Posch B, El-Baz M, Mokhtar AA, Susani M, Ghoneim MA & Marberger M et al (2001). Bilharzial related, organ confined, muscle invasive bladder cancer: prognostic value of apoptosis markers, proliferation markers, p53, E-cadherin, epidermal growth factor receptor and c-erbB-2.*J.Urol;* 165(5):1481-1487.

Herr, H.W.; Bochner, B. & Dalbagni, G.(2002). Impact of the number of lymphnodes retrieved on outcome in patients with muscle invasive bladder cancer. *J.Urol* 167:1295.

Hicks, R. M. (1980). Nitrosamines as possible etiological agents in Bilharzial bladder cancer. *Banbury Rep.* 12:455–471.

Hollstein, M.; Sidransky, D.; Vogelstein, B. & Harris, C. C. *(1991).* P53 mutations in human cancers. *Science* 253:49–53.

Ibrahim, A. S. (1986). Site distribution of cancer in Egypt: twelve years experience (1970–1981), Cancer prevention in developing countries. *Pergamon Press, Oxford, UK. p.* 45–50.

Ibrahim, A. & Khaled H. (2006).Urinary Bladder Cancer. *MECC Monograph,* 97- 110.

Jemal A., Bray F., . Center M., Ferlay J, Ward E. & Forman D.(2011): Global cancer statistics *CA Cancer J Clin;* 61; 69-90.

Johansson, S. L. & Cohen, S. M.(1997). Epidemiology and etiology of bladder cancer. *Semin Surg Oncol* 13:291-298.

Jung, M. & Messing, E M. D. (2000) Molecular Mechanisms and Pathways in Bladder Cancer Development and Progression *Cancer Control,* .7 (4), 325 - 333.

Kadlubar, F. F. & Badawi, A. F. (1995).; Genetic susceptibility and carcinogen-DNA adduct formation in human urinary bladder carcinogenesis. *Toxicol Lett.* 82-83:627-632.

Kaderlik, KR. & Kadlubar, FF.(1995) Metabolic polymorphisms and carcinogen-DNA adduct formation in human populations. *Pharmacogenetics*..5:S108-S117.

Karim-Kos HE, de Vries E, Soerjomataram I, Lemmens V, Siesling S & Coebergh JW.*(2008)*Recent trends of cancer in Europe: a combined approach of incidence, survival and mortality for 17 cancer sites since the 1990s. *Eur J Cancer.* 44:1345-1389.

Khaled H.M, Aly M.S & Magrath I. T.*(2000).* Loss of Y chromosome in Bilharzial bladder cancer. *Cancer Genet Cytogenet 117:32-36.*

Khafagy, M. M.; EL-Bolkainy, M. N. & Mansour, M. A. (1972). Carcinoma of the Bilharzial bladder. A study of the associated mucosa lesions in 86 cases. *Cancer, 30: 150-159.*

Koraitim, M.M., Metwalli, N.E., Atta, MA. & El-Sadr, A.A.(1995).Changing age incidenc and pathological types of schistosoma-associated bladder carcinoma. *J Urol* 154: 1714-1716.

La Vecchia, C., B. Nagri, B. D'Avanzo, R. Savoldelli, and S. Franceshi.(1991). Genital and urinary tract diseases and bladder cancer. *Cancer Res.* 51:629–631.

Lehman, J.S. Farid, Z.; Smith, J.H.; Bassily, S & El-Masry, NA. (1973). Urinary schistosomiasis in Egypt: clinical, radiological, bacteriological and parasitological correlations. *Trans R Soc Trop Med Hyg*.67: 384-399.

Leissner J, Ghoneim M..A, Abol-Enein H, Thüroff J.W, Franzaring L, Fisch M & Schulze H, et al. (2004) Extended radical lymphadenectomy in patients with urothelial bladder cancer: results of a prospective multicenter study. *J Urol.* 171(1):139-144.

Linnenbach, A.J., Robbins, S.L., Seng B.A., Tomaszewski, J.E. Pressler, L.B & Markowitz, S.B. (1994). Urothelial carcinogenesis. *Nature* 367, 419-420.

Lokeshwar, VB., Habuchi, T., Grossman, HB, Murphy, WM., Hautmann, SH. & Hem street, GP., 3rd, et al(.2005). Bladder tumor markers beyond cytology: International Consensus Panel on bladder tumor markers. *Urology.* 66(6 Suppl 1):35-63.

Lotan, Y & Roehrborn, CG. *(2003) Sensitivity* and specificity of commonly available bladder tumor markers versus cytology: results of acomprehensive literature review and meta-analyses. *Urology*. 61(1):109- 113.

Mohkatar N. Gouda I., Adel I. (2007). Cancer pathology registry (2003-2007), 2nd edn. The National Cancer Institute at Cairo University, Cairo Egypt.

Mostafa, M. H.; Helmi, S.; Badawi, A. F.; Tricker, A. R.; Spiegelhalder, B & Preussman, R. (1994). Nitrate, nitrate and volatile N-nitroso compounds in the urine of *Schistosoma mansoni* infected patients.*Carcinogenesis*15:619–625.

Mostafa M.H, Sheweita S.A & O'Connor PJ (1999) Relationship between schistosomiasis and bladder cancer. *Clin Microbiol Rev*. 12: 97-111.

Michaud, D.S., Platz, E.A. & Giovannucci, E. (2007).Gonorrhoea and male bladder cancer in a prospective study. *Br J Cancer*; 96: 169-71.

Mitra, AP, Birkhahn, M, Penson, DF & Cote, RJ. (2009) Molecular screening for bladder cancer. Waltham, MA: UpToDate; [cited October 01, 2009.]; Available from: http://www.uptodate.com.

Mitra, AP (2010) Urine cytologic Analysis: Special Techniques for Bladder Cancer detection:*Connection* 169-177.

Mostofi, F.K. (1975). Pathology of malignant tumors of the urinary bladder. In: The Biology and. Clinical Management of Bladder Cancer. E. H. Cooper & R. E. Williams, eds., Blackwell Scientific Publications, Oxford, London, Edinburgh, Melbourne, pp. 87-109.

Osman, I, .Scher, H.I. Zhang, ZF., Pellicer, I. Hamza, R & Eissa, S.et al.(1997) Alterationsaffecting the p53 control pathway in bilharzial-related bladder cancer. *Clin Cancer Res;* 3:531-536.

Orlow, I., Lianes, P., Lacombe, L., Dalbagni, G., Reuter, V.E. & Cordon- Cardo, C. (1994). Chromosome 9 allelic losses and microsatellite alterations in human bladder tumors. *Cancer Res*. 54, 2848-2851.

O'Brien, P. J. (1988). Radical formation during the peroxidase- catalisedmetabolism of carcinogens and xenobiotics. The reactivity of these adicals with GSH, DNA and unsaturated fatty lipid. *Free RadicalBiol. Med*. 4: 216–226.

Parkin MD, Bray F, Ferlay J, Pisani P (2005) Global cancerstatistics, 2002. *Cancer J Clin* 55:74–108.

Parkin DM.(2006). The global health burden of infection-associated cancers in the year 2002. *Int J Cancer*. 118:3030-3044.

Pycha A, Mian C, Posch B, Haitel A, El Baz M & Ghoneim MA, et al.1(998). Numerical aberrations of chromosomes 7, 9 and 17 in squamous cell and transitional cell cancer of the bladder: a comparative study performed by fluorescence in situ hybridization. *J Urol*.160:737-40.; 7:1269-1274.

Reznikoff C.A., Belair C.D., Yeager T.R., Savelieva E., Blelloch R.H., Puthenveettil J.A. & Cuthill S. (1996). A molecular genetic model of human bladder cancer pathogenesis. *Semin. Oncol*. 23, 571-584.

Sanchez-Carbayo, M., Urrutia, M., Gonzalez de Buitrago, JM. & Navajo, JA..(2001) Utility of serial urinary tumor markers to individualize intervals betwecystoscopies in the monitoring of patients with bladder carcinoma. *Cancer*; 92:2820-2828.

Stein, l.P. Lieskovsky, G.Cote, R & Goshen, S.(2001). Radical cystectomy in the treatment of invasive bladder cancer: long term results in 1054 patients.*Clin Onc*. 19:2001-2006.

Stein, J. Grossfield, C & Ginsberg, D. et al. (1998) Prognostic markers in bladder cancer. A contemporary review of the literature. *J Urol*; 160:645-659.

Steiner, G, .; Schoenberg, MP & Linn, J.F., et al. (1997) Detection of bladder cancer recurrence by microsatellite analysis of urine. *Nat Med*.:3:621-624.

Sliverman D, Devesa S, Moore L & Rothman N. Bladder cancer. (2006).In: Schottenfeld D, Fraumeni FJ eds. Cancer Epidemiology and Prevention. 3rd ed. *Oxford: Oxford University Press*; :1101-1027.

Seripa, D., Parrella, P., Gallucci, M., Gravina, C., Papa, S., Fortunato, P., Alcini, A.Flammia, G., Lazzari, M. & Fazio, V.M. (2001). Sensitive detection of transitional cell carcinoma of the bladder by microsatellite analysis of cells exfoliated in urine. *Int. J. Cancer* 95, 364-369.

Simoneau A.R., Spruck C.H., Gonzalez-Zulueta M., Gonzalgo M.L., Chan M.F., Tsai Y.C., Dean M., Steven K., Horn T. & Jones P.A.(1996). Evidence for two tumor suppressor loci associated with proximal chromosome 9p to q and distal chromosome 9q in bladder cancer and the initial screening for GAS1 and PTC mutations. *Cancer Res*. 56, 5039-5043.

Tamimi, Y., Bringuier, P. P. Smit, F. Bokhoven, A. Abbas, A. Debruyne, F. M. & Schalken, J. A. (1996). Homozygous deletions of p16INK4 occur frequency in bilharziasis-associated bladder cancer. *Int. J. Cancer* 68:183–187.

Theodorescu D. (2003). Molecular pathogenesis of urothelial bladder cancer. *Histol Histopathol* 18: 259-274.

Urinary Tumor Markers for Bladder Cancer Corporate Medical Policy (2011).1 - 6 available from www.bcbsnc.com/.../medicalpolicy/urinary_tumor_markers_for_bladder.

Utting , M., Werner , W., Dahse, R., Schubert , J. & Junker, K. (2002). Microsatellite analysis of free tumor DNA in urine, serum, and plasma of patients: a minimally invasive method for the detection ofbladder cancer. *Clin. Cancer Res*. 8, 35-40.

Weintraub, M. Khaled, HM. Abdel-Rahman, Z, .Bahnasi, A. Eissa, S & Venzon, DJ. et al (1995) p53 mutations in Egyptian bladder cancer. *Int J Oncol*. 7:1269-74.

Wiener, H. G., Vooijs, G. P., van't Hof-Grootenboer, B. (1993).Accuracy of urinary cytology in the diagnosis of primary and recurrent bladder cancer. *Acta Cytol*.; 37(2):163-169.

Weiner, D.P., Koss, L.G., Sablay, B & Freed S.Z.(1997). The prevalence and significance of Brunn's nests, cystitis cystica and squamous metaplasia in normal bladders.*Vrit.J.Urol* 122:317.

Wishahi, M; Mikhail, N. E & Akl, M. (2000*)* c-erbB-2 Expresion in transitional and squamous cell carcinoma of schistosomal urinary bladder:An immunohistochemicaL and clical Study. *Egyptian Journal of* Surgery 19, (4), 255-262.

World Health Organization [homepage on the Internet]. Country Profiles, (2000) Available http://www.emro.who.int/emrinfo/index.

Xu, HJ.; Cairns P. & Hu SX, et al.(1993).Loss of RB protein expression in primary bladder cancer correlates with loss of heterozygosity at the RB locus and tumor progression. *Int J Cancer*. 53:781-784.

Yamamoto, S.; Chen, T.; Murai, T.; Mori, S.; Morimura, K. Oohara, T.Makino, S; Tatematsu, M.; Wanibuchi, H. & Fukushima, S. (1997). Geneticinstability and *p53* mutations in metastatic foci of mouse urinary bladder carcinomas induced by *N*-butyl-*N*-(4-hydroxybutyl) nitrosamine. *Carcinogenesis* 18:1877–1882.

Zaghloul M, Nouh A., Moneer M; Al-Baradie M; Nazmy M & Yunis A. (2008). Time-Trend in Epidemiological and Pathological Features of Schistosoma-Associated Bladder Cancer. *Journal of the Egyptian Nat.Cancer.* 20, (2), 168-174.

Zahran, M.M., Kamel, M, Mooro, H. & Issa, A. (1976) Bilharziasis of the urinary bladder and Ureter, comparative histopathologic Study. *Urology* 8:73.

Zhang, J. Zheng, S., Fan, Z., Gao, Y., Di, X. Wang, D., Xiao, Z. Li, C., An, Q. & Cheng, S. (2001). A comparison between micro satellite analysis and cytology of urine for the detection of bladder cancer. *Cancer Lett.* 172, 55-58.

Zekri A., El-Kabany M & Khaled HM. (1995). Concordance between PCR amplifiable HPV DNA and the presence of inclusion bodies in bilharzial bladder cancer among Egyptians.*Cancer Mol Biol;* 2:441-7.

Zlotta, A & Schulman, C. (2000). Biological markers in superficial bladder tumors and their prognostic significance. *Urol Clinics of North America;* 27:179-189.

Part 5

Epidemiology

8

Imported Schistosomiasis

J. Uberos and A. Jerez-Calero
Pediatrics Service, Universitary Hospital "San Cecilio", Granada
Spain

1. Introduction

Schistosomiasis is a parasitic disease caused by a trematode helminth of the genus *Schistosoma*. Of the latter, only six species affect humans: *S. haematobium, S. mansoni S. japonicum S. intercalatum, S. mekongi* and *S. malayensis*. It is also termed bilharziasis, after its discoverer, the German doctor Theodor Maximilian Bilharz. In 1851, during his work at the Egyptian Department of Hygiene, he discovered this new class of helminth in the vena cava blood of patients who had died of haematuria.

2. Biological cycle of the genus *schistosoma*

Schistosoma has a cylindrical body, ending in two oral suckers. The adult forms are hematophagous, and are found in the venous plexuses, especially the mesenteric or perivesical, in the definitive host, where the male-female pairing takes place. The female migrates to the capillaries and venules, where 100-1000 eggs a day may be deposited. These eggs, in turn, migrate through the walls of the vessels in which they were deposited, reaching the tissues and then either the intestinal lumen or the urinary bladder lumen. Finally, they emerge in the faeces or the urine, respectively. There are two main forms of schistosomiasis: intestinal and urogenital. Among the species that parasitise humans, only *S. haematobium* affects the urogenital apparatus, with the other species normally producing intestinal parasitisation.

Transported in the faeces or urine, the embryo eggs contaminate stagnant water in rivers, lakes and irrigated fields, where in a few hours they hatch and release the miracidia. The latter penetrate and parasitise certain snails that inhabit the fresh water and constitute the intermediary host. Each species of *Schistosoma* parasitises a particular genus of snail, as follows:

- **S. Haematobium:** Bulinus, Physopis, Planorbis.
- **S. mansoni:** Biomphalaria.
- **S. japonicum:** Oncomelania.
- **S. mekongi:** Tricula aperta.
- **S. intercalatu:** Bulinus.
- **S. malayensis:** Tricula aperta.

Within the snail, they mature for approximately 6 weeks to become cercariae (with a bifurcated tail and penetration glands), which are then released back into the water. Humans can become infected by walking, bathing or washing in water contaminated by cercariae, which adhere to the skin and penetrate it. In this process, they lose their tails and are transformed into schistosomulae, which reach the bloodstream and are systemically distributed, reaching the lungs and finally the liver, where they mature into the adult form and attach themselves in their definitive location, the mesenteric or vesical venous plexuses, and thus the cycle is completed. The period between the cercariae penetrating the skin and the beginning of egg production from adult worms is 4-7 weeks. Adult worms can live in the venous plexuses for 20-30 years. Direct transmission between persons does not take place, as the participation of the snail in the biological cycle of this trematode is absolutely necessary.

3. Geographic distribution

Schistosomiasis is the second most prevalent tropical disease, after malaria, and has been included in the World Health Organisation list of 'forgotten' tropical diseases. Its geographic distribution varies according to the species of *Schistosoma*, but it is endemic in 74 countries. Recent studies have calculated that over 95% of cases are concentrated in Africa, especially in sub-Saharan Africa (80%), which is explained by the particular socio-ecological conditions prevailing in these areas, with widespread poverty and a virtual absence of populational health systems. Other endemic areas include Central and South America, the Middle East, and SE Asia (Gryseels et al., 2006).

Worldwide, 800 million people are at risk and over 200 million have been infected, most of them in poor communities without access to clean drinking water or adequate sanitation. Of these, 20 million suffer severe consequences of the infection, although, on the other hand, 120 million are asymptomatic. It has been estimated that intestinal schistosomiasis causes, in Africa alone, over 200,000 deaths a year (130,000 due to portal hypertension).

These are agricultural populations, where contact with infected fresh water occurs constantly, when people walk in stagnant water, or swim in rivers or lakes. The construction of new dams and the extension of irrigation systems are known to multiply the risk of contracting this disease (Steinmann et al., 2006). Children, who may play in infected water, and who often suffer a hygiene deficit, are particularly vulnerable. Also at risk are women who carry out domestic tasks such as washing clothes in these waters. It has been estimated that in chronic cases of vaginal schistosomiasis, the risk of HIV infection is multiplied three-fold (Ndhlovu et al., 2007).

The WHO strategies for controlling schistosomiasis are centred on reducing cases of the disease via periodic, focused treatment with praziquantel. This is a cheap and effective drug, costing only €0.08 per dose. Nevertheless, it may still be expensive for the health administrations of some developing countries. Outbreaks of schistosomiasis can be identified by haematuria screening of schoolchildren and, in cases of epidemic, treating the entire community at risk. Annual doses of praziquantel are sometimes recommended in these areas at high risk of re-infection, and contribute to reducing the severity of symptoms among the chronically sick, and minimising the consequent multi-organ dysfunction. In Egypt, China and Uganda, in just a few years, this approach has reduced the prevalence and intensity of parasitisation, and anaemia (Global Network for Neglected Tropical Diseases; Hotez et al 2010).

Therefore, the international community must be made aware of the social and economic magnitude of the problem. International donations are urgently needed to control this disease, which by its prevalence and severity is greatly hampering the economic advance and sustainable development of many African countries (Baker et al., 2010). Nevertheless, praziquantel is not a panacea, and actions in endemic countries should also include integrated strategies aimed at the identification, monitoring and surveillance of these tropical diseases which, because they are so infrequent in developed countries, are frequently overlooked or ignored (Utzinger et al., 2010). This is the background to the creation of the Global Network for Neglected Tropical Diseases, an initiative aimed at supporting developing countries in their fight against 'forgotten' diseases that affect 1400 million people all over the world. This organisation was inaugurated in 2006 and has its headquarters at the Sabin Vaccine Institute in Washington.

In Africa, refugee movements and migration toward cities, as well as to countries in the developed world, are introducing this disease into previously unaffected areas. Increasing population numbers and the corresponding greater demand for energy and water often give rise to development plans and environmental actions that also contribute to increasing the transmission of the disease. The boom in ecotourism and journeys outside controlled areas are also provoking an increase in the number of tourists with imported schistosomiasis, among all the neglected tropical diseases (López-Vélez et al, 2008).

The GeoSentinel Surveillance Network carried out a transversal study of affected travellers who had visited endemic schistosomiasis areas between 1997 and 2008. Confirmed cases were communicated in 12 countries belonging to this worldwide surveillance network. In a total sample of 25,240, some 410 persons (16 per thousand) were found to be suffering from schistosomiasis; 37% were European, 24% North American, 24% Asian and 15% from Oceania. Over 80% of those affected had acquired this disease in Africa, mainly in sub-Saharan Africa. There were some differences depending of demographic characteristics and the type of travel. Male travelers and travelers < 45 years of age were more likely to be diagnosed with schistosomiasis relative to another illness. When the data were controlled for age and sex, those traveling for missionary or other volunteer work were twice as likely to be diagnosed with schistosomiasis as were tourist and other types of travelers. Business travelers were less likely to be diagnosed with schistosomiasis than were tourists and other types of travelers. Individuals traveling as expatriates, regardless of the type of travel, were twice as likely to be diagnosed with schistosomiasis as those staying for shorter times and staying in hotels. Having a pre-travel consultation was also associated with being diagnosed with schistosomiasis. Sixty-three percent of the 401 ill returned travelers with schistosomiasis presented to a GeoSentinel clinic within six months after travel with a median time-to-presentation of six weeks (IQR 2–12 weeks; The median duration of travel for this group was 13 weeks (IQR 4–33 weeks). One hundred ten (27%) travelers presented to a GeoSentinel clinic more than 6 months after travel. Time-to-presentation was between 6 months and two years for 73 (18%), three to four years for 16 (4%), and five or more years for 18 (4%). 41% of the 319 travelers who were asymptomatic at presentation, were diagnosed with schistosomiasis. The most commonly reported symptoms Gastrointestinal symptoms were fever, genitourinary symptoms, and fatigue. Returned travelers with schistosomiasis were more likely to present with fever than those who were ruled-out for schistosomiasis. Those with *S. haematobium* and *S. mansoni* infections presented with more respiratory symptoms than did those ruled-out for schistosomiasis. Moreover, returned travelers with schistosomiasis who were seen within six months of travel more often presented with fever and respiratory symptoms compared with those who presented later (Nicolls et al., 2008).

Imported travel-related infections were studied in a retrospective and descriptive study of travelers returning from the tropics and attended at the Tropical Medicine Unit, Infectious Diseases Department of Hospital Ramon y Cajal in Madrid (Spain) during the period January 1989 to November 2006. The total number of ill travelers analyzed was 2,982; 1387 traveled to Sub-Saharian Africa and 44 of them were diagnosed with schistosomiasis (3%). A total of 98% of patients with schistosomiasis had traveled to Sub-Saharian Africa and only 2% to other geographical areas. (Zamarrón et al, 2010)

Many centres in Australia routinely screen African refugees for schistosomiasis using serology, and in some cases with faeces and urine examination for schistosome ova. There were a seroprevalence of 38% for 653 African refugee adults and children arriving in Australia, predominantly from Liberia, Burundi, Tanzania and Sudan. A multivariate analysis of the Newcastle data showed that schistosomiasis serology was much more likely to be positive in those from East Africa (OR 14.5) and West Africa (OR 5.5) than from the Sudan region (OR 1.0). (Davis et al., 2007) In those who had faeces and urine examination in these cohorts, urinary schistosomiasis is uncommon, with >95% of those with positive microscopy having S. mansoni in faeces (Australasian Society for Infectious Diseases, 2009).

4. Clinical signs

The clinical manifestations of the disease are produced by the body's inflammatory reaction to the eggs and larvae, as the adult worm eludes the humeral and cell-mediated immune response. In the blood vessels, attempts at migration through the walls may produce haemorrhages and inflammatory processes. When larvae become lodged in the intestinal or vesical tissues, they may provoke granulomas, which in time become calcified. In the intestinal forms, some of the eggs are transported to the portal venous plexuses and may become trapped in the liver, producing periportal fibrosis.

4.1 Acute schistosomiasis

In the cercariae entry zone, pruriginous skin lesions of a macular or macular-papular type may appear, the so-called "swimmer's itch". In persons who have previously been exposed and therefore are sensitised, itching may persist and wheals may be suffered for some days. In endemic zones, this cercarial dermatitis may remain unnoticed.

Katayama fever is a systemic hypersensitivity reaction that appears at 2 to 6 weeks after exposure to and penetration by the cercariae. It is relatively infrequent among the endemic population (due to infradiagnosis or intrauterine sensitisation) and more common among persons who have not been previously exposed, such as tourists who come into contact with contaminated water. It is provoked mainly by the species *S. mansoni* and *S. japonicum*, and less frequently so by *S. haematobium*. The most obvious symptoms coincide with the egg-depositing phase and consist of fever, shivering, swollen lymph nodes, headaches, abdominal pain, bloody diarrhoea and painful swelling of the liver. In addition, respiratory symptoms such as coughing, chest pain or breathing difficulties are often encountered. This process is normally self-limiting in time, with a progressive improvement after several weeks. Only complications derived from massive infestation may lead to death (approximately 0.5% of symptomatic cases).

4.2 Chronic schistosomiasis

Lesions arising from chronic infection are due to eggs that remain trapped in the tissues over a long period of time. These eggs release proteolytic enzymes that typically provoke eosinophilic and granulomatous inflammatory reactions, which are progressively followed by fibrotic deposits. This commonly affects individuals who are continually exposed to infection in poor rural areas. Apart from digestive or urinary manifestations, other less common locations have been reported, such as the lungs, the genitals or the brain.

Among children, the clinical presentation of chronic schistosomiasis varies widely, although cases with a high degree of parasitisation normally present anaemia, malnutrition and delayed growth. Many of these paediatric cases are reversible with appropriate treatment. Moreover, the vertical transmission of the disease by pregnant women has been reported.

4.3 Urogenital schistosomiasis

This condition is produced solely by the species *S. haematobium*. Haematuria is a classical, initial sign of urogenital schistosomiasis. In advanced cases, a frequent sign is urinary-bladder fibrosis, which may in turn provoke hydronephrosis. Symptoms and signs include dysuria, urgent urination, terminal microscopic and macroscopic haematuria, secondary urinary infections and non-specific pelvic pain. Approximately half of all infected children develop moderate-severe pathology of the urinary tract, including pyelonephritis, urethral hydronephrosis, vesical pseudo-papillomas, nephrotic syndrome, etc. Women with urogenital schistosomiasis may present genital lesions, vaginal haemorrhages, dyspareunia or vulvar nodules. Vaginal alterations provoked by chronic schistosome infection may triple the risk of HIV infection. Among men, it may cause disorders of the seminal vesicles and of the prostate and consequent male infertility. Chronic renal insufficiency and squamous cell carcinoma of the bladder are other possible long-term complications.

4.4 Intestinal schistosomiasis

This is produced by the species *S. mansoni, S. japonicum, S. intercalatum* and *S. mekongi*. The areas where it is most commonly found are the mucous membranes of the large intestine and the rectum, where it produces a granulomatous inflammation, with pseudopolyps and microulcerations. Clinical manifestations include colicky abdominal pain, diarrhoea and, sometimes, gastrointestinal blood loss.

4.5 Hepatic schistosomiasis

Hepatic alterations may range from mild inflammation to severe fibrosis. The initial inflammation appears as a periportal pre-sinusoidal reaction to the presence of the eggs and is an important cause of hepatomegaly among children and adolescents (it appears in up to

80% of infected children). In the initial stages, most cases remain asymptomatic. Chronic hepatic schistosomiasis or fibrosis develops years after the original infection and is found more in young adults with intensive, long-term infections and perhaps a certain degree of genetic predisposition. It is the result of a massive deposit of collagen in the periportal spaces, which produces pipe-shaped pathognomonic periportal fibrosis, as described by Symmer (5-10% of patients). In advanced phases, hepatomegaly is frequent, as are ascites and portal hypertension, which with their secondary complications may lead to death (King and Dangerfield-Cha, 2008). Associated with these cases, in addition, may be splenomegaly, esophageal varices and severe haematemesis.

Sometimes other organs are compromised by the systematic embolisation of eggs or following anomalous migration of the adult schistosome. In the lungs, it is not uncommon for this to cause coughing, breathing difficulties and, finally, pulmonary hypertension or cor pulmonale. In the nervous system, the medulla may be the site of infection by *S. mansoni* or *S. haematobium*, provoking transverse myelitis or affecting the medullary cone and the cauda equina. Encephalic effects are only produced by *S. japonicum* and usually involve epileptic symptoms or diffuse encephalitis, following the formation of cerebral granulomas.

5. Diagnosis

In Spain and in other countries bordering the Mediterranean, immigration has increased in recent years. According to data published by the Spanish National Institute of Statistics, in the year 2000 the immigrant population constituted 2.7% of the population, while in 2007, there were 4.5 million immigrants, making up 12.7% of the population. Over 50% of the immigrant population comes from areas with a high prevalence of schistosomiasis: 39% from Latin America and 14% from sub-Saharan Africa (Instituto Nacional de Estadística, 2010). In Spain and other European countries, the absence of intermediate hosts, together with generally good healthcare conditions, makes infection here almost impossible, and there is no risk of transmission within the population. The high prevalence of schistosomiasis in some countries in sub-Saharan Africa, together with rising rates of immigration, has led to more and more cases of urinary schistosomiasis being reported in many European countries. Investigation of cases of long-term haematuria often reveals a background of journeys to endemic areas, and in such cases a fresh urine examination may be requested. These data demonstrate the need to consider schistosomiasis in the differential diagnosis of hematuria in daily practice in primary care in developed countries. There are references to urinary schistosomiasis among immigrants arriving from endemic areas or following prolonged stays in the above countries, involving contact with contaminated water (Uberos et al., 2010).

During the stage of larval invasion or migration, clinical symptoms respond to the laying of eggs and the formation of soluble antigens. This is characteristic of *S. mansoni* and may last up to three months. It is characterised by periportal fibrosis, portal hypertension and enlargement of the liver and spleen, with high fever, fatigue, urticaria, swollen lymph nodes and eosinophilia. There may also be abdominal pain, weight loss and diarrhoea. The presence of eosinophilia among the immigrant population is almost always due to infection by helminths (Corachan, 2002). Eosinophilia is defined as a total eosinophil count exceeding

$440x10^6$/ml. Various studies (Bierman et al., 2005) have estimated that eosinophilia affects 40-65% of patients. When the egg-laying stage is attained, the clinical pattern is characterised by fever, coughing, shivering, urticaria, abdominal pain, adenopathy and enlarged spleen, which occurs at 1 to 2 months following infection and may last for over 3 months. This symptomatic complex is known as the Katayama syndrome.

Months or years after the beginning of parasitisation there may occur granulomatous reactions and fibrosis in the organs affected, including mild effects in the gastrointestinal tract with epigastralgia and diarrhoea, or chronic polyps, bloody diarrhoea, haematemesis and enlarged spleen. In the urogenital tract, *S. haematobium* is associated with haematuria, pollakiuria, suprapubic pain and thickening of the vesical wall, hydroureter or hydronephrosis. Cases of neuroschistosomiasis have also been reported. Histological lesions of the schistosomes result from the deposition of eggs in the tissues, where they may provoke the formation of granulomas, hyperplasia of the mucous membranes and the formation of nodules and polyps that tend to ulcerate and bleed.

In many cases, there is haematuria, with the emission of several drops of fresh blood at the end of every urination. In general, no fever or dysuria is reported. In Spain, the existence of parasitisation by *S. haematobium* is frequently revealed when patients seek treatment for persistent haematuria, which is addressed by serial urine culture and empirical antibiotic treatment. In these cases, careful consideration of the patient's background, together with evidence of journeys made in recent months to endemic zones, should guide the physician's diagnosis.

Classic parasitological techniques (analysis of sediment) are available to any laboratory, are easy and cheap, but time consuming and require experience of the observer. They also have a low sensitivity for diagnosis. Direct parasitological diagnosis is performed by examination of eggs in the faeces (the Kato-Katz technique) or in 24-hour urine. The presence of eggs in the intestinal mucosa may also be investigated, by biopsy. At present, the Kato-Katz technique is the most frequently recommended, and this is preferred by the WHO both for individual diagnostic studies and for epidemiological investigation. Moreover, it is used to determine the prevalence and intensity of soil-transmitted helminthiasis. In addition, it is useful for establishing the relation between the number of eggs in the faeces and the quantity of adult parasites in the infected host. This information is essential for determining the parasite load in the patient.

Schistosomiasis may be hard to diagnose in patients with a low parasite load and scant excretion of eggs, when microscope identification is difficult. Live parasites produce and excrete many protein compounds in the different phases of the parasitic cycle. Immunodiagnostic techniques are based on the detection of these proteins or antibodies formed against them, being more sensitive than conventional ones. The detection of circulating antigens difference between active and past infection, and correlate with the intensity of infection, morbidity and severity.

Serological diagnosis may be useful for cases of acute schistosomiasis in areas where it is not endemic (Tarp et al., 2000). When serological results are positive, another search for *Schistoma* eggs should be made. When the results of the serological examination are negative, it can be assumed that in non-endemic areas the risk of schistosomiasis is very low. The determination of antibodies allows early diagnosis of the disease. While not opposed to an actual infection of another pass, since the antibodies can be kept at high titers for months or even years. Serology requires a period of six weeks for positivisation.

Serological diagnosis can be carried out using indirect immunofluorescence techniques and ELISA. The following in vivo precipitation techniques are applied:

a. Vogel-Minning technique (circum-cercarial precipitin test - CCPT). With this technique, the cercariae are brought into contact with the patient's serum. If the serum produces specific antibodies, the presence of a highly specific precipitate can be observed, due to the intervention of cercarial metabolic antigens.
b. Oliver-Gonzalez technique (circum-oval precipitin test - COPT). This technique is identical to the previous one, except that live eggs are used.

By means of these techniques, it is possible to determine the evolution of the disease. For example, for recent schistosomiasis, the CCPT technique is used.

Image testing (ultrasound imaging, urography, etc.) can be very useful. For digestive schistosomiasis, rectal or liver biopsy and colonoscopy may also be useful. Most methods used to evaluate the success of interventions, such as egg counting, measure the level of infection but do not provide direct evidence of the pathological changes induced by the infection. Ultrasound is an excellent tool for assessing the secondary pathological alterations produced by the infection. The prevalence and severity of the pathological lesions detected by ultrasound are related to the intensity of the infection, evaluated by the quantity of eggs eliminated in the faeces or urine. In endemic zones, the maximum rate of morbidity is observed among children aged 7-14 years, while in non-endemic zones, the disease is diagnosed in all series following an evolution of 2-3 months. The lesions most often diagnosed by ultrasound include hydronephrosis, the presence of intravesical masses, thickening of the bladder wall and calcification, with the appearance of hydronephrosis being associated with the poorest prognosis. Some series have identified lesions to the female genital apparatus, with masses identifiable by ultrasound examination. An association has been shown between epidermoid carcinoma of the bladder and *S. haematobium* (Corachan, 2002).

Ultrasound may be useful for diagnosing periportal fibrosis and portal hypertension (dilation of the portal and splenic veins and the portosystemic collaterals). Treatment for intestinal schistosomiasis generally produces an improvement in the signs of infection, including reduced bloody diarrhoea, intestinal polyposis, hepatosplenomegaly and periportal fibrosis.

6. Treatment

Following confirmation of urinary schistosomiasis, the treatment normally prescribed is oral praziquantel at a dose of 600 mg/12 h, in two doses. The analytical analysis is repeated, 15 days following this treatment, by determining the eosinophil count in blood and by a serial examination of fresh urine samples, on three consecutive days, with the presence of *S. haematobium* in urine being discounted when haemogram results are normal. *S. haematobium* is the most frequent cause of haematuria in countries where this disease is endemic. All protocols for treating immigrant children include the search for *S. haematobium* when persistent haematuria is reported. We believe this search should be expanded to cases of persistent haematuria when there is a case history of bathing or swimming in rivers in zones endemic for *S. haematobium*. The existence of haematuria is related with the presence of viable eggs in the bladder wall, which in long-term processes is in turn related with the presence of granulomas in the vesical submucosa and the distal part of the urethra (Tzanetou et al., 2007). In cases of repeated, severe infection, the urethral mucosa are also affected, and this may evolve to obstructive uropathology and hydronephrosis. The preferred treatment in this case is praziquantel at a dose of 40 mg/kg/day, in two doses at intervals of 12 hours. At this dose, the cure rate at six weeks is 88%. The administration of a second dose of praziquantel at 4-6 weeks increases the cure rate to 100% (Midzi et al., 2008). To prevent resistance, some authors recommend a dose of praziquantel at 60 mg/kg/8 h, for three days (Botros et al., 2005). During their immature stages, the schistosomes are moderately resistant to praziquantel, becoming more sensitive on maturity, when the eggs are laid. This means that during the first 10-12 weeks following infection by *S. haematobium*, praziquantel may not be effective (Botros et al., 2005). As an alternative treatment for *S. haematobium*, metrifonate or niridazol may be applied.

Metrifonate is a reversible competitive inhibitor of the acetylcholinesterase enzyme, including the human enzyme. As such, it is a parasympathetic mimetic agent that prolongs the action of the parasympathetic nervous system, and in which the neurotransmitter is acetylcholine. It performs selective, variable schistosomocidal activity against *S. haematobium*, provoking its partial metabolisation into dichlorvos, an active anti-cholinesterase compound. The cholinesterase of the schistosome is more susceptible to this metabolite than that of the human host, but at the recommended treatment dose, transitory reductions in cholinesterase activity, both in plasma and in erythrocytes can be observed. Despite early concerns expressed about its possible toxicity, metrifonate is well tolerated and has been widely employed, with good results in important treatment programmes. A dose of 7.5 mg/kg, taken on three occasions, at intervals of two weeks, produces a 40-80% cure rate. Mass chemotherapy should not be undertaken in communities recently exposed to insecticides or other agricultural chemicals with an anti-cholinesterase action. Treated patients should not be given depolarizing neuromuscular blocking agents such as suxamethonium until at least 48 hours have elapsed from the time of metrifonate administration. If necessary, to alleviate the symptoms of cholinergic activity, atropine sulphate can be used as a specific antidote (for adults, 1 mg every six hours). This measure does not impair the anti-parasitic action.

Niridazol is absorbed slowly from the gastrointestinal tract in 10-15 hours. It metabolises rapidly during its first pass through the liver, and its metabolites are eliminated in equal quantities in the urine and faeces. Schistomocidal activities are produced because niridazol is not metabolised in the blood. The normal dose for adults infected with *S. haematobium* or *S. mansoni* is 25 mg/kg/day, for seven days. For children infected with *S. haematobium*, the treatment duration may be reduced to 5 days if a daily dose of 30-35 mg/kg is administered. Children infected with *S. mansoni* should be treated with 25 mg/kg/day for seven days. In bilharziasis caused by *S. japonicum*, the daily dose for both adults and children is 20-25 mg/kg for five days.

As the recommended treatment for intestinal schistosomiasis (*S. mansoni*), both in the acute phase and when the liver and spleen are affected, we propose oxamniquine. This is a tetrahydroquinoline derivative with selective, variable schistosomocidal activity against *S. mansoni*. Male schistosomes are more susceptible than females, but the females that survive cease to lay eggs after exposure to oxamniquine and become irrelevant from a pathological standpoint. Some varieties are resistant, especially in South America, although these respond to subsequent treatment with praziquantel. Oxamniquine is well absorbed when administered orally and generally metabolises to inactive acid metabolites that are eliminated in the urine. It is well tolerated and has been widely used with good results in control programmes carried out in South America.

7. Control measures against schistosomiasis

The aim of control programmes is to reduce morbidity. In 1922, after the discovery of the role played by snails in transmission of the disease, strategies were developed consisting in the primary control of snails in highly endemic areas. From 1960, new technologies were discovered to achieve the same goal; on the one hand, niclosamide, was applied to eliminate the snails, and on the other, praziquantel was found to be a safe treatment option with few secondary effects. Countries such as Egypt, with high rates of endemic schistosomiasis, have developed control programmes including annual checkups for school-age children and treatment for all suspected cases, together with programmes to control snail infestation by the drainage and cleaning of all rivers and canals (Salem et al., 2011). Thanks to these measures, by the end of 2002, the prevalence of *S. mansoni* had been reduced to 2.7%, from the value of 14.8% recorded in 1993. Similarly, the prevalence of *S. haematobium* fell from 6.6% in 1993 to 1.2% in 2006. This method reduced morbidity, but in other areas, improved water supply has also led to low levels of prevalence.

In countries of origin, it seems reasonable that the primary objective in the control of schistosomiasis consists in reducing morbidity, or at least severe forms of the disease. The imported forms of the disease appears early diagnosis key to disease, in environments where the low prevalence of the disease complicates the diagnosis. The importance of history, focusing on the existence of previous residence or travel in endemic areas seems essential.

In the communities of African immigrants, is often found that more than one family member is parasitized and hematuria, if not too intensive, is an inconspicuous sign for the patient or their relatives. This fact illustrates the need to subject these patients to a series of systematic reviews of health in destination countries to establish not only the diagnosis of imported diseases as the present one, but also those others present in our midst and very frequent in the geographic area of origin.

8. References

Baker, M.C., E.Mathieu, F.M.Fleming, M.Deming, J.D.King, A.Garba, J.B.Koroma, M.Bockarie, A.Kabore, D.P.Sankara, and D.H.Molyneux. 2010. Mapping, monitoring, and surveillance of neglected tropical diseases: towards a policy framework. *Lancet* 375:231-238.

Bierman, W.F., J.C.Wetsteyn, and G.T.van. 2005. Presentation and diagnosis of imported schistosomiasis: relevance of eosinophilia, microscopy for ova, and serology. *J. Travel. Med.* 12:9-13.

Botros, S., L.Pica-Mattoccia, S.William, N.El-Lakkani, and D.Cioli. 2005. Effect of praziquantel on the immature stages of Schistosoma haematobium. *International Journal for Parasitology* 35:1453-1457.

Corachan, M. 2002. Schistosomiasis and international travel. *Clin. Infect. Dis.* 35:446-450.

Gryseels, B., K.Polman, J.Clerinx, and L.Kestens. 2006. Human schistosomiasis. *Lancet* 368:1106-1118.

Global Network for Neglected Tropical Diseases. http://www.globalnetwork.org/ Acces June, 16 2011.

Hotez P, Engels D, Fenwick A, Savioli L. 2010.Africa is desperate for praziquantel. Lancet. 376, Issue 9740: 496-8

Instituto Nacional de Estadística. Encuesta nacional de inmigrantes 2007. www.ine.es/inebmenu/mnu_migrac.htm . Acces June, 16 2010.

López-Vélez R, Pérez Molina JA, Zamarrón P, Pérez de Ayala A. Enfermedades infecciosas importadas por viajeros internacionales a los trópicos. 2008. Ministerio de Sanidad y Consumo. Gobierno de España.

King, C.H., and M.Dangerfield-Cha. 2008. The unacknowledged impact of chronic schistosomiasis. *Chronic Illn.* 4:65-79.

Midzi, N., D.Sangweme, S.Zinyowera, M.P.Mapingure, K.C.Brouwer, N.Kumar, F.Mutapi, G.Woelk, and T.Mduluza. 2008. Efficacy and side effects of praziquantel treatment against Schistosoma haematobium infection among primary school children in Zimbabwe. *Transactions of the Royal Society of Tropical Medicine and Hygiene* 102: 759-766.

Ndhlovu, P.D., T.Mduluza, E.F.Kjetland, N.Midzi, L.Nyanga, S.G.Gundersen, H.Friis, and E.Gomo. 2007. Prevalence of urinary schistosomiasis and HIV in females living in a rural community of Zimbabwe: does age matter? *Trans. R. Soc. Trop. Med Hyg.* 101:433-438.

Nicolls, D.J., L.H.Weld, E.Schwartz, C.Reed, S.F.von, D.O.Freedman, and P.E.Kozarsky. 2008. Characteristics of schistosomiasis in travelers reported to the GeoSentinel Surveillance Network 1997-2008. *Am. J. Trop. Med Hyg.* 79:729-734.

Zamarrón Fuertes P, Pérez-Ayala A, Pérez Molina JA, Norman FF, Monge-Maíllo B, Navarro M, López-Vélez R. Clinical and epidemiological characteristics of imported infectious diseases in Spanish travelers. J Travel Med. 2010 Sep;17(5): 303-9.

Davis JS, Webber MT. A prospective audit of 215 newly arrived African refugees. J Paediatr Child Health 2007;42:A11

Australasian Society for Infectious Diseases. Diagnosis, management and prevention of infections in recently arrived refugees. Dreamweaver Publishing Pty Ltd. 2009. ISBN 978-0-9750-483-4-4.

Salem, S., R.E.Mitchell, A.El-Alim El-Dorey, J.A.Smith, and D.A.Barocas. 2011. Successful control of schistosomiasis and the changing epidemiology of bladder cancer in Egypt. *BJU. Int.* 107:206-211.

Steinmann, P., J.Keiser, R.Bos, M.Tanner, and J.Utzinger. 2006. Schistosomiasis and water resources development: systematic review, meta-analysis, and estimates of people at risk. *Lancet Infect. Dis.* 6:411-425.

Tarp, B., F.T.Black, and E.Petersen. 2000. The immunofluorescence antibody test (IFAT) for the diagnosis of schistosomiasis used in a non-endemic area. *Trop. Med. Int. Health* 5:185-191.

Tzanetou, K., G.Adamis, E.Andipa, C.Zorzos, K.Ntoumas, K.Armenis, G.Kontogeorgos, E.Malamou-Lada, and P.Gargalianos. 2007. Urinary tract Schistosoma haematobium infection: a case report. *J Travel. Med* 14:334-337.

Uberos, J., M.Gamarra, E.Prados, and E.Narbona-Lopez. 2010. Importance of anamnesis in the diagnosis of urinary schistosomiasis.. *An. Pediatr.* (Barc.) 73:214-216.

Utzinger, J., E.K.N'goran, C.R.Caffrey, and J.Keiser. 2010. From innovation to application: Social-ecological context, diagnostics, drugs and integrated control of schistosomiasis. *Acta Trop.* (doi:10.1016/j.actatropica.2010.08.020).

9

Epidemiology of Schistosomiasis Mansoni in Brazil

Maria José Conceição and José Rodrigues Coura
[1]Faculdade de Medicina da Universidade Federal do Rio de Janeiro-UFRJ,. Doctor- Serviço de Doenças Infecciosas e Parasitárias-Hospital Universitário Clementino Fraga Filho, Departamento de Medicina Preventiva da Faculdade de Medicina- UFRJ, Professor from Curso de Pós-Graduação em Doenças Infecciosas e Parasitárias-UFRJ
[2]Fundação Oswaldo Cruz- Fiocruz- Ministério da Saúde-Brasil. Laboratório de Doenças Parasitárias
Brasil

1. Introduction

The present chapter emphasized the historical aspects of *Schistosoma mansoni* infection in Brazil. It was introduced in the state of Bahia, possibly during the traffic of slaves infected by the parasite, and the disordered migratory movements from Northeast region towards the Southeast and South regions contributed significantly for infection expansion; another contributing factor was the sugar cane culture. The sectional and longitudinal surveys pointed out high levels of prevalence and morbidity due to aspects related to race, age, sex, occupation, parasite load, specific treatment and reinfection. Treatment with oxamniquine has been shown non-responsive in groups of patients, and the use of praziquantel for more than three decades has begun to reveal therapeutic failure. Support for the researches about new drugs is critical. The decrease in the prevalence rates as well as in the severe forms, though without reaching the transmission control goals, should be considered an alert sign for schistosomiasis not being neglected in the country.

The Brazilien authors have concluded in different endemic areas of Brazil that the indices of prevalence and morbidity are reducing, however the transmission control keeps the same high levels. On recommend the implementation of multiple measures as people should continue to receive treatment, improve sanitation conditions, potable water supply, and education in health, besides to avoid the frequent reinfections.

2. Key results

This chapter aims to provide some advances in reducing the rates of prevalence and morbidity of Schistosomiasis mansoni in many areas in Brazil, including Minas Gerais, Bahia, Pernambuco, Alagoas, Paraíba, Rio Grande do Norte and Sergipe, since these areas present high prevalence and severe hepatosplenic clinical forms.

The introduction of a Special Program for Schistosomiasis Control based on mass chemoprophylaxis, in 1976, changed the disease course. Sectional and longitudinal studies

developed by Brazilian researchers have contributed considerably for that purpose, due to specific treatment, education for health, and use of molluscicides in some areas.
Reinfection has been identified as one of the main factors related to the failure of infection transmission control.

3. Objectives

This chapter aims to analyze:
1. The source of infection by *S. mansoni* in Brazil, and the factors that led to its expansion toward vast areas of the territory,
2. The contribution of studies developed by Brazilian authors in different endemic areas and their impact on disease current situation,
3. Specific treatment with Oxamniquine or Praziquantel, and patients that present treatment failure.

4. Research methods

The research methods used for preparing this Chapter were based on articles written by our group and by other authors in literature on the topic Epidemiology of Schistosomiasis in Brazil, which were published in journals, national and international books, Master and Ph.D thesis, available at Internet, at Oswaldo Cruz Foundation-Fiocruz Libraries, and at the Faculty of Medicine of Federal University of Rio de Janeiro-UFRJ. Protocols and records used in clinic and in endemic areas, with the inhabitants clinical specifications and socio-economic conditions, with the sanitary situation of residences, maps with residences numbers, water streams localization and the specification of the productive seasons of mollusks of genus *Biomphalaria spp*. It also employed the statistical analysis methods for evaluating whether the results obtained presented significant differences.

4.1 The source of infection by *S. mansoni* in Brazil, and the factors that led to its expansion toward vast areas of the territory

Data on infection by *Schistosoma mansoni* in Brazil, a disease that affects around six million people, have obtained, since its initial phase, high emphasis in international scientific literature, due to the great number of affected municipalities. The increasing infection rates are directly related to the disorderly migratory movements that brought many inhabitants, especially those from the northeastern states towards the southeastern and south regions, creating new foci of infection in areas yet unaffected (Neiva 1947). The presence of the intermediate hosts *Biomphalaria glabrata, B. tenagophyla* and *B. straminea* in these regions facilitated the maintenance of the infection. It was emphasized the high prevalence, besides the severity and diversity of clinical forms, affecting mainly the age groups that were in productive phase. A follow-up study of fifteen-years was carried out in a locality of Paracambi.
It is estimated that, in Brazil, the disease has been introduced in Bahia, soon after the country discovery (1500), through the commerce of slaves infected by the parasite. Pirajá da Silva (1908) is considered the discoverer of *Schistosoma mansoni* in South America, after assisting an infected patient, at Bahia. Since 1904, he observed a lateral spicule in the worm eggs found in the feces of his patients, differently from the terminal spicule seen in eggs of *Schistosoma haematobium,* registered at that time, in Egypt, in patients with hematuria,

characterizing schistosomiasis haematobium. Lutz confirmed its initial discovery as he found out, during the autopsies of patients who passed away due to severe infection by *S. mansoni,* female mated worms, in the portal vein, with egg-endowed lateral spicule. In 1919, Lutz described the evolving forms of the parasite.

Uncontrolled migration may be related to outbreaks of *S. mansoni* focus in the northeast of the State of Santa Catarina (Schlemper Junior et al. 1996), and in the Southern most Brazilian State, Rio Grande do Sul (Graeff-Teixeira et al. 1999).

The transmission of *S. mansoni* infection in some touristic rural places in endemic areas of Minas Gerais was detected in 17 people with toxemic form of the disease, after a bath in a swimming pool, where there was infected *B. glabrata* (Enk et al. 2004). Also in Minas Gerais, Massara et al. (2008) confirmed the diagnosis of schistosomiasis infection in visitors who frequented ecotourism area. In a touristic beach of Pernambuco, Brazil, Barbosa et al. (2001) described an outbreak of acute schistosomiasis.

A follow-up study of fifteen-years was carried out in a locality of State of Rio de Janeiro, aiming to evaluate *S. mansoni* prevalence between 1360 inhabitants. The results showed 1.0%, of positivity. The authors concluded that over the years, it remained as a low prevalence area (Igreja et al. 2010). Other areas in the Rio de Janeiro State, also presented low infection levels reached and maintained by *Nectomys squamipes* rodents (Soares et al. 1995).

4.2 The contribution of studies developed by Brazilian authors in different endemic areas and their impact on the current situation of disease

Since 1908 there was two main stages regarding the disease study in Brazil. One aimed to detect the prevalence of infection and its clinical manifestations, and the other intended to understand the evolution of infection in the different areas over the years, as well as the main determining factors for the severity of clinical forms. Penna, cited by Lutz (1916), reported the infection in the School for Sailors, in Rio de Janeiro, which received students coming from Bahia, Sergipe, Alagoas and Rio Grande do Norte, but mostly from Sergipe and Pernambuco (Lutz and Penna, 1918).

After that Maciel (1925), studying a group of sailors, found higher rates in those originated from Alagoas (34.6%), in comparison to those from Sergipe (32.7%), Bahia (23%), and finally Minas Gerais (2.9%). Cançado (1929) defined the main foci of infection in Minas Gerais. In 1937, Gilberto Freyre analyzed the main foci of infection in Pernambuco and Bahia, and the interference of sugar cane culture zones on the infection expansion, highlighting the intense migratory movements and the impact of disease spreading. He emphasized ¨the dissemination route¨ toward Southeast and South regions, through infected individuals coming from the Northeast, Bahia and Minas Gerais.

Different epidemiological investigations unfolded, as Martins & Versiani (1938) in Minas Gerais; Meira (1947) in migrants settled in São Paulo; Pellon & Teixeira (1950) in students of 11 states (they were the first to delimit the endemic areas in the country); and Pessoa & Barros (1953) who conducted a survey with 1500 inhabitants of Sergipe.

Longitudinal studies were initiated by Jansen (1946), who assessed the prevalence of *S. mansoni* in a population of Pernambuco, between 1937 and 1941, and started to treat children and adults with antimonial drugs. Sette (1953), in a review of the same group, from 1942 to 1951, revealed that 1.7% of treated individuals developed hepatosplenic form, while this rate reached 9.9% in the untreated group. Brener and Mourão (1953) worked in five different areas of Minas Gerais, which were reviewed ten years later, by Katz & Brener (1966). These authors found that less than 10% of hepatointestinal forms evolved to hepatosplenic forms, and among these, 25% had decompensation. Klöetzel & Klöetzel (1958), and Klöetzel (1966), in a municipality of Pernambuco, followed inhabitants evolutionarily, correlating severe clinical forms to higher parasite load. He concluded, in an original way, that chemoprophylaxis, in children and adolescents under severe risk of infection, constituted an effective measure for preventing progression to severe clinical forms. In 1958, Barbosa (1966) began to study four localities in Pernambuco, and only in one of them he introduced sanitation measures and use of molluscicides. In comparison with the others, it was observed a significant reduction of infection. Prata & Bina (1968) in Bahia, found no decrease in prevalence after five successive reviews.

Since 1974, Coura et al. (1984) conducted evolutionary surveys, involving 3782 inhabitants from four counties of Rio Doce and Jequitinhonha Valleys, Minas Gerais, of which 47.3% were infected and 78.4% were treated, with infection recurrence and reduction of parasite load in all municipalities. Also in Minas Gerais, Conceição & Borges-Pereira (2002), Conceição et al. (2007), following up, in evolutionary terms, individuals for a period up to 30 years, in the longer term study conducted in Brazil, found out that there were decrease in prevalence and hepatosplenic forms, although without success in the transmission control, attributed to reinfections. These results corroborate the conclusions presented by Andrade (1998) pointing out a remarkable improvement in the scenario of disease prevalence and severe forms in Brazil.

Klöetzel (1992) in a district of Alagoas concluded that the transmission was primarily peridomestic through the pollution of open ditches and some collections of water that required modest investments for the control. The measures have brought about the decline in the prevalence of schistosomiasis in the Northeast Brazil.

In Minas Gerais, from 2008 to 2010, in two areas located in Rio Doce and Jequitinhonha Valleys, Carlôto (2011) showed in a total of 288 and 257 inhabitants, 22,9% and 20,2 %, respectively, of infection. It was emphasized the high prevalence rates, mainly in males and young people, besides a low intensity of infection, and the lack of sanitary conditions that indicated towards immediate control actions in both areas, including education in health.

In a recent study carried out in one area of Maranhão, Brazil, Santos & Melo (2011) observed a schistosomiasis prevalence of 3.2% and 8.3 % of positivity in *B. glabrata*, raising control measures in the area. Drumond et al. (2010) have emphasized the program of surveillance for schistosomiasis control in Minas Gerais, Brazil, and the improvement related to the morbidity. Clinical and histopathological contributions came from the studies of Lenzi et al. (1998), Cheever et al. (2002), and Lambertucci et al. (2005), respectively. An important advance in the understanding of the intermediate hosts of the infection has been achieved by Carvalho et al. (2008), and Paraense (2008).

In the Fig. 1 are represented the nineteen States of Brazil with transmission of *S. mansoni* infection. The states of Northeast present the highest levels of prevalence alongside the states of Bahia and Minas Gerais. Some states have foci of infection, and are not endemic areas, like Rio Grande do Sul, Santa Catarina, Paraná, São Paulo, Distrito Federal, Rio de Janeiro, Piauí, Maranhão and Pará.

Figure 2 shows the prevalence of *S. mansoni* in a municipality of Minas Gerais, Brazil, studied by our working group up for more than thirty years, is observed on an ongoing basis the highest prevalence rates in males compared to females.

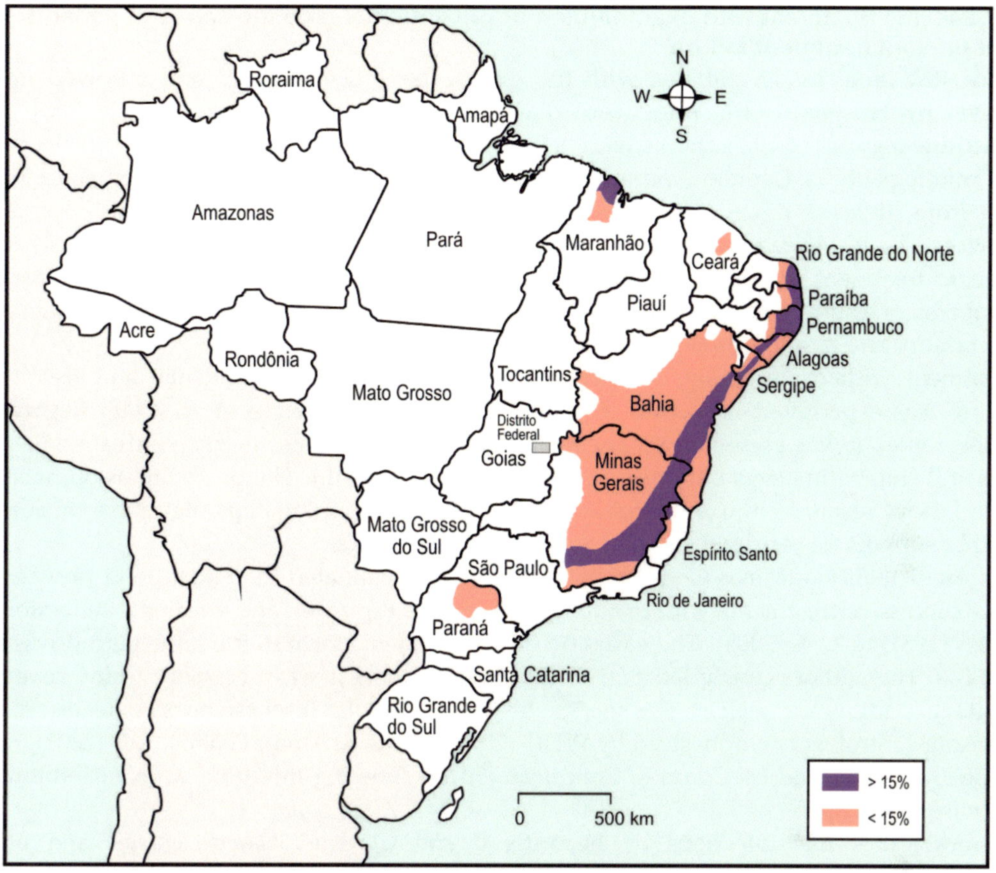

Fig. 1. States of Brazil with transmission of *S. mansoni* infection

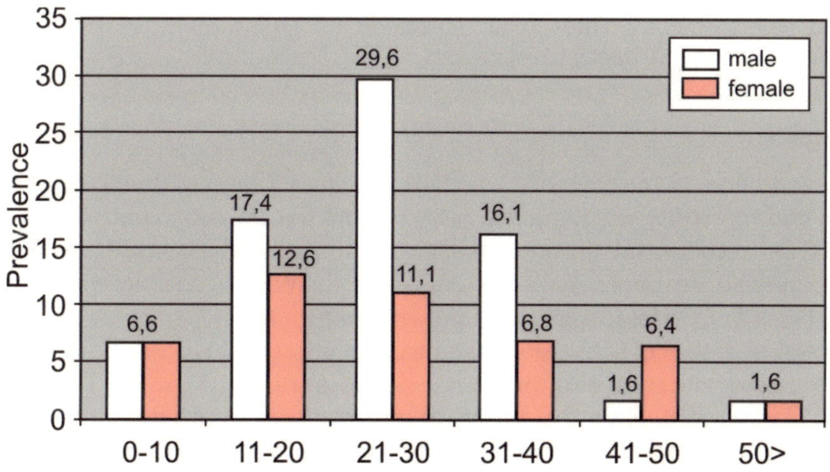

Fig. 2. Prevalence of *Schistosoma mansoni* in a Municipality of Minas Gerais, Brazil, according to age and gender.

4.3 Specific treatment with oxamniquine or praziquantel, and the cases of patients that present treatment failure

Since 1978 until today, patients with the disease have been treated and followed up at University Hospital-UFRJ. They were diagnosed in the period from 1985 to 2001 and constitute a group of 102 patients with hepatosplenomegaly, of which 63% were male, from the municipality of Capitão Andrade, Minas Gerais (n=26), where we worked since 1973, and from different Brazilian regions (n=76). It must be emphasized that young patients between 11 and 14 years old, with splenomegaly, showed regression of the spleen, only with specific treatment. In the other cases, surgical indications were due to gastrointestinal hemorrhage resultant from esophageal varices rupture, hypersplenism, abdominal pain and discomfort, and hypogonadism (Conceição et al. 2002).

Treatment with oxamniquine showed no response in 10.3% of patients, and treatment failure was experimentally confirmed (Katz et al. 1973, Conceição et al. 2000). Regarding praziquantel, it was presented a patient that underwent to three successive treatments and was still eliminating eggs of *S. mansoni* (Conceição et al. 2010). The publications on patients with lack of response to oxamniquine and, more recently, to praziquantel must encourage further support for researches on the synthesis of new drugs.

In a municipality of Minas Gerais, Sarvel et al. (2011) evaluated the variation of prevalence after successive treatments with oxamniquine and praziquantel, and verified a reduction of 70.4% (1981) to 1.7% (2005). The variation of hepatosplenic form in the same period was 7% to 1.3%. The authors concluded that to reach best results it was necessary to improve the sanitary conditions as well as give specific treatment. Similar discussions on schistosomiasis mansoni control were emphasized by WHO (2002), Coura & Amaral (2005), Rey (2007), Katz & Coelho (2008), and by Coura & Conceição (2010), showing the Brazilian contribution on the clinical therapy.

Co-morbidities like infections by hepatitis B and C virus, *Salmonella spp.* and other enterobacteria may add worse prognostic in the clinical evolution of schistosomiasis. The follow-up study of ten patients, including one who was eleven years old, infected by *S. mansoni* and *Salmonela infantum,* revealed prolonged fever, abdominal pain, diarrhoea, hepato and splenomegaly. There was regression of symptoms after treatment of both infections (Conceição et al. 2009).

5. Conclusion

The Brazilien authors have concluded in different endemic areas of Brazil that the indices of prevalence and morbidity are reducing, however the transmission control keeps the same high levels. On recommend the implementation of multiple measures as people should continue to receive treatment, improve sanitation conditions, potable water supply, and education in health, besides to avoid the frequent reinfections.

The transmission control of Schistosomiasis mansoni infection in Brazil did not improve and that has been showed in nineteen different endemic areas of the country and in areas with focal transmission. Although the levels of prevalence and morbidity have presented reduction, on emphasize the necessity of the widest prevention measures acting on all elements of the natural history of disease: the agent, host and environment. Preventing schistosomiasis has been overlooked and created health problems, mainly with the population of the rural areas.

6. References

Andrade Z 1998. The situation of hepatosplenic Schistosomiasis in Brazil. Mem Inst Oswaldo Cruz 93 (Suppl. I): 58-75.

Barbosa 1966. Morbidade da Esquistossomose. Estudo em quatro localidades no Estado de Pernambuco. Rev Bras Malar D Trop 3: 3-159.

Barbosa CS, Domingues ALC, Abath F, Montenegro SML, Guida U, Carneiro J. 2001. Epidemia de esquistossomose aguda na praia de Porto de Galinhas, Pernambuco, Brasil. Cad. Saúde Pública. 17: 725- 8.

Brener Z, Mourão OG. 1953. Inquéritos clínico-epidemiológicos em focos endêmicos de esquistossomose mansoni. Rev Bras Malar D Trop 8: 519-526.

Cançado JR. 1947. Contribuição ao estudo da Esquistossomose mansônica no Brasil. Dados relativos à má distribuição de renda no Brasil. Rev Bras. Med. 31 (1): 31 -35.

Carlôto AE. 2011. Avaliação Diagnóstica da Infecção por *Schistosoma mansoni* em duas áreas rurais de Minas Gerais: Comunidade São João, no Vale do Jequitinhonha, e Capitão Andrade, no Vale do Rio Doce. MSc Thesis. Curso de Pós-Graduação em Doenças Infecciosas e Parasitárias da Faculdade de Medicina da UFRJ. 57 pp.

Carvalho OS, Amaral RS, Dutra LV, Scholte RGC, Guerra MAM. 2008. Distribuição Espacial de *Biomphalaria glabrata, B. straminea e B. tenagophila*-Hospedeiros Intermediários de *Schistosoma mansoni* no Brasil. In: Carvalho OS, Coelho PMZ, Lenzi HL (org.), *Schistosoma mansoni e esquistossomose: uma visão multidisciplinar*, Editora Fiocruz, 1ª ed. Rio de Janeiro, p. 493-518.

Cheever AW, Lenzi JA, Lenzi HL, Andrade ZA. 2002. Experimental models of Schistosoma mansoni infection. Mem Inst Oswaldo Cruz. 2002. 97(7): 917-40.

Conceição MJ, Argento CA, Corrêa A.. 2000. Study of *Schistosoma mansoni* Isolates from Patients with Failure of Treatment with Oxamniquine. Mem Inst Oswaldo Cruz, Rio de Janeiro, Vol. 95(3): 375-380.

Conceição MJ, Borges-Pereira J 2002. Influence of specific treatment on the morbidity of schistosomiasis mansoni in an endemic area of Minas Gerais, Brazil. Mem Inst Oswaldo Cruz 97: 755-757.

Conceição MJ, Borges-Pereira J, Coura JR 2007. A thirty years follow-up study on schistosomiasis mansoni in a community of Minas Gerais, Brazil. Mem Inst Oswaldo Cruz 102: 1007-1009.

Conceição MJ, Pereira NG, Pereira JB, Carlôto AE, Melo EV. 2010. Não-Resposta de Paciente Infectado com *Schistosoma mansoni* a três Tratamentos Sucessivos com Praziquantel e Estudo Experimental em Camundongos com Repetição de Falha ao Tratamento. Rev Soc Bras Med Trop. 43 (Supl. I): 186-187.

Conceição MJ, Pereira NG, Vasques CHS, Rodrigues DP, Frota AC, Carlôto AE,Coura JR. 2009. Estudo de 10 Casos de Enterobacteriose Septicêmica Prolongada observados no Serviço de Doenças Infecciosas e Parasitárias-UFRJ e no Instituto de Pediatria Martagão Gesterira-IPPMG. Rev. Soc Bras Med Trop 42 (Supl.1): 206-207

Coura JR, Amaral RS 2004. Epidemiological and control aspects of schistosomiasis in Brazilian endemic areas. Mem Inst Oswaldo Cruz 99 (Suppl. I): 13-19.

Coura JR, Conceição MJ 2010. Specific Schistosomiasis treatment as a strategy for disease control. Mem Inst Oswaldo Cruz, Rio de Janeiro, Vol. 105(4): 598-603.

Coura JR, Conceição MJ, Pereira JB 1984. Morbidade da esquistossomose mansoni no Brasil. III. Estudo evolutivo em uma área endêmica no período de dez anos. Mem Inst. Oswaldo Cruz 79: 447-453.

Drumond SC, Pereira SRS, Silva LCS, Antunes CMF, Lambertucci JR. 2010. Schistosomiasis control program in the state of Minas Gerais in Brazil. Mem Inst Oswaldo Cruz, Rio de Janeiro, 105(4): 519-523.

Enk MJ, Caldeira RL, Carvalho OS, Schall VT. Rural tourism as risk factor for the transmission of schistosomiasis in Minas Gerais, Brazil. Mem Inst. Oswaldo Cruz 2004, 99 (Suppl 1):105-8.

Graeff-Teixeira C., Anjos CB, Oliveira VC, Velloso CFP, Fonseca MBS, Valar C, Moraes C, Garrido CT, Amaral RS, 1999. Identification of a transmission Focus of *Schistosoma mansoni* in the Southern most Brazilian State, Rio Grande do Sul Mem Inst Oswaldo Cruz, Rio de Janeiro, Vol. 94(1): 9 -10.

Igreja R.P, Gusmão MF, Barreto MGM, Paulino MT, Silva JF, Seck OK, Gonçalves M.M.L, Soares MS. 2010. A 15 - year follow-up study on schistosomiasis in a low-endemic area in Rio de Janeiro State, Brazil. J. Helminth. 84: 229-233.

Jansen G 1946. Profilaxia experimental da esquistossomose de Manson. Mem Inst Oswaldo Cruz 44: 549-578.

Katz N 2008. Terapêutica clínica na esquistossomose mansoni. In OS Carvalho, PMZ Coelho, HL Lenzi (org.), *Schistosoma mansoni e esquistossomose: uma visão multidisciplinar*, Editora Fiocruz, 1ª ed. Rio de Janeiro, p. 850-870.

Katz N, Brener Z. 1966. Evolução clínica de 112 casos de Esquistossomose mansoni observados após 10 anos de permanência em focos endêmicos de Minas Gerais. Rev Inst Med Trop S Paulo 8: 139-142.

Katz N, Chaves A, Pellegrino J 1972. A simple device for quantitative stool thick-smear technique in schistosomiasis mansoni. Rev Inst Med Trop S Paulo 14: 397-400.

Katz N., Coelho PMZ 2008 Clinical therapy of schistosomiasis mansoni: The Brazilian contribution. Acta Tropica 108 (2-3): 72-78

Klöetzel K. 1966. Morbidity in chronic splenomegaly due to Schistosomiasis mansoni: follow- up study in a Brazilian population .Trans.Roy.Soc.Trop.Med. Hyg , 1967 61 (6) : 803- 805

Klöetzel K. 1992. Some personal views on the control of schistosomiasis mansoni. Mem Inst Oswaldo Cruz. 87 (Suppl 4): 221- 226.

Klöetzel K, Klöetzel J. 1958. The hepatosplenic syndrome in Manson's schistosomiasis; notes on a series of 119 cases. Rev Bras Med. 15 (3):172-8.

Lambertucci JR, Silva LCS, Voieta I. 2005. Esquistossomose e Doenças Associadas. In: Coura JR. Dinâmica das Doenças Infecciosas e Parasitárias. Ed. Guanabara Koogan, 1ª ed, p. 789 -806.

Lenzi HL, Kimmel E, Schechtman H, Pelajo-Machado M, Romanha WS, Pacheco RG, Mariano M, Lenzi JA. Histoarchitecture of schistosomal granuloma development and involution: morphogenetic and biomechanical approaches. Mem Inst Oswaldo Cruz 93 (Suppl. 1): 143-151.

Lutz, A., 1919. O Schistosomum mansoni e a schistosomatose segundo observações feitas no Brasil. Mem. Inst. Oswaldo Cruz 11, 121–155.

Maciel H. 1925 Contribuição ao estudo da distribuição geográfica da schistosomose. . Imprensa Naval, Rio de Janeiro, 147 pp.

Martins AV, Versiani W. 1938. Schistosomose mansoni em Belo Horizonte. Brasil Médico, 52: 471-472.

Massara CL, Amaral GL, Caldeira RL, Drumond SC, Enk MJ, Carvalho OS. 2008. Schistosomiasis in an ecotourism area in Minas Gerais State, Brazil.Cad. Saúde Pública, Rio de Janeiro, 24 (7) :1709-1712.

Meira JA. 1947. Esquistosomíase mansoni: subsídio ao estudo de sua incidência e distribuição geográfica no Brasil - lista bibliográfica brasileira sobre a esquistosomose mansoni (doença de Manson-Pirajá da Silva). Arq. Fac. Hig. Saúde Públ.. Univ. São Paulo, 1 (1): 5 -146.

Neiva AH. 1947. Aspectos geográficos da imigração e colonização do Brasil. Rev. Bras. Geog. 9: 249- 270.

Paraense WL. 2008. Histórico do gênero *Biomphalaria*-Morfologia e Sistemática morfológica. In: Carvalho OS, Coelho PMZ, Lenzi HL. Schistosoma mansoni-Esquistossomose, uma visão multidisciplinar.Ed. Fiocruz. 1ª ed, Cap.8, p. 288 -307.

Pellon AB, Teixeira I. 1950. Distribuição geográfica da esquistossomose mansônica no Brasil. Ministério da Educação e Saúde, Rio de Janeiro, 24 pp.

Pessoa SB, Barros PR.1953. Notas sobre a epidemiologia da esquistossomose mansônica no Estado de Sergipe. Rev Med Cir São Paulo *13*: 147-154.

Pirajá da Silva MP. 1908. A esquistossomose na Bahia. Arquivo sobre Parasitologia 13: 281-300.

Prata A, Bina JC. 1968. Development of hepatosplenic form of schistosomiasis. Gazeta Médica da Bahia 68: 49-60.

Rey L. 2007. Parasitologia.Schistosoma e Esquistossomíase-Epidemiologia e Controle. ed. Guanabara Koogan, 1ª ed. p 475- 566.

Santos AM, Melo ACFL. 2011. Schistosomiasis prevalence in Tutóia village, Maranhão, Brazil. Rev Soc Bras Med Trop 44(1): 97-99.

Sarvel AK, Oliveira AA, Silva AR, Lima ACL, Katz N. 2011. Evaluation of a 25-Year-Program for the Control of Schistosomiasis . PLoS Neglected Diseases. 5 (3): e 990

Schlemper Junior BR, Ferreira Neto JA, São Thiago PT, Bressan C, Amarante AR. 1996 The southern known limit of occurrence of *Schistosoma mansoni* Sambon 1907 in Brazil was the northeast of the State of Santa Catarina, Brazil. Rev Soc Bras Med Trop 29: 411-418).

Sette H.1953. *O tratamento da esquistossomose à luz da patologia hepática (Estudo clínico)*. Thesis, Universidade Federal de Pernambuco, Recife, 220 pp.

Soares MS, Barreto MG, da Silva CL, Pereira, JB, Moza PG, Rey L, Calçado MS, Lustoza A, Maspero R. 1995. Schistosomiasis in a low prevalence area: incomplete urbanization increasing risk of infection in Paracambi, R.J., Brazil. Mem. Inst. Oswaldo Cruz 90: 451-458.

WHO-World Health Organization 2002. Prevention and control of schistosomiasis and soil-transmitted helminthiasis.World Health Organization Tech Rep Ser 912(I-VI): 1-57.

10

Ecological Aspects of *Biomphalaria* in Endemic Areas for Schistosomiasis in Brazil

Marco Antônio Andrade de Souza[1] and Alan Lane de Melo[2]
[1]*Departamento de Ciências da Saúde, Centro Universitário Norte do Espírito Santo, Universidade Federal do Espírito Santo*
[2]*Departamento de Parasitologia, Instituto de Ciências Biológicas, Universidade Federal de Minas Gerais*
Brazil

1. Introduction

Schistosomiasis is a disease caused by trematodes belonging to family Schistosomatidae. Within this family, only genus *Schistosoma* has species that parasitize humans. It is accepted that the genus *Schistosoma* was brought to the Americas during the Atlantic slave trade and with Eastern and Asian immigrants. However, only *Schistosoma mansoni* Sambon, 1907, settled here certainly due to the presence of susceptible intermediate hosts, freshwater planorbid snails belonging to the genus *Biomphalaria* and to environmental conditions similar to the region of origin (Morgan et al., 2001). Of the major endemic diseases that occur in Brazil, schistosomiasis is widely distributed, being considered as a serious medical and socio-economic problem. Brazil is considered one of the endemic foci of the disease, with active transmission in at least 16 states, despite the variability of data regarding its prevalence in different regions of the country (Cunha, 1970; Katz & Peixoto, 2000). Since human activity plays a significant role in expanding the territory colonized by hosts of *S. mansoni*, human migration has contributed to the expansion of schistosomiasis to developing regions. In Brazil, the first centuries of territory occupation were marked by the presence of scattered populations in coastal areas, increased by the first expeditions, called colonial exploratory expedition, in the seventeenth century. The discovery of gold and precious stones in the eighteenth century in the current states of Minas Gerais, Mato Grosso, Goiás and Bahia contributed to the increase in population, and encouraged the opening of roads, which significantly strengthened the relationships of these areas with the sources of supplies. Many cities that emerged in function of these and other activities have become more important with the intensification of trade, such as port cities. The nineteenth century opened up new perspectives for the settlement of the Brazilian territory, also marked by the beginning of the territory mechanization with the construction of railroads, telegraph and the first shipping companies, resulting in urbanization process in the country (Ferreira, 1959; L.A. Souza, 2004). The phenomenon of urbanization itself only emerged in the mid twentieth century. After the 50s, as a result of industrialization, economic ties and the urban factor became correlated. A new logic in the organization of Brazilian society was established. Economic and social innovations are enormous as they are associated, in this context, to the demographic revolution, the rural exodus and the integration of the territory by transport and communications. Cities of all kinds and with different functional levels emerged (Chiavenato, 1999). Industrialization, agriculture mechanization and the rural exodus are also responsible for the fact that some Brazilian cities received enormous population contingents in search of jobs and access to various services, people without qualification and perspectives. The phenomenon of *favelizações* (social phenomenon that occurs in urban centers where there is growth and proliferation of slums) was intensified during this period, where population clusters settled without any technical and administrative control in the suburbs of metropolitan areas. The 1970s was also marked by the construction and expansion of roads and by the creation of a modern telecommunications system, which enabled a greater fluidity in the territory, besides allowing the unification of the market nationwide (Brazilian Institute of Geography and Statistics [IBGE], 2000). The effects of the urbanization process and the deployment of large urban centers could be perceived by the shortage of spaces favorable to the territorial occupation and the increasing difficulty of exploitation of natural resources. The disordered growth led to major environmental disturbances, which can be evidenced by the spread of diseases, initially restricted to certain areas, for different regions of Brazil. In this context, schistosomiasis stands out, which is a disease associated to the livelihood of people, and has advanced in the country by human migrations into different directions. Although the first record of human infection with *S. mansoni* in Brazil has been reported by Pirajá da Silva (1908), the importance of schistosomiasis in the country was only evidenced when Pellon & Teixeira (1950, 1953), conducting the first major national parasitological survey, showed the prevalence of the disease in 612 of 877 localities surveyed in Northeastern Brazil and state of Minas Gerais. The presence of schistosomiasis was later reported in Northern Brazil and in other states in Southern and Southeastern Brazil. Until today, schistosomiasis is increasingly spreading to new regions of the country (Araújo et al., 2007; Barbosa et al., 1996, 2010; Graeff-Teixeira et al., 1999, Paredes et al., 2010). The disease is a major public health problem in Brazil, and it is estimated that schistosomiasis affects 4.6% of the population, approximately 8,000,000 individuals, and in the states of Minas Gerais, Pernambuco and Espírito Santo, approximately 2.9 million people are infected (Katz & Peixoto, 2000; Paraense et al., 1983). The country's tropical climate allows, in most Brazilian states, the development of ecological conditions necessary for its transmission. The enormous variety of aquatic habitats, which play the role of nurseries for transmitter snails, high temperatures and intense lighting contribute to the maintenance and spread of this disease. In addition, the concentration of susceptible human hosts, living in unsanitary conditions, lack of health education and public sanitation, are key factors for the establishment of transmission foci, providing the contamination of sites, where susceptible snails reproduce, by feces containing viable eggs of *S. mansoni* and thus contributing to the maintenance of schistosomiasis and the expansion of its area of occurrence. Men become infected when in contact with contaminated water during their normal daily or leisure activities (Figure 1). When in contact with the host's skin, cercariae, which are infective larvae, adhere to it through mucoprotein substance secreted by their acetabular glands. After penetration, the resulting larvae known as schistosomula, adapt to the physiological conditions of the internal environment, and are carried from the skin to the lungs primarily by the blood vascular system, with likely participation of the lymphatic system (Wilson et al., 1978, 1986). Thus, progressively and regardless of route, these larvae pass through the pulmonary arteries and veins and when they reach the portal venous system, either by blood or transtecidual route, the parasites complete their development and sexual maturation. This

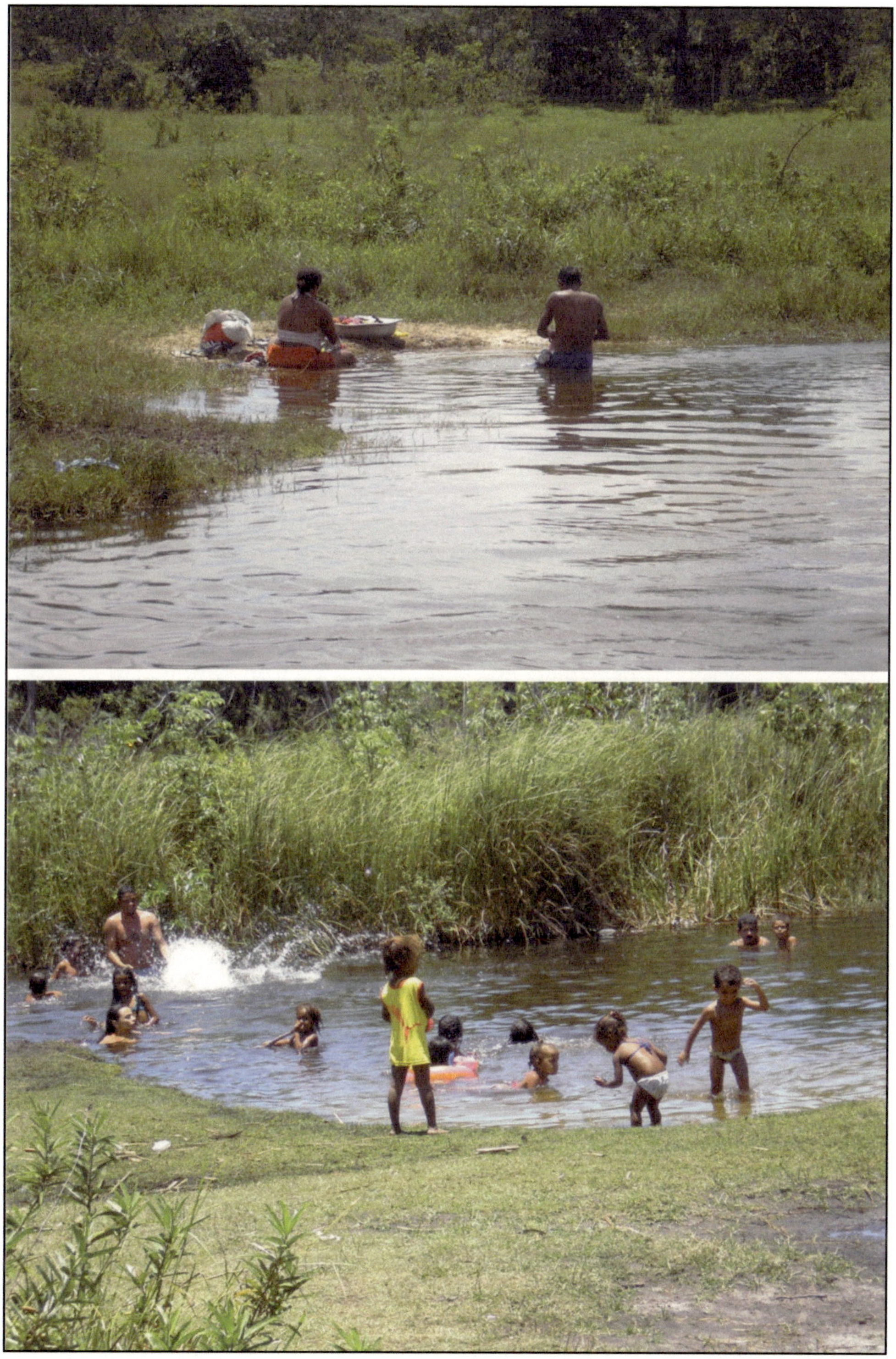

Fig. 1. Human activities on water collections: Work and leisure

cycle takes approximately 28 days. After mating, they migrate against the current towards the branches of the inferior mesenteric vein. Around the 35th day (which may occur between the 27th and 48th day of infection), they begin to lay about 300 or more eggs per day for each pair of parasites, depending on the vertebrate host, starting up a new cycle (Melo & Coelho, 2000). Among the planorbid snails that occur in Brazil, main species of *Biomphalaria* (*B. glabrata, B. tenagophila* and *B. straminea*) are considered natural vectors of *S. mansoni*, whose distribution varies according to each region. According to Paraense (1984), in Northeastern and Southeastern Brazil, the most important species is *Biomphalaria glabrata* (Say, 1818), due to its distribution amplitude and transmission efficiency, being responsible for much of outbreaks in the states of Minas Gerais and Espírito Santo (Giemsa & Nauck, 1950a, 1950b; Lambertucci et al., 1987; C.P. Souza et al., 2001). On the other hand, it is important to emphasize that in part of Southeastern and Southern Brazil, the main intermediate host species is *B. tenagophila* (Orbigny, 1835) (Paraense, 1972, 1984; Telles et al., 1991). *B. straminea* (Dunker, 1848), despite being the species found in almost all watersheds of Brazil and adapted to climate variations, its natural infection occurs predominantly in the Northeastern states (Barbosa et al., 1996). Distribution and infection rates of these planorbid snails are correlated to disease distribution, and the presence of aquatic habitats suitable for the survival of these snails is governed by climatic and environmental factors such as vegetation, temperature, precipitation, characteristics of water bodies, topography and soil use. Any change in one of these factors may change the distribution of snails and therefore the dynamics of schistosomiasis transmission. Since the environment plays an important role in this dynamics, the assessment of habitat diversity provides an opportunity to examine the levels of human impacts on watershed areas (Galdean et al., 2000), constituting an important tool in environmental monitoring programs (Callisto et al., 2001). Thus, this study aims to examine some ecological aspects relevant for the identification of risk areas for schistosomiasis transmission in Brazil, using impact assessment protocols that enable determining and classifying sites for collection of *Biomphalaria*, such as areas under natural conditions, altered or impacted.

2. Study areas

The studies were conducted in 147 sites of the municipality of Mariana, located in the central region of Minas Gerais, about 110 Km distant from Belo Horizonte, in 9 sampling stations in the Carne de Vaca beach, municipality of Goiana (Pernambuco), distant about 70 km from Recife and in 41 sites in seven municipalities from northern state of Espírito Santo as follows: Boa Esperança, Conceição da Barra, Montanha, Mucurici, Ponto Belo, Pedro Canário and Pinheiros (Figure 2), taking into account, for the determination of sampling sites, the human presence and the existence of water collections, with antropogenic impact or not. Freshwater environments occurring in the localities and their systems were characterized as lotic (consisting of collections of running water, streams, waterfalls and rivers) and lentic (consisting of collections of waters with little flow, such as lakes, ponds, puddles, artificial ponds and swamps). Thus, uses and conservation conditions were identified and a protocol for assessing the habitat diversity (Callisto et al., 2002), with modifications (Table 1), which allows evaluating the impact of human action on aquatic environment through a specific score for the study areas (Galdean et al., 2000), was used. In all sites selected, geographic coordinates were obtained with the aid of a GPS device.

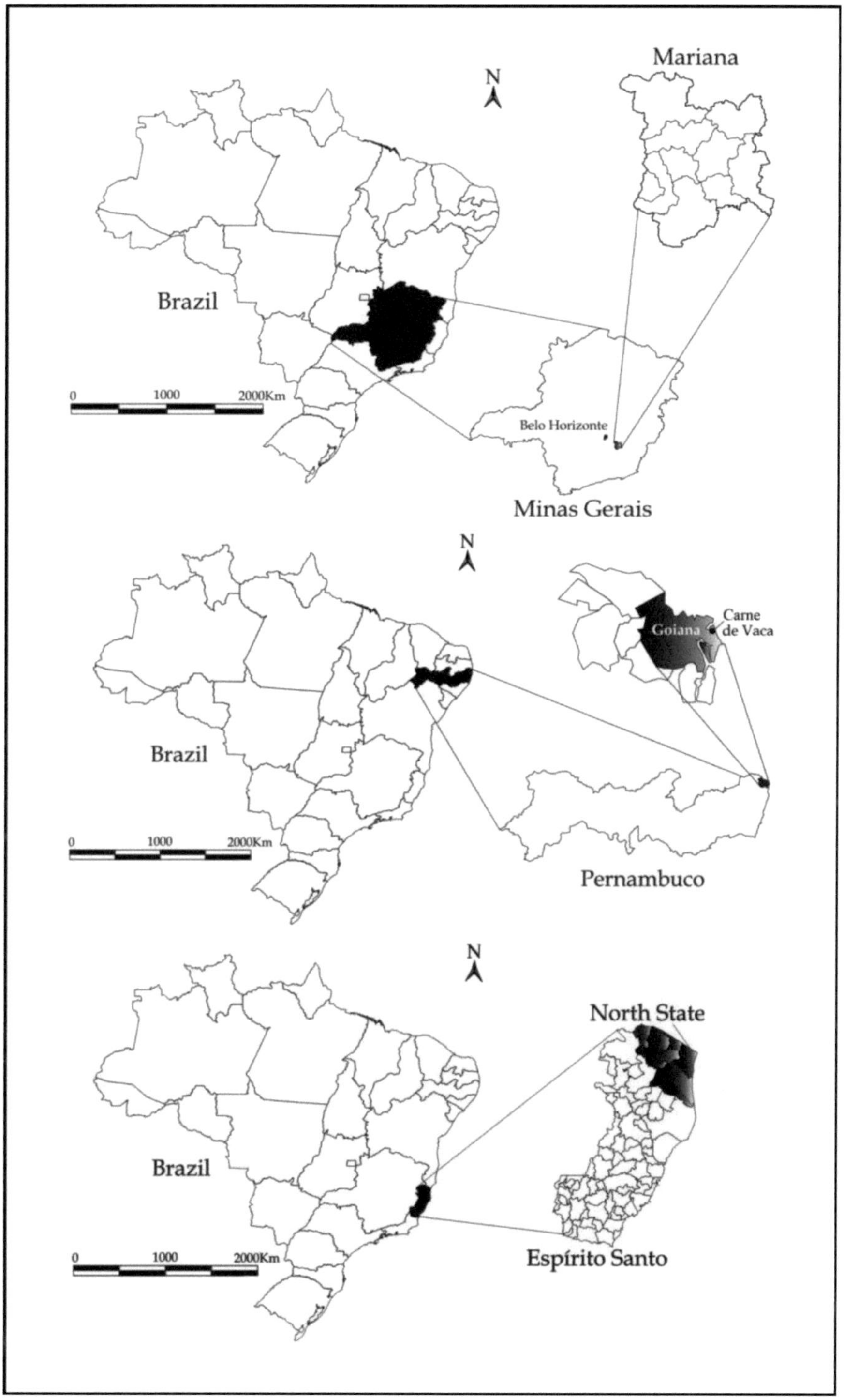

Fig. 2. Study areas: Mariana, Carne de Vaca beach and municipalities in northern state of Espírito Santo

Location:	Date of collection:		
Time of collection:	Time (situation of the day):		
Collection mode (Collector):	Water pH:		
Type of environment: Stream ( ) River ( ) Lake ( ) Pond ( ) Waterfall ( )			
Parameters	**Score**		
	4 points	*2 points*	*0 point*
1- Type of occupation at the margin of water bodies (main activity)	*Native vegetation*	*Pasture/ Agriculture/ Monoculture/ Reforestation*	*Residential/ Commercial/ Industrial*
2- Erosion near the margin of rivers and silting of the riverbed	*Absent*	*Moderate*	*Accentuated*
3-Anthropic alterations	*Absent*	*Alterations of domestic origin (sewage, garbage)*	*Alterations of industrial / urban origin (factories, iron and steel industry, canalization, reuse of the river course)*
4- Vegetal coverage in the riverbed	*Partial*	*Total*	*Absent*
5- Water odor	*None*	*Sewage (rotten egg)*	*Oil / Industrial*
6- Water oiliness	*Absent*	*Moderate*	*Abundant*
7- Water transparency	*Transparent*	*Turbid*	*Opaque or colorful*
8- Odor of the sediment (bottom)	*None*	*Sewage (rotten egg)*	*Oil / Industrial*
9- Bottom oiliness	*Absent*	*Moderate*	*Abundant*
10- Type of bottom	*Rocks/rubble*	*Mud/sand*	*Cement / canalized*

Note: 4 points (natural situation), 2 and 0 points (slightly or deeply altered).

Table 1. Rapid assessment of habitat diversity in watershed areas, modified from the protocol of the Environmental Protection Agency (EPA), USA, 1987 (Callisto et al. 2002;)

3. Collection of snails

Two monthly snail collections were performed between 2004 and 2010 using a hand net (netting), made with nylon (50 cm of width, 40 cm in height, 30 cm of opening, with mesh of 1 mm ^{2}), adapted to wooden or steel end of 150 cm in length (Figure 3). An individual sampling effort of 30 minutes per scanning, was applied at each 10 (ten) meters in each of the selected sampling stations (Souza et al., 2006). All material collected was packed in plastic bags, labeled and transported to the laboratory, where the snails were sorted, macroscopically observed for preliminary analysis of the species, counted, measuring the diameter of the shells and placed in small plastic containers with 10 ml capacity containing 5 ml of water free of chlorine. Then, they were left overnight to be evaluated before and after direct artificial photostimulation (60 W lamp), to verify the occurrence of cercarial emergence. On the next day, after examination without photostimulation, they were examined after exposure to light for two hours (Figure 4). This procedure was repeated weekly for 90 days. After this period, the snails that were negative were crushed between glass plates for the detection of possible larval stages (Coutinho, 1950). From each batch of snails collected, about 10% of live individuals were removed and sacrificed in water at 70°C. The soft tissues were fixed in Railliet - Henry and dissected under a stereomicroscope (Paraense & Deslandes, 1955). For the identification of species, conchological and morphological parameters were considered according to Paraense (1975).

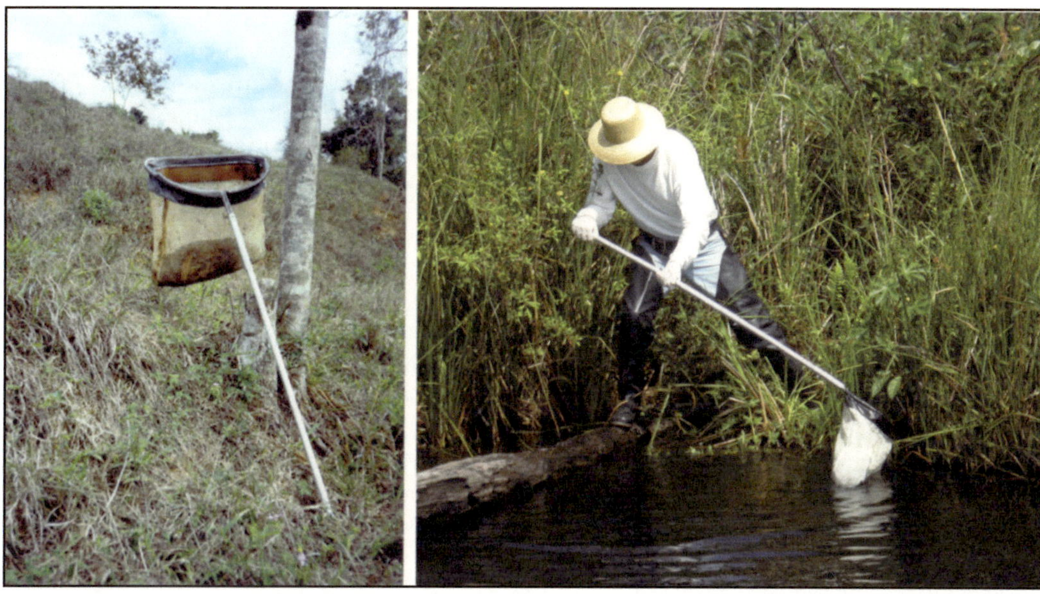

Fig. 3. Hand net (netting) used for the collection of snails (left); Procedures for the collection of snails through scanning (right)

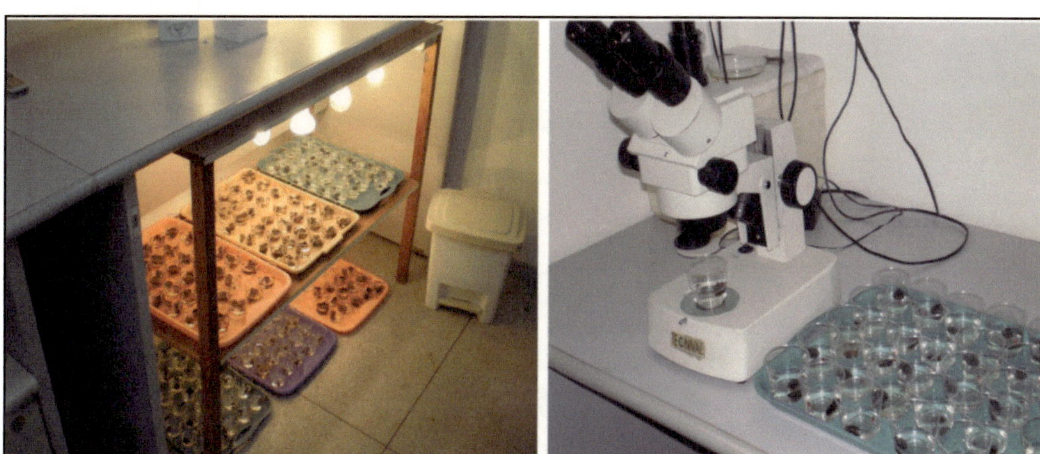

Fig. 4. Direct artificial photostimulation (left); analysis of cercarial emergence in stereomicroscope (right)

4. Remarks and discussion

The assessment of habitat diversity provides an opportunity to examine the levels of human impacts on watershed areas (Galdean et al., 2000), and constitutes an important tool in environmental monitoring programs (Callisto et al., 2001). Residential occupation on banks of water courses (leading to moderate and severe erosion processes and silting of the riverbed), alterations of domestic origin such as garbage and sewage (an important source of organic matter for the development of snails) and the presence of vegetation cover on the river bed, very favorable to the fixing of snails in the freshwater environment stand out as the most relevant (Figures 5 and 6). The use of assessment protocols in each location allowed analyzing the collection sites with the determination of areas in natural conditions, altered or impacted. Impacted areas were considered as those whose scores achieved by the protocol for the assessment of habitat diversity reached up to 20 points. Altered areas scored between 20 and 36 points, and over 36 points, areas in natural conditions (Figures 7a, b, c). Among the sampling stations established in the municipality of Mariana, MG, Carne de Vaca beach, PE, and municipalities in northern state of Espírito Santo, the presence of *Biomphalaria* was directly related to sites with anthropogenic changes (Figure 8). Approximately 5928 snails from Mariana were analyzed, all *B. glabrata* with positivity rate of 2.19%. In this municipality, *B. tenagophila* and *B straminea* were not found. In Carne de Vaca beach, Pernambuco, 4435 *B. glabrata* were analyzed, with an infection rate of 0.44%. On the other hand, in municipalities from northern state of Espírito Santo, 732 *B. glabrata* and 921 *B. straminea* were analyzed, and so far none of them were positive for *S. mansoni*. The collection of snails was performed using a hand net (netting), adapted to wooden or steel end according to Souza et al. (2006). This procedure was proposed as an alternative to traditional metal scoop (WHO, 1965), keeping in mind that in some areas, quantifying is not feasible and in another area, qualitative study fits well to the work objectives. The use of netting consists of scanning previously established collection waters, providing better coverage of the study area, in less time. Associating positive sites with the protocol for rapid assessment of habitat diversity, it was observed that the presence of snails infected by *S. mansoni* is

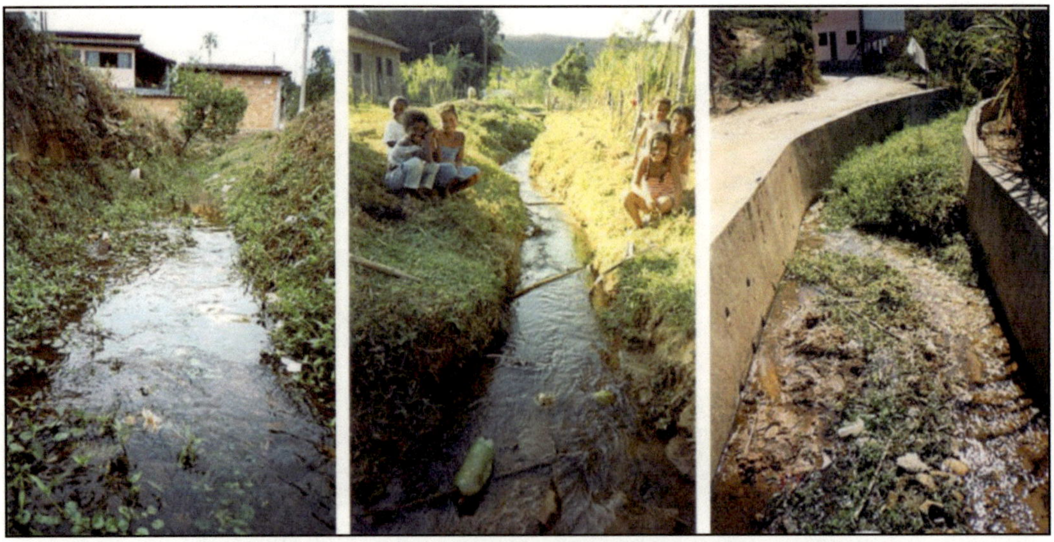

Fig. 5. Sampling stations in the city of Mariana, MG. Anthropic disturbances

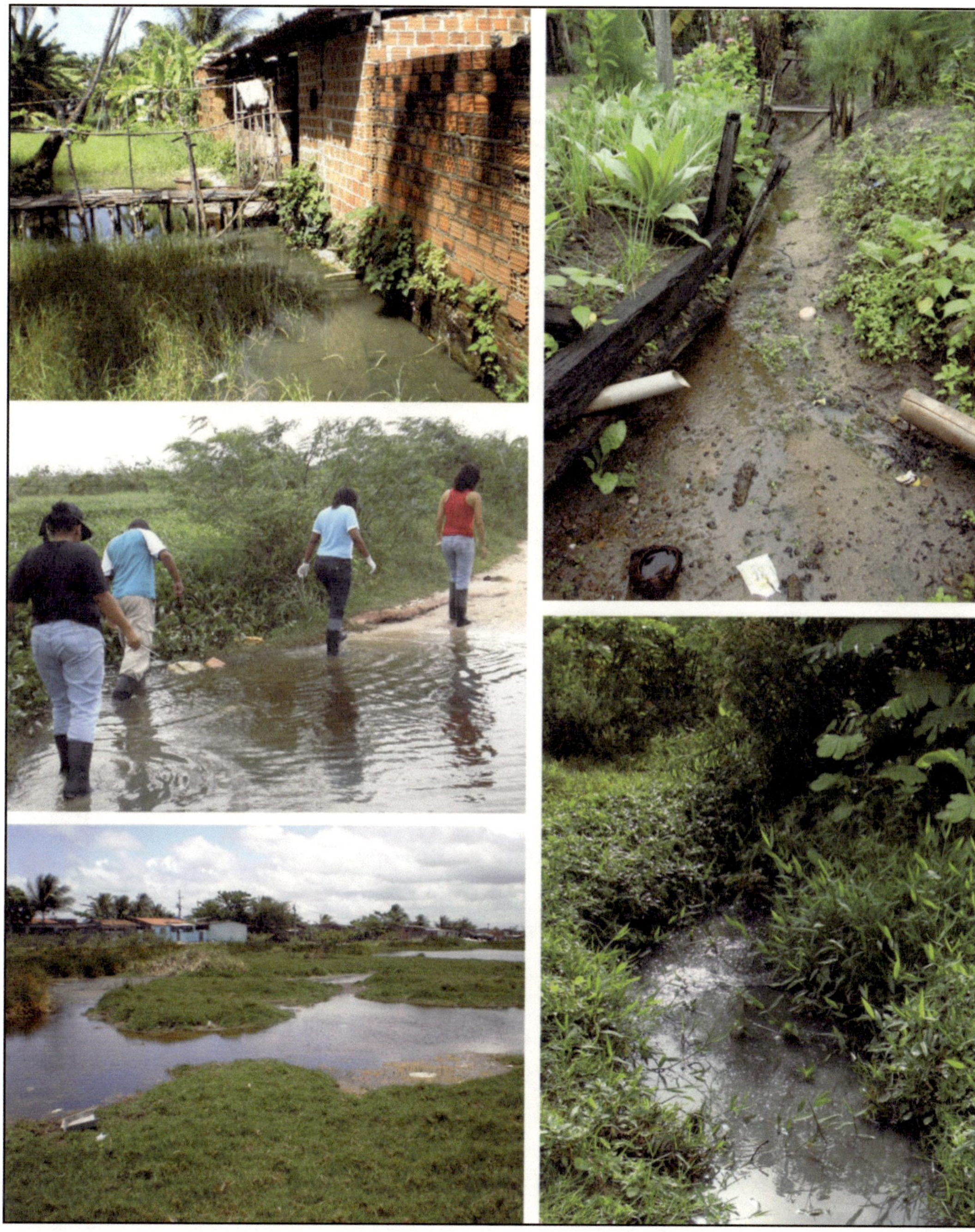

Fig. 6. Sampling stations in Carne de Vaca beach, PE (left) and northern state of Espírito Santo (right). Anthropic disturbances

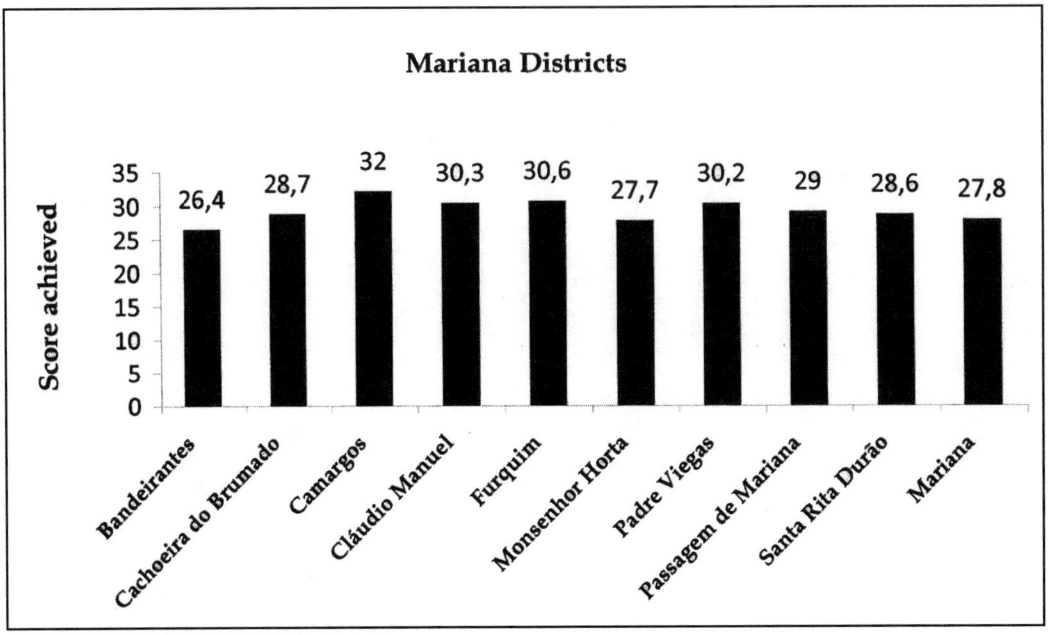

Fig. 7a. Rapid assessment of habitat diversity. Collection sites in the municipality of Mariana, Minas Gerais state. Impacted areas: up to 20 points; Altered areas: > 20 < 36 points; Natural areas: > 36 points

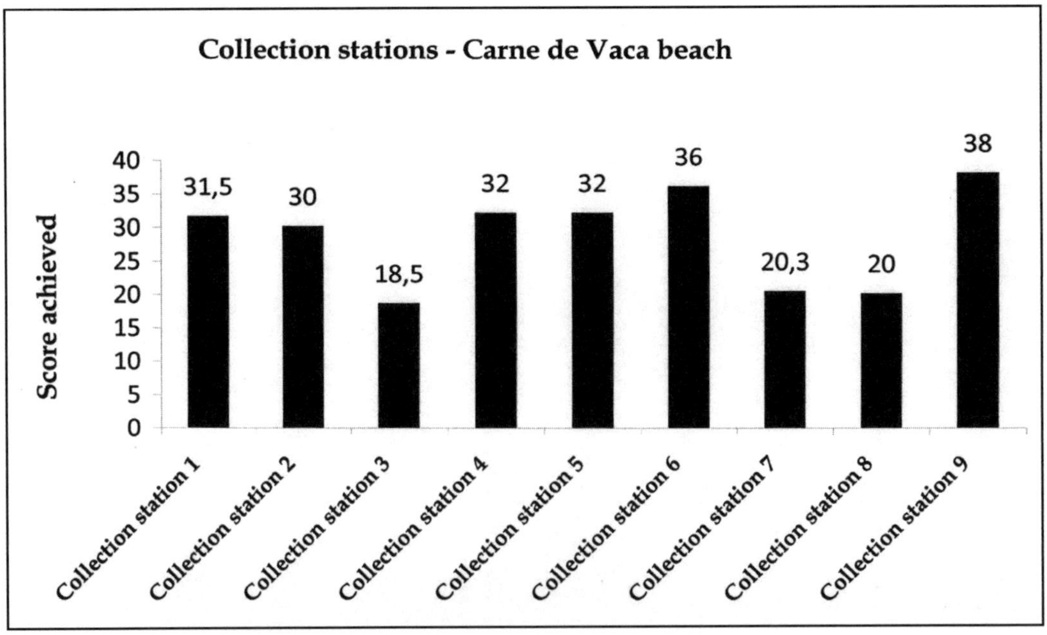

Fig. 7b. Rapid assessment of habitat diversity. Collection stations in Carne de Vaca beach, PE. Impacted areas: up to 20 points; Altered areas: > 20 < 36 points; Natural areas: > 36 points

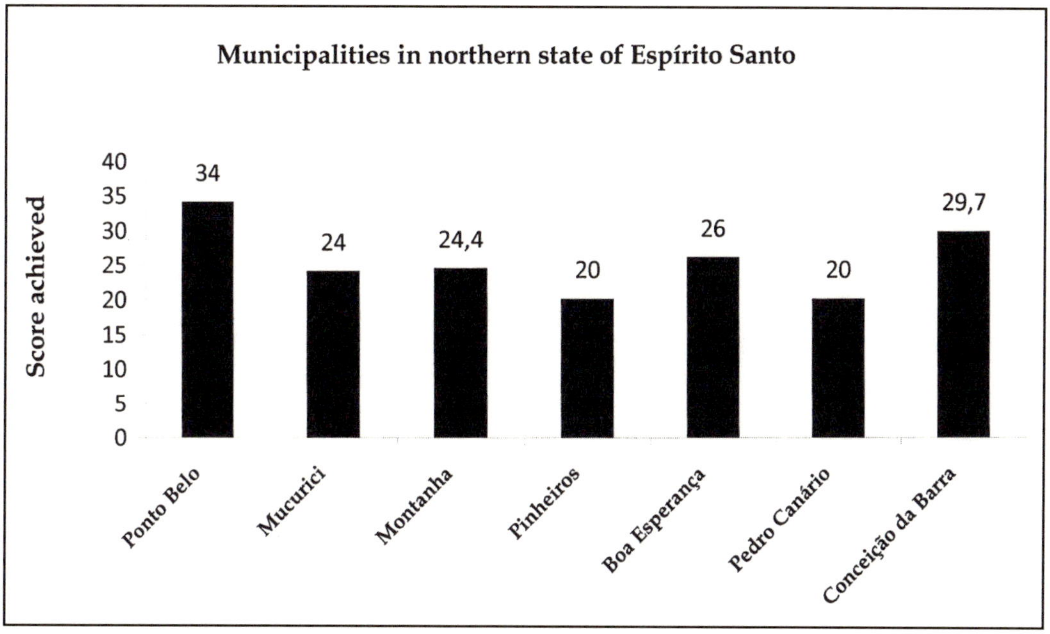

Fig. 7c. Rapid assessment of habitat diversity. Collection sites in municipalities from northern state of Espírito Santo. Impacted areas: up to 20 points; Altered areas: > 20 < 36 points; Natural areas: > 36 points

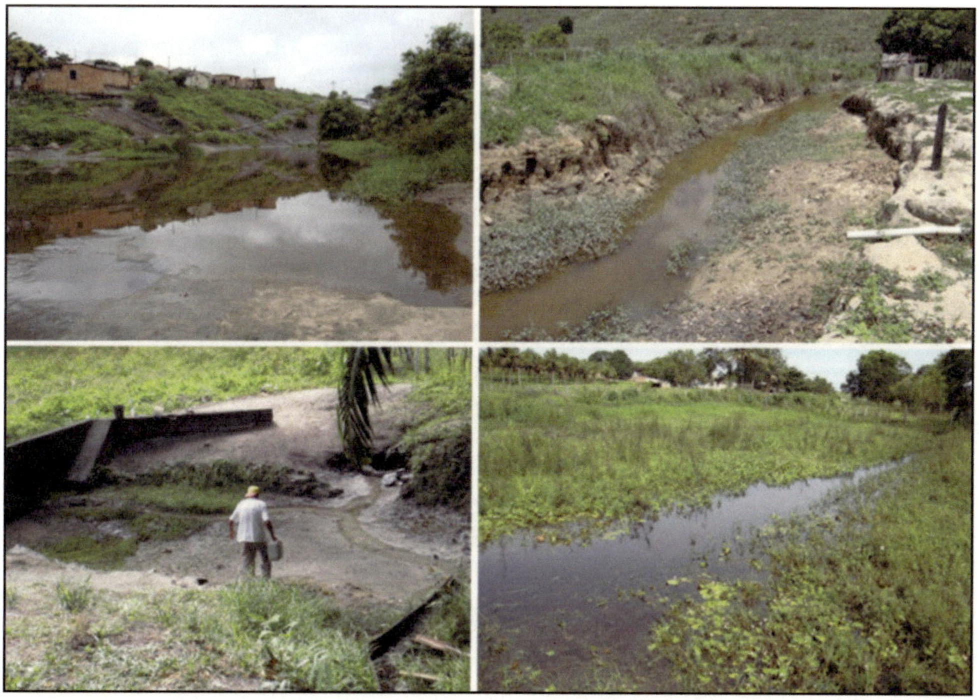

Fig. 8. Collection sites with the presence of snails *Biomphalaria*. Mariana (both pictures on top), Carne de Vaca (left) and northern state of Espírito Santo (right)

directly related to impacted areas and areas altered by human activity. Of the 10 districts from the municipality of Mariana, in 6 of them (Cachoeira do Brumado, Cláudio Manuel, Furquim, Monsenhor Horta, Santa Rita and Mariana), the gathering of snails infected by *S. mansoni* was directly related to the presence of anthropogenic changes. This characteristic also applies to the Carne de Vaca beach, where the presence of *B. glabrata* infected by *S. mansoni* was observed in sampling stations II, VII and VIII (Figures 7a, 7b). Similarly, although no infected snails were found in the northern Espírito Santo, its presence was also related to impacted areas, especially in the municipalities of Ponto Belo, Mucurici, Montanha, Pinheiros, Boa Esperança and Pedro Canário. Among the environment analyzed, it seems that the highest prevalence of infected snails was found in lotic environments, demonstrating the dispersal of snails and therefore the disease in these municipalities. The present study also assessed some geographical variables of these municipalities, relating them to areas positive for *S. mansoni*. The greatest number of localities with the presence of positive snails showed prevalence of grassland and pastures as vegetal cover, represented by regions devoid of trees and areas cleared by human activity (Baltazar & Raposo, 1993). Analyzing the morphological territorial units (relief), it was observed that the positive sites were those with predominant smooth undulated relief, with predominance of slopes below 35%, with softer slopes and floodplains. Floodplains are areas of materials from larger relieves, represented by the bottom of the more open valleys. They have elevations below 600 m ((Environmental urban plan of Mariana [PDUAM] 2003), which is a factor consistent with the hypsometric analysis performed in the municipalities in which the largest number of locations positive for *S. mansoni* was between 500 and 600 m. Although representing only 3.5% of the total area of these municipalities, floodplains are important because they have conditioned the development of many villages, either due to the concentration of placer gold, or to the flatter relief or the soil fertility (PDUAM, 2003). In both units, better conditions for urban development were observed, and consequently, there were increased human activities. During the study period, comprising in all locations, dry and rainy seasons, it was found that the smallest planorbid snails, whose shell diameters ranged from 1 to 6 mm, were found in greater amounts during the dry season, suggesting a lower dispersion in this season and higher during the rainy season, which favors the expansion of the distribution area of snails and in consequence of the disease. The pH measured in the study areas ranged from 5.5 to 8.4 in the most impacted environments and with high concentration of organic matter, especially environments with lower water flow (lotic environments), such as irrigation ditches or small deviations from the natural course. Although *Biomphalaria* had been found in some wooded and well-preserved environments, in some other areas, with prevalence of grassland and pasture and devoid of trees, in general, snails were more abundant in lentic environments. However, most areas considered foci of transmission were concentrated close to urban populations, which have contact with aquatic environments for leisure or domestic activities, and show higher population density of snails, probably due to anthropogenic input of nutrients that results in higher pH, favouring the growth of aquatic vegetation (algae and macrophytes) such as some Cyperaceae (*Eleocharis* spp.), Araceae (*Pistia stratioides*), Lemnaceae (*Lemna* sp.), Nymphaeacaeae (*Nymphaea* sp.), Pontederiaceae (*Eichhornia* spp. and *Heteranthera reniformis*), Salviniaceae (*Salvinia molesta*) and, consequently, providing shelter and food for snails. Moreover, the bed of most breeding spots and foci was almost muddy and some were sometimes covered with sand, sometimes with fine mud, favouring the camouflage of snails. The heterogeneity in the study areas was also verified, for example, in relation to climate (rainy season from October to March in the Southeastern region and from May to July in the Northeastern region) and almost all temperatures above 25°C, topography, vegetation and altitude (from 0 to ~ 800 m a.s.l.) and the presence of snails and other aquatic gastropod mollusks, thus making a more precise characterization of the breeding spots difficult. In fact, similar results were obtained by Pieri (1995). The presence of fish (mainly *Australoheros Cf. facetus* and *Tilapia* spp.), *Pomacea canaliculata* and *Melanoides tuberculata* apparently did not change the dynamics of the planorbid population. It is noteworthy that in higher areas and in places with higher anthropogenic contribution, high densities of *Physa* spp. associated with *B. glabrata* were found. Other predators mainly hirudinea (*Helobdella* sp.) and several species of aquatic heteroptera in large amounts were also associated with snails without, however, apparently be pushing their population (Souza et al., 2006).

5. Conclusions and perspectivies

In the dynamics of schistosomiasis transmission, environment plays a crucial role. Among the environment analyzed, lotic environments, those represented by collections of running waters, contributed with the greatest number of locations worked (143), while lentic environments, those represented by collections of waters with little flow, contributed with 54. Among the lotic environments, streams stood out, with 119 occurrences in municipalities. According to the score obtained using the protocol for rapid assessment of habitat diversity, it appears that almost all municipalities in the areas under study are within areas in altered situation as a result of disordered development process, also observed in most municipalities in Brazil. This fact is very relevant, considering that the presence of diseases is directly related to environmental degradation and human activity, as observed by Souza et al. (2006, 2008), which reflects the need for combined public policies to prevent their transmission. Among these diseases, schistosomiasis stands out, which control can only be achieved through multidisciplinary engineering, sanitation and healthy actions knowledge. This endemic condition has important epidemiological, parasitological, ecological and malacological determinants and only combined efforts in different areas could lead to the development of effective control. However, health agencies responsible for applying this knowledge in health care should be empowered to implement control procedures adequately. Outbreaks of the disease should be epidemiologically characterized, municipal managers and health agents should be appropriately trained to diagnose, plan and implement appropriate control measures to each situation and prevent future outbreaks, based on the following actions:

- Identification of breeding spots containing naturally infected snails.
- Classification of the focus area according to the risk factors involved.
- Reduction of the relative abundance of vector snails through the environmental manipulation of breeding spots.
- Identification of individuals with history of infection reported by reports of specific symptoms.
- Identification of carriers of the infection based on parasitological examination.
- Chemotherapy treatment of infected individuals with consequent reduction of the prevalence and severity of the disease in affected localities.

6. Acknowledgments

To Prof. Karina Carvalho Mancini for assembling digital photographs.
To Geological Engineer Leonardo Andrade de Souza from Zemlya Consulting and Services for the preparation of cartographic maps.
To technicians from the National Health Foundation (FUNASA) João Afonso, Luiz do Rosário and Sebastião Alves dos Santos for assistance in field work.
To governmental agencies DECIT/SCTIE, CNPq, FAPES, SESA, UFES, for granting financial support for the conduction of studies.

7. References

Araújo, K. C. G. M.; Resendes A. P. C.; Souza-Santos R.; Silveira Júnior J. C. & Barbosa C. S. (2007). Análise espacial dos focos de *Biomphalaria glabrata* e de casos humanos de esquistossomose mansônica em Porto de Galinhas, Pernambuco, Brasil, no ano 2000. *Cadernos de Saúde Pública,* vol.23, pp. 409-417.

Baltazar, O. F. & F. O. Raposo. (1993). Levantamentos Geológicos Básicos do Brasil, Mariana. Folha SF. 23- XB - 1. *Centro de Pesquisa em Recursos Minerais. Estado de Minas Gerais.* Escala 1: 100.000. Brasília, pp. 196.

Barbosa, C. S.; Silva, C. B. & Barbosa, F. S. (1996). Esquistossomose: reprodução e expansão da endemia no estado de Pernambuco no Brasil. *Revista de Saúde Pública,* vol.30, pp. 609-616.

Barbosa, C. S.; Araujo, K. C.; Sevilha, M. A.; Melo, F.; Gomes, E. C. S. & Souza-Santos, R. (2010). Current epidemiological status of schistosomiasis in the state of Pernambuco, Brazil. *Memórias do Instituto Oswaldo Cruz,* vol.105, No.4, pp. 549-554.

Callisto, M.; Moreno, P. & Barbosa, F. A. R. (2001). Habitat diversity and benthic functional trophic groups at Serra do Cipó, Southeast Brazil. *Revista Brasileira de Biologia,* vol.61, pp. 259-266.

Callisto, M.; Ferreira, W. R.; Moreno, P.; Goulart, M. & Petrucio, M. (2002). Aplicação de um protocolo de avaliação rápida da diversidade de hábitats em atividades de ensino e pesquisa (MG-RJ). *Acta Limnologica Brasiliensia,* vol.14, pp. 91-98.

Coutinho, J. O. (1950). Índices de infestação natural dos planorbídeos pelas cercárias do *Schistosoma mansoni* na cidade do Salvador-Bahia. *Anais da Faculdade de Medicina de São Paulo,* vol.25, pp. 29-53.

Chiavenato, I. (1999). *Teoria geral da administração: abordagens prescritas e normativas da administração,* Macgraw-Hill do Brasil, ISBN 85-352-0423-7, São Paulo, Brasil.

Cunha, A. S. (1970). *Esquistossomose mansoni*, Sarvier/USP, São Paulo, Brasil, 435p.

Environmental Protection Agency. EPA. (1987). *Biological criteria for the protection of aquatic life*. Columbus: Division of water quality monitoring and assessment, surface water section,. 120 p.

Ferreira, J. P. (1959). *Mariana.* In Enciclopédia dos municípios do Brasil, Minas Gerais, (1957 - 1960), J. P. Ferreira, (Ed), pp. 49-57, Rio de Janeiro, Brasil.

Galdean, N.; Callisto, M. & Barbosa, F. A. R. (2000). Lotic ecosystems of Serra do Cipó, southeast Brazil: water quality and a tentative classification based on the benthic macroinvertebrates community. *Aquatic Ecosystem Health and Management,* vol.3, pp. 545-552.

Giemsa, G. & Nauck, E. G. (1950a). Uma Viagem de Estudos ao Espírito Santo. II *Boletim Geográfico. CNG-IBGE*, Ano VIII, No.89. pp. 560-575.

Giemsa, G. & Nauck, E. G. (1950b). Uma Viagem de Estudos ao Espírito Santo. III *Boletim Geográfico. CNG-IBGE*, Ano VIII, No.90. pp. 653-701.

Graeff-Teixeira, C.; Anjos, C. B.; Oliveira, V. C.; Velloso, C. F. P.; Fonseca, M. B. S.; Valar, C.; Moraes, C.; Garrido, C. T. & Amaral, R. S. (1999). Identification of a transmission focus of *Schistosoma mansoni* in the southernmost brazilian state, Rio Grande do Sul. *Memórias do Instituto Oswaldo Cruz*, vol.94, pp. 9-10.

Instituto Brasileiro de Geografia e Estatística. IBGE. (October 2000). *Municípios Brasileiros*, Available from: http://www.ibge.gov.br/cidadesat/default.php.

Katz, N. & Peixoto. S. V. (2000). Análise crítica da estimativa do número de portadores de esquistossomose mansoni no Brasil. *Revista da Sociedade Brasileira de Medicina Tropical*, vol.33, pp. 303-308.

Lambertucci, J. R.; Rocha, R. S.; Carvalho, O. S. & Katz, N. (1987). A esquistossomose mansoni em Minas Gerais. *Revista da Sociedade Brasileira de Medicina Tropical*, vol.20, pp. 47-52.

Melo, A. L. & Coelho, P. M. Z. (2000). *Schistosoma mansoni*. In: *Parasitologia Humana*, D. P. Neves; A.L. Melo; O. Genaro; P.M. Linardi, (Eds), pp. 174-193, Atheneu, São Paulo, Brasil.

Morgan, J. A. T.; Dejong, R. J.; Snyder, S. D.; Mkoji, G. M. & Loker, E. S. (2001). *Schistosoma mansoni* and *Biomphalaria*: past history and future trends. *Parasitology*, vol.123, pp. 211-228.

Paraense, W. L. & Deslandes, N. (1955). Observations on the morphology of *Australorbis nigricans*. *Memórias do Instituto Oswaldo Cruz*, vol.53, pp. 121-124.

Paraense, W. L. (1972). Fauna planorbídica do Brasil. In: *Introdução à Geografia Médica do Brasil*, C.S. Lacaz; G.R. Baruzzi; J.R.W. Siqueira (Eds), pp. 213-239, USP, São Paulo, Brasil.

Paraense, W. L. (1975). Estado atual da sistemática dos planorbídeos brasileiros. *Arquivos do Museu Nacional do Rio de Janeiro*, vol.55, pp. 105-128.

Paraense, W. L.; Aires De Alencar, J. T. & Corrêa, L. R. (1983). Distribuição de planorbídeos e prevalência da xistossomose mansoni no Estado do Espírito Santo. *Memórias do Instituto Oswaldo Cruz*, vol.78, pp. 373-384.

Paraense, W. L. (1984). Distribuição dos caramujos no Brasil. In: *Modernos Conhecimentos sobre Esquistossomose Mansônica. Suplemento dos Anais de 1983 e 1984 da Academia Mineira de Medicina*, F.A. Reis; J. Faria; N. Katz (Eds), pp. 117-128, Minas Gerais, Brasil.

Paredes, H.; Souza-Santos, R; Resendes, A. P. C.; Souza, M. A. A.; Albuquerque, J.; Bocanegra, S.; Gomes, E. C. S. & Barbosa, C. S. (2010). Spatial patter, water use and risk level assciated with the transmission of schistosomiasis on the north coast of Pernambuco, Brazil. *Cadernos de Saúde Pública*, vol.26, pp. 1013-1023.

Pellon, A. B. & Teixeira, I. (1950). Distribuição geográfica da esquistossomose mansônica no Brasil. Publicação do Ministério da Educação e Saúde, Departamento Nacional de Saúde, Divisão de Organização Sanitária, Oitavo Congresso Brasileiro de Higiene, Rio de Janeiro, 1950.

Pellon, A. B. & Teixeira, I. (1953). O inquérito helmintológico escolar em cinco estados da região leste, sul e centro. Publicação do Ministério da Educação e Saúde,

Departamento Nacional de Saúde, Divisão de Organização Sanitária, XI Congresso Brasileiro de Higiene, Curitiba, 1953.

Pirajá da Silva, M. A. (1908). Contribuição para o estudo da Schistosomiase na Bahia. Vinte observações. *Publicações do Brazil-Médico*, vol.22, pp. 451-454.

Plano Diretor Urbano Ambiental de Mariana. PDUAM. (2003). *Relatório Diagnóstico de Mariana.* Mariana: Equipe Consultora do Plano Diretor, 350 p.

Pieri, O. S. (1995). Perspectivas no controle ambiental dos moluscos vetores da esquistossomose. In: *Tópicos em Malacologia Médica,* F.S. Barbosa, (Ed), pp. 239-252, Fiocruz, Rio de Janeiro, Brasil.

Souza, C. P.; Caldeira, R. L.; Drummond, S. C.; Melo, A. L.; Guimarães, C. T.; Soares, D. M. & Carvalho, O. S. (2001). Geographical distribution of *Biomphalaria* snails in the state of Minas Gerais, Brazil. *Memórias do Instituto Oswaldo Cruz,* vol.96, pp. 293-302.

Souza, L. A. (2004). Diagnóstico do meio físico como contribuição ao ordenamento territorial do município de Mariana. Dissertação (mestrado em Engenharia Civil - área de concentração - Geotecnia) - Departamento de Engenharia Civil - Escola de Minas da Universidade Federal de Ouro Preto, Ouro Preto, Minas Gerais, Brasil, 182p.

Souza, M. A. A.; Souza, L. A.; Machado-Coelho, G. L. L. & Melo, A. L. (2006). Levantamento malacológico e mapeamento das áreas de risco para transmissão da esquistossomose mansoni no município de Mariana, Minas Gerais, Brasil. *Revista de Ciências Médicas e Biológicas,* vol.5, No.2, pp 132-139.

Souza, M. A. A.; Barbosa, V. S.; Wanderlei, T. N. G. & Barbosa, C. S. (2008). Criadouros de *Biomphalaria,* temporários e permanentes, em Jaboatão dos Guararapes, PE. *Revista da Sociedade Brasileira de Medicina Tropical,* vol.41, No.3, pp. 252-256.

Teles, H. M. S.; Pereira, P. A. C. & Richinitti, L. M. Z. (1991). Distribuição de *Biomphalaria* (Gastropoda, Planorbidae) nos estados do Rio Grande do Sul e Santa Catarina, Brasil. *Revista de Saúde Pública*, vol.25, pp. 350-352.

Wilson. R. A.; Draskau. T.; Miller. P. & Lawson. R. J. (1978). *Schistosoma mansoni*: The activity and development of the schistosomulum during migration from the skin to the hepatic portal system. *Parasitology*, vol.77, pp. 57-73.

Wilson, R. A.; Coulson, P. S. & Dixon, B. (1986). Migration of the schistosomula of *Schistosoma mansoni* in mice vaccinated with radiation-attenuaed cercariae, and normal mice: An attempt to identify timing and site of parasite death. *Parasitology,* vol.92, pp. 101-16.

WHO. (1965). Snail control in the prevention of bilharziasis. *Monograph series,* No.50, 255p.

Out of Animals and Back Again: Schistosomiasis as a Zoonosis in Africa

Claire J. Standley[1], Andrew P. Dobson[1] and J. Russell Stothard[2]
[1]*Princeton University*
[2]*Liverpool School of Tropical Medicine*
[1]*USA*
[2]*UK*

1. Introduction

Schistosomiasis is one of the world's most widely distributed and prevalent parasitic diseases, with approximately 700 million people at risk of infection. The vast majority of human cases of the disease are found in Africa, with distribution in virtually all corners of the continent, bar the Sahara and Namib deserts and the depths of the Congo jungle (Hotez et al., 2009). Pre-prubescent children, and particularly boys, are the age group most at risk from adverse clinical symptoms and are frequently targeted for treatment interventions, yet even with readily available drugs (namely praziquantel), the pervasiveness of the intermediate host snails and the ease at which re-infection occurs has hampered attempts to manage the disease in many places (Standley et al., 2009, Fenwick, 2009). Less widely recognized is that some species of *Schistosoma,* including several which commonly affect man, can also be infective in other mammalian species, and particularly in non-human primates. Given current high levels of research interest into emerging zoonotic diseases, the status of schistosomiasis as a zoonotic infection is in need of re-appraisal, especially in light of advances in application of molecular epidemiological methods; it has been 20 years since the last formal review was published (Ouma and Fenwick, 1991), with earlier appraisals fully half a century ago (Nelson, 1960, Nelson et al., 1962). By comparing historical accounts to on-going, cutting edge research using molecular tools, it will be possible to gain an insight into the dynamics of schistosomiasis in human and other hosts and whether this relationship is changing as a result of anthropogenic activities. As such, this chapter provides an overview of zoonoses involving schistosomiasis, focusing on Africa where the burden of the disease is highest, and also discusses the ways in which this information can be integrated into more effective conservation management and human disease control strategies. The emphasis will be on the most common forms of human schistosomiasis and how animals not only may suffer clinical manifestations from infection, but may also act as reservoirs for schistosomiasis, thus confounding control efforts that focus mainly on the treatment of humans.

2. Overview of schistosomiasis as a global infection of wildlife and domestic animals

There are many species of *Schistosoma* that are only known from animal infections. Out of the 22 currently recognized species, only eight have been reported from humans (Table 1), and of these, only three are heavily implicated as diseases of public health importance. The rest of the genus *Schistosoma* is only known from animal infections, and specifically mammals; the various species have adapted to a wide variety of taxa, with some specializing on one species while others have a wide definitive host range. For the purposes of examining cross-over of parasitic infections between humans and animals and vice versa, the term 'zoonosis' is used throughout this chapter to describe transmission in both directions. Figure 1 shows a phylogeny of the genus *Schistosoma*, with main geographic distributions and primary definitive hosts marked.

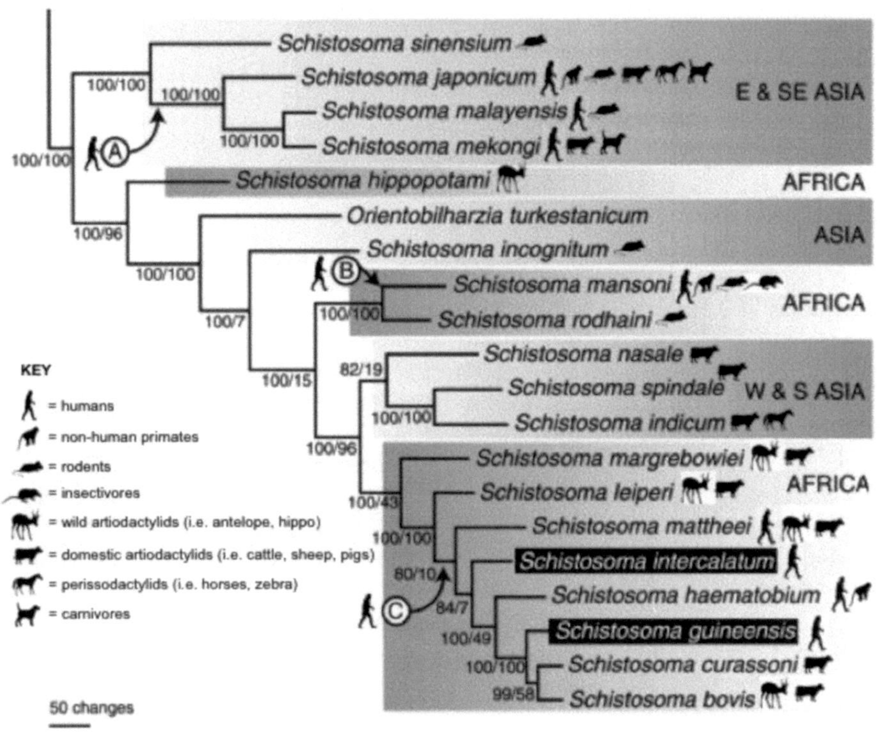

Fig. 1. Phylogeny of *Schistosoma*, as recognized in 2006 (*S. kisumuensis* was described in 2009; Hanelt et al., 2009). Known naturally infected definitive host groups are shown by the icons. The points 'A', 'B' and 'C' indicate the three suggested points where species adapted to infect humans; molecular clock estimates place the date of each divergence at roughly 3.8 MYA (millions of years ago) for point A and less than 1 million years ago for points B and C (Morgan et al., 2005, Webster et al., 2006, Attwood et al., 2008). The lines marked 'H' demonstrate clades with known hybridization between species (see section 4.1). Figure adapted from Webster et al. (2006).

2.1 *Schistosoma* infections of animals in Asia and Latin America

Although this chapter specifically focuses on the role of schistosomes as zoonotic infections in Africa, it is worth considering the distribution of the genus elsewhere in the world and the various animal definitive hosts the various species utilize, for comparison. In Asia, schistosomes from the *Schistosoma indicum* group (including *S. indicum*, *S. spindale* and *S. nasale*) are commonly found in domestic animals such as ungulates, horses, pigs and

Schistosoma species	Distribution	Natural definitive host species (excluding humans)	Human public health importance
S. mansoni	Africa, Middle East, South America, Caribbean	Non-human primates (including apes), rodents, insectivores, artiodactylids (waterbuck), procyonids (raccoon)	High
S. haematobium	Africa, Middle East	Non-human primates (not apes), artiodactylids (pigs, buffalo)	High
S. intercalatum	Central Africa (D.R. Congo only)	Possibly rodents	Low
S. guineensis	West Africa (Lower Guinea)	Possibly rodents	Low
S. mattheei	Southern Africa	Non-human primates (not apes), artiodactylids (cattle, antelope)	Low
S. japonicum	East Asia (China, Philippines, Indonesia)	Non-human primates, artiodactylids (water buffalos in particular), carnivores, rodents, perissodactylids (horses)	High
S. mekongi	SE Asia (Vietnam, Cambodia, Laos, Thailand)	Carnivores (dogs), artiodactylids (pigs)	Moderate
S. malayensis	Peninsular Malaysia	Rodents (van Mueller's rat)	Low

Table 1. The eight species of schistosome reported in humans. *Schistosoma guineensis* was only described in 2003, and so many past references to *S. intercalatum* may have actually been referring to *S. guineensis*. References include Fenwick (1969), Pitchford (1977), Loker (1983), Christensen et al. (1983), Pagès et al. (2003), and Standley et al. (2011).

possibly dogs. *Schistosoma indicum* is associated predominantly with artiodactylids, infecting a wide range of species, although perissodactylids have also been found naturally infected (Loker, 1983). *Schistosoma nasale* appears specialized to cattle, causing the veterinary condition known as 'snoring disease' (Bont et al., 1989). *Schistosoma spindale*, like *S. indicum*, appears to have a relatively low host specificity (Haas et al., 1990), though again it is mainly found in ungulates.

Species from the *Schistosoma japonicum* group are also widely recovered from different groups of animals, with *S. japonicum* itself described from perissodactylids, artiodactylids (particularly water buffalo), carnivores, rodents and primates (He et al., 2001). *Schistosoma mekongi*, conversely, is limited to humans and dogs, with pigs also possibly a natural host (Crosby and Garnham, 2009). Rodents have been successfully infected experimentally but there is no indication that these serve as natural definitive hosts (Byram and Von Lichtenberg, 1980). *Schistosoma malayensis*, the third member of the *S. japonicum* group, is rarely found in humans, with van Mueller's rat (*Rattus muelleri*) the usual definitive host in nature. Basal to this group are *S. ovuncatum* and *S. sinesium*, both of which utilize the common rat (*Rattus rattus*) as definitive hosts (Baidikul et al., 1984, Lockyer et al., 2003).

Schistosoma incognitum forms its own group (Webster et al., 2006); dogs, pigs and rats have been identified as naturally infected (Bunnag et al., 1983, Sinha and Srivastava, 1960), while in addition, rabbits and macaque monkeys have been experimentally determined to be susceptible.

The two remaining groups of *Schistosoma* species, the *S. mansoni* group and the *S. haematobium* group, are historically confined to Africa and the Middle East. However, *S. mansoni* is also found in Latin America, introduced via the slave trade from Africa (Desprès et al., 1993). Concerted public health initiatives have eliminated schistosomiasis as a human health concern in many Latin American and Caribbean locations (Hotez et al., 2008, Steinmann et al., 2006). However, transmission of *S. mansoni* in this region remains widespread, due to the susceptibility of other animals to the infection. Specifically, it is rodents that are now the primary definitive host in many parts of Latin America and the Caribbean. An interesting effect of this host switch has been the change of cercarial shedding patterns; those adapted to infecting humans tend to have peak cercarial emergence time at midday, whereas those adapted to rodents show maximum shedding at dawn and dusk, corresponding to the times of day when rodents are most active t water sources (Alarcón De Noya et al., 1997, Theron and Combes, 1995). This behavioural plasticity may explain how schistosomes can optimize infection in a wide variety of different host species.

2.2 *Schistosoma* of animals in Africa

In Africa, species of *Schistosoma* belong either to the *S. mansoni* group, characterized by eggs with lateral spines, or the *S. haematobium* group, identified by terminal spines on the eggs. Unlike the Asian schistosomes, the eponymous species of these two groups are most commonly found in humans and exact a huge public health burden on many communities and regions. However, as in Asia, there are other species within these groups that primarily affect non-human animals; this section will outline the other species of *Schistosoma* that are found in Africa, which are known as infection of domestic and wild animals, while the rest of the chapter deals with accounts of 'human' schistosome species as infections of animals.

The other species that make up the *Schistosoma haematobium* group are *S. intercalatum*, *S. guineensis*, *S. bovis*, *S. mattheei*, *S. margrebowiei*, *S. leiperi*, *S. curassoni* and the recently-described *S. kisumusensis* (Hanelt et al., 2009, Webster et al., 2006). *Schistosoma intercalatum* and *S. guineensis* primarily infect humans (Table 1). The remaining species, with the exception of *S. kisumuensis*, usually parasitize artiodactylid ruminants, with some most commonly found in domestic ungulates whereas others are more frequently observed in wild bovids. Between them, they are distributed over most of sub-Saharan Africa. *Schistosoma bovis* and *S. mattheei* are both principally parasites of domestic cattle; *S. bovis* is located throughout Africa but primarily north of 10° south, and it is replaced by *S. mattheei* south of this latitude (Nelson et al., 1962). In addition to domestic cattle, both *S. bovis* and S. *mattheei* have been naturally found in a variety of other artiodactylids as well as horses, zebras and rodents (Hanelt et al., 2010, Pitchford, 1977). There are even reports of these species from humans and baboons, although usually alongside a mixed infection with either *S. mansoni* or *S. haematobium*. *Schistosoma mattheei* was recently confirmed using molecular methods from a free-ranging baboon troop in Zambia (Weyher et al., 2010).

Sympatric to *Schistosoma bovis* in parts of Western Africa is *S. curassoni*, which is also naturally found in cattle, as well as sheep and goats (Ndifon et al., 1988, Vercruysse et al., 2003). In sub-Saharan Africa, *S. leiperi* and *S. margrebowiei* are two broadly sympatric species known as 'antelope' schistosomes, although they both have been observed to be transmissible through a wide range of artiodactylids, including domestic livestock. Both are also reported from horses and zebras; in addition, there is one account of eggs of *S.*

margrebowiei being recovered from a human rectal biopsy in Mali, mixed with *S. haematobium* and *S. mansoni* (Pitchford, 1959a). The egg morphology of *S. margrebowiei* is unique among African schistosomes (Christensen et al., 1983); although experimental passage has never been successful, other infections have also been reported from Zambia (Giboda et al., 1988), suggesting that while humans may contract incidental infections with *S. margrebowiei*, infections are not viable in man. *Schistosoma kisumuensis* is unique among the 'non-human' *S. haematobium* group species in being exclusively an infection of small mammals, such as rodents and insectivores; it was very recently described, using molecular methods, from western Kenya, and as such is not included in the 2006 phylogeny on which Figure 1 is based (Hanelt et al., 2009).

The *Schistosoma mansoni* group has traditionally been classified to consist only of three other species: *S. hippopotami*, *S. edwardiense* and *S. rodhaini*. *Schistosoma hippopotami*, on the basis of recent molecular analysis, has since been re-classified as basal to all African schistosomes (Webster et al., 2006); *S. hippopotami* and *S. edwardiense* are also unusual in only having been found in a single species of definitive host: the African hippopotamus (*Hippopotamus amphibius*). *Schistosoma rodhaini*, on the other hand, is primarily an infection of rodents, although there are past reports of dogs and even a serval cat being naturally infected in Central Africa (Pitchford, 1977, Schwetz, 1954). More recently, insectivore species around Lake Victoria have also been observed to be infected with *S. rodhaini* (Hanelt et al., 2010); baboons have been successfully experimentally infected, but only when also co-infected with *S. mansoni* (Nelson and Teesdale, 1965). The literature only mentions one reported case of a natural infection of *S. rodhaini* in a human, from what is now DR Congo (D'haenens and Santele, 1955); however, given the age of the reference and its isolation in the literature, it may be suggested that it is a case of false diagnosis of *S. mansoni*.

3. Accounts of 'human' schistosomiasis in African animals

Of the 12 species of *Schistosoma* found in Africa, only four are regularly reported as infections of humans; these are *S. mansoni*, *S. haematobium*, *S. intercalatum* and *S. guineensis* (see Table 1). Of these, the overwhelming majority of human cases are caused by the first two; indeed, *S. guineensis* was only first described in 2003, following from a molecular appraisal and as such, many older records of infections of *S. intercalatum*, especially if reporting from the Lower Guinear region (countries such as Nigeria, Cameroon, Equatorial Guinea, São Tomé and Gabon), may actually be referring to what would now be known as *S. guineensis* (Pagès et al., 2003). As such, throughout this chapter, these two will be considered together, as *S. intercalatum/guineensis*. The following section examines both past and present records of human forms of schistosomiasis in animals, evaluates how hybridization of non-human schistosomes may result in emerging zoonotic threat, and finally describes methods for determining the extent and validity of a cross-over of schistosome infection between humans and animals or vice versa.

3.1 Historical records of *Schistosoma mansoni*, *S. haematobium* and S. *intercalatum/guineensis* in African animals

Schistosomiasis has long been reported as a human parasitic disease in Africa: eggs of *Schistosoma haematobium* have been observed from mummies in Egypt, dating back to more than a millennium BCE (Lambert-Zazulak et al., 2003). Moreover, molecular evidence has suggested a similar length and geography for the evolution of *Schistosoma* in Africa to that of modern *Homo sapiens*, suggesting a very ancient association between humans and schistosomes (Despres et al., 1992). The distribution of the four main types of human schistosome (*S. haematobium, S. mansoni, S. intercalatum* and *S. guineensis*) covers vast swathes of Africa and Madagascar, including areas of high human density such as the West African coast, the Sahel and the southern and eastern highlands (Figure 2). High population density of humans is accompanied by large numbers of domestic livestock, putting such animals, as well as others that are associated with human activity, at risk of contracting diseases such as schistosomiasis. Moreover, many of these regions are known to possess high biodiversity of non-domesticated animals, which may also be exposed to transmission.

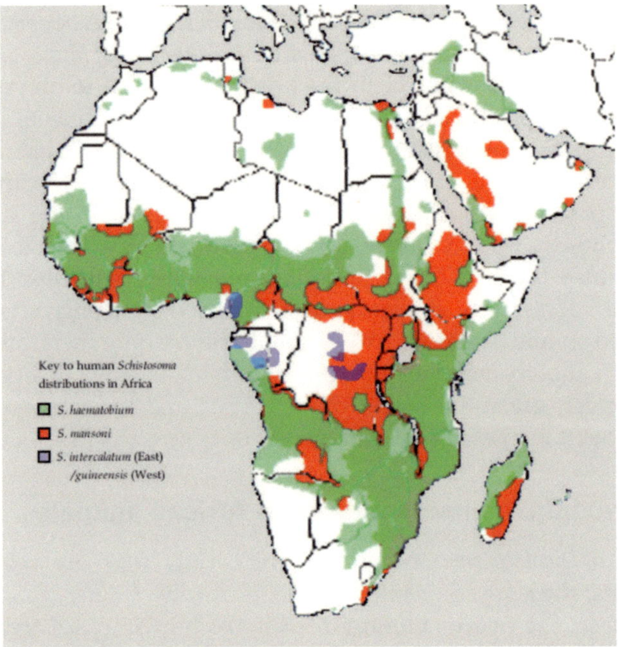

Fig. 2. Map of distribution of human *Schistosoma* species in Africa, Madagascar and the Middle East. Redrawn from www.path.cam.ac.uk (University of Cambridge, Dept. of Pathology)

Although interest in tropical medicine and parasitology had been first extensively stimulated by European troops returning home from stations in Africa after the First World War, it was the creation of the World Health Organisation after World War II which led to concerted and coordinated research programmes involving tropical diseases (Sandbach, 1976, Sturrock, 2001). These programmes included detailed surveys of human communities for incidence, prevalence and intensity of a range of infectious diseases, including schistosomiasis; in many cases, domestic and wild animals were also explicitly included in these surveys. Other cases of animal infections were reported *ad hoc*, either based on veterinary concern or commercial interest.

The explicit focus on concurrently surveying animals alongside human communities dwindled in the 1970s; the emphasis on chemotherapeutic control of schistosomiasis led to resources being targeted at mass drug administration and human treatment programmes. However, the emergence of interest in conservation issues resulted in re-energised monitoring of wild animals populations, and the continued, if sporadic, reporting of cases of human parasites in wild animals. The modern, molecular, era has transformed the way in which zoonotic infections are identified and analysed, as will be discussed further in section 4; moreover, the status of animals as reservoirs of human schistosomiasis, as the situation was in the 1960s and 1970s, has been comprehensively covered by Nelson and colleagues (1960, 1962) and R. J. Pitchford (1977), respectively. More recently, Ouma and Fenwick (1991) reviewed schistosomiasis as a zoonosis in Africa; as such, there is little need to re-review and the following paragraphs will briefly summarise and update these earlier works regarding the main discoveries of schistosomiasis in non-human hosts in Africa in the last years of the 20th century and first decade of the 21st century.

3.2 Recent reports of *Schistosoma mansoni*, *S. haematobium*, and *S. intercalatum/guineensis* in non-human animals in Africa

Pitchford's (1977) checklist of natural hosts of *Schistosoma mansoni, S. haematobium* and *S. intercalatum* included a range of wild and domestic animals throughout Africa, although primates were considered the main mammal groups affected for all three, with *S. mansoni* also being an important infection of rodents (Table 1). These two groups will be considered separately in subsequent sub-sections.

In addition, for *Schistosoma mansoni* Pitchford lists two records of shrews (insectivores) being found naturally infected in the wild and two instances of eggs being found in artiodactylids, though the eggs were dead and thus these ruminants cannot be considered naturally viable hosts (Pitchford et al., 1974). Nelson et al. (1962) also report on a case of *S. mansoni* eggs, mixed with *S. rodhaini*, being found in a dog in Kenya; other similar discoveries of *S. mansoni* eggs in dogs has been attributed to ingestion of human feces containing parasite eggs, and hatching of the specimens in dogs does not seem to produce viable miracidia (Mango, 1971). Moreover, laboratory experiments conducted a few years earlier did not find dogs, or indeed carnivores in general, susceptible to infection, supporting the hypothesis that these incidental observations should not be the basis for considering dogs natural hosts of *S. mansoni* (Kuntz and Malakatis, 1955a, Stirewalt et al., 1951).

More recently, shrews were found naturally infected with *Schistosoma mansoni* at a marsh site in Kenya, near Lake Victoria, confirming earlier reports of their likely susceptibility (Hanelt et al., 2010). In terms of infections in artiodactylids, adult *S. mansoni* worms were recovered from a small number of cattle in Sudan during a survey in the 1980s; eggs were not recovered from the stool so viability of the infection cannot be confirmed (Karoum and Amin, 1985). The same survey failed to find signs of infection in local dogs, sheep and goats, despite 70% prevalence of infection in resident school-age children.

Schistosoma haematobium, in contrast to *S. mansoni*, has long been considered almost exclusively a primate, disease, mainly due to the paucity of observations of natural infections in other taxa (Nelson et al., 1962, Vianna Martins, 1958). Pitchford (1977) lists only a handful of reported cases from artiodactylids, including domestic pigs and sheep (the latter mixed with *S. mattheei* infection) and a single female Cape buffalo. Vianna Martins (1958) elucidates the low susceptibility of sheep and rodents to *S. haematobium*, describing comprehensive surveys of these taxa in highly endemic areas of human infection in Iraq and D.R. Congo, and finding no trace of infection. To the authors' knowledge, modern surveys have thus far not found naturally-acquired, non-hybrid *S. haematobium* infections in mammals other than primates or rodents; like *S. mansoni*, carnivores do not appear to be readily susceptible to infection with *S. haematobium* in the laboratory so there is little reason to assume they are more permissive under natural conditions (Kuntz and Malakatis, 1955b). Like *Schistosoma haematobium, S. intercalatum/guineensis* are considered primarily to be infections of man, and have rarely been reported from other taxa. Pitchford (1977) only lists primate records of natural infection, and in his review of the life history of schistosomes, Loker (1983) puts a question mark next to possible infections of rodents and artiodactylids with *S. intercalatum* (*S. guineensis* had yet to be described); Christensen et al. (1983) fully dismiss bovids as significant natural hosts of *S. intercalatum*, along, in fact, with *S. mansoni* and *S. haematobium*. Similarly, a recent review of the status of *S. intercalatum* in Central Africa fails to mention reports of this parasite in non-human mammals (Ripert, 2003); as such, as with *S. mansoni* and *S. haematobium*, it is suggested that attention should focus on rodents and non-human primates as primarily at risk from *S. intercalatum/guineensis*.

3.2.1 Schistosomiasis in African rodents

Given the broad and excellent experimental susceptibility of a range of rodent species to infection with all four of the above-mentioned 'human' schistosomes, it would come as no surprise to observe natural infections in this taxon. Moreover, the high biodiversity and abundance of rodent species especially around human settlements, lends them importance as potential reservoirs of human schistosomiasis, even if their egg excretion rates are relatively low. Understanding the role this group of mammals plays in the transmission of schistosomiasis, therefore, may be an important step towards maintaining control of the disease in human communities, as has been suggested in other locations where rodents are significant definitive hosts, such as Latin America and the Caribbean (Modena et al., 2008).
As it happens, the vast majority of reports relate to infections with *Schistosoma mansoni* alone; given that a variety of rodents have been known to be experimentally susceptible to *S. haematobium* (Gear et al., 1966), suggesting further scrutiny of this taxon be a research objective. In the literature, a single adult male worm of *S. haematobium* was reported from a Nile rat in Egypt in the 1970s (Mansour, 1973); given that the rodent was co-infected with *S. mansoni*, and no terminally-spined eggs were recovered from any of the surveyed rats, this observation may well be a misidentification (Morand et al., 2006). An earlier single report of *S. haematobium* in a rodent has likewise since been considered erroneous (Pitchford, 1959b). Similarly, there is a paucity of information on infections with *S. intercalatum* in rodents; a single historical report exists of a natural infection of a rodent with *S. intercalatum*, despite sympatric species of rodents known to be experimentally susceptible (Imbert-Establet et al., 1997).
Schistosoma mansoni, as mentioned above, is relatively commonly observed in African rodents, although usually at lower prevalence levels than seen in Latin American or Caribbean transmission settings (Hanelt et al., 2010). Historical accounts of natural infections in rodents are mainly based around a series of comprehensive surveys undertaken in D.R. Congo in the 1950s, which revealed presence of *S. mansoni* in six genera of rodents (Schwetz, 1954, 1956). At this time, the form of *S. mansoni* found in rodents was considered to be a separate variant to the human form, and was described as *S. mansoni* var. *rodentum*. More recent analyses have shown using molecular tools that there is gene flow between the parasites found in rodents and in man, suggesting that the form observed in rodents subtly changes its morphology in response to different host environments (Steinauer et al., 2008b); this work was done on rodent populations in Western Kenya, where several other reports of *S. mansoni* in rodents from recent years have originated

(Hanelt et al., 2010, Steinauer et al., 2009, Steinauer et al., 2008a). Rodents have also been found infected with *S. mansoni* throughout the rest of Africa, with more reports from Kenya (Kawashima et al., 1978, Nelson et al., 1962), South Africa (Pitchford and Visser, 1962), Senegal (Duplantier and Sène, 2000), Sudan (Karoum and Amin, 1985) and Egypt (Arafa and Massoud, 1990, Mansour, 1973).

3.2.2 Schistosomiasis in non-human primates in Africa

Whereas rodent infections with humans schistosomiasis are relatively constrained to *Schistosomiasis mansoni,* natural infections in non-human primates are known also from *S. haematobium* (Pitchford, 1977). Moreover, given the close geographical and genetic proximity of many primate species to humans, it is no surprise that these are the group of mammals most likely to be at risk from infection with human diseases of all kinds, including schistosomes, and infections with other trematode genera have been observed in free-ranging primate populations in Africa (Murray et al., 2000, Sleeman et al., 2009). In addition, as human populations grow at a rapid rate and communities push ever further into remote forest locations, they are coming into contact with relatively pristine primate habitats, thus potentially putting new species at risk of exposure to schistosomiasis infection. Given the endangered and threatened status of many of Africa's primate populations, these examples of human to wildlife transmission of parasites are of grave concern to primate conservation managers. As such, and particularly considering the vast amount of research attention awarded to wild primate populations, it is surprising that until recently, relatively little concerted effort has been undertaken to characterize and diagnose parasitic infections in non-human primates. Fortunately, the early years of the 21st century have witnessed renewed interest in questions of zoonotic transmission of diseases, and thus a number of surveys have since reported on the observation of *Schistosoma* in a variety of non-human primates. The methods for identifying these infections and confirming their transmission will be discussed in the next section; here, it suffices to outline past reports of human schistosomiasis in non-human primate species, as well as more current accounts.

It is worth mentioning initially that *Schistosoma intercalatum/guineensis* has never been recently observed as a natural infection in non-human primates. This may be because on the whole, these parasites are distributed in relatively dense tropical forest regions, where primate species tend to be arboreal and are less likely to come into contact with terrestrial infected water sources. Evidence for this hypothesis comes from the observation that several primate species, including some which are distributed in the same countries as *S. intercalatum/guineensis,* are experimentally susceptible to infection (Cheever et al., 1976, Kuntz et al., 1980, Kuntz et al., 1978b). However, these species might not be exposed to the parasite, due to habitat preference or behaviour; for example, the Patas monkey is known to be a good experimental host of *S. intercalatum* (Kuntz et al., 1978a), and is found in parts of Central and West Africa, but tends to inhabit savannah habitats which might not be suitable for *Bulinus forskalii* or *Bulinus africanus* group snails, the intermediate snail hosts of *S. guineensis* and *S. intercalatum,* respectively. Wright et al. (1978) indeed suggested that the forest/non-forest interface might be a barrier to transmission. Given that chimpanzees are also known to be susceptible (Kuntz et al., 1978b), are ground-dwelling, and are distributed in patches throughout the region where *S. intercalatum/guineensis* are found, future parasitological surveys of *Pan troglodytes* and *P. paniscus* (the bonobo) should bear in mind the possibility of encountering *S. intercalatum/guineensis.*

Schistosoma haematobium, in contrast, has been reported as a natural infection of non-human primates, although *S. mansoni* is still the more common human schistosome in this taxon. Based on the collated records presented by Ouma and Fenwick (1991), by the early 1990s both parasites had been observed in vervet monkeys (*Cercopithecus aethiops*, also known as grivet monkeys), Sykes monkeys (*C. mitis*) and baboons (*Papio* spp.). These accounts have spanned Africa; they include surveys from Kenya, Tanzania, Uganda, Zimbabwe, Senegal and Ethiopia. In addition, a chimpanzee imported into the USA from Senegal was diagnosed with *S. haematobium* (De Paoli, 1965), although at the time of Ouma and Fenwick's review (1991) no *S. mansoni* had ever been observed as a natural infection of any ape other than humans. It is no coincidence that all of these localities are known areas with high endemic prevalence of schistosomiasis in human communities, suggesting that a combination of environmental transmission suitability and high levels of infection in humans is putting non-human primates at risk of exposure to schistosomiasis.

As such, it should come as no surprise that human-mediated landscape change and population growth may explain the increasing number of observations of human schistosomiasis in non-human primates in recent years. By far the most common reported non-human primate host has been the baboon, and the dominant parasite in these instances has been *Schistosoma mansoni*, although one observation of a baboon infected with *S. haematobium* was made from South Africa in the 1990s (Appleton and Henzi, 1993). Observations have been equally as widespread in the last two decades as in earlier years, with accounts of infection from Kenya (Hahn et al., 2003, Munene et al., 1998, Muriuki et al., 1998), Tanzania (Muller-Graf et al., 1997, Murray et al., 2000), Ethiopia (Legesse and Erko, 2004, Phillips-Conroy, 1986), Senegal (Howells et al. 2011, Mcgrew et al., 1989) and Nigeria (Weyher et al., 2006); baboons have also recently been implicated as potential reservoir hosts for *S. mansoni* in parts of the Arabian peninsula (Ghandour et al., 1995, Zahed et al., 1996). In several of these cases, as well as other incidences of parasite transmission between humans and non-human primates, it has been suggested that forest fragmentation, increased proximity of humans to wild habitats and the emerging reliance of wild primates on human settlements for food (such as through crop-raiding) is at least partially responsible for increased exposure and risk of these animals contracting 'human' diseases (Gillespie and Chapman, 2008, Weyher et al., 2006). A worrying trend is that national park and forest reserve areas, which might have been expected to afford a degree of protection against zoonotic transmission of infections, also seem to show signs of human to animal transfer of parasites, as has been seen in Mahale Mountains National Park and Gombe Stream National Park, to name but two examples.

Of note is the observation that while baboons in many locations have been shown to be infected with *Schistosoma mansoni*, other sympatric non-human primate species were described as free of the parasite. This is particularly interesting given that in several cases, these sympatric primate species are known to be susceptible to *S. mansoni* infection, and have even been observed naturally infected in the wild. For example, in their survey of three species of wild primate in Kenya, Munene et al. (1998) positively identified *S. mansoni* infections in baboons but not in local vervet or Sykes monkeys, despite earlier accounts of these species being infected, also in East Africa (Nelson, 1960). Similarly, Legesse and Erko (2004) observed schistosomiasis infection in baboons in Ethiopia, but not in sympatric vervet monkeys. Infected baboons have also been reported from two localities, Fongoli in Senegal and Gombe Stream National Park in Tanzania, which are also inhabited by troops of chimpanzees; despite extensive parasitological surveys, these chimpanzees have never convincingly displayed positive infection with *S. mansoni* (Bakuza and Nkwengulila, 2009, Howells et al., 2011, Muller-Graf et al., 1997, Murray et al., 2000). There is an isolated, unpublished account, from the early 1990s, of *S. mansoni* eggs being recovered from chimpanzee stool in Gombe Stream NP (Nutter, 1993); however, since both earlier and ensuing examinations failed to reconfirm the finding, it may be that this report is a case of mislabeled samples, and the stool had actually belonged to a baboon.

Likewise, there are locations where chimpanzees are known to inhabit areas that have high levels of schistosomiasis transmission to humans, and yet appear not to have been exposed to the disease; one such location is Rubondo Island, where prevalence in humans in island communities nearby is very high, and snails shedding *Schistosoma mansoni* cercariae have been observed in the shallow waters fringing the island itself (Standley et al., 2010). However, despite extensive parasitological surveys, the chimpanzees, vervet monkeys and guerezas (*Colobus guereza*) that inhabit the island have not been reported as infected (Petrášová et al. 2010, Petrzelkova et al., 2006), based on stool examinations; it would be interesting to also include serological tests for exposure, which offer much greater levels of sensitivity.

The relative absence of natural infections of *Schistosoma* species in chimpanzees has long suggested that despite their close phylogenetic relationship to humans, chimpanzees are perhaps not naturally susceptible to the parasite, or do not access infected water sources in ways which would expose them to infection. This assumption has been resolutely refuted through the confirmation of naturally acquired infections of *S. mansoni* in wild-born, semi-captive chimpanzees on Ngamba Island, a sanctuary for rescued and orphaned chimpanzees (Standley et al., 2011). Over the course of four surveys in three years, 11% of chimpanzees tested for *S. mansoni* infection were stool-positive for eggs, which were later hatched and used to infect *Biomphalaria* snails, proving their viability. Chimpanzees were also observed close to the water's edge on a number of occasions, indicating behavioural risk of exposure (Figure 3). Of more concern is recent evidence of significant liver pathology in these chimpanzees, comparable to humans progressing towards chronic infection status; this observation was made by using ultrasound imagery, a technology never before used, to the authors' knowledge, for diagnosis of clinical schistosomiasis in naturally-infected

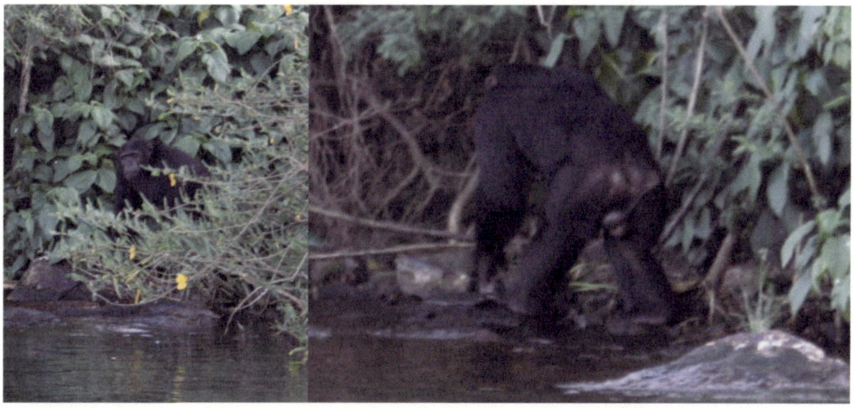

Fig. 3. The above photographs show Kalema, a chimpanzee resident on Ngamba Island. These chimpanzees are regularly observed walking through shallow water; snails shedding *Schistosoma mansoni* cercariae have been collected from near this location, indicating the exposure risk of these chimpanzees to schistosomiasis (photographs taken by C. J. Standley).

non-human primates (C. J. Standley and J. R. Stothard, manuscript in preparation). These new discoveries of infections in semi-wild animals indicate the importance of continued surveys in order to catch new and emerging cases of transmission of parasites between humans and wild animal populations. In addition, there may be cases in which schistosomes themselves change in ways in which enables them to infect a wider variety of hosts; examples of this, along with a further analysis of the methods for diagnosing and evaluating risk of zoonotic transmission of schistosomiasis, will be considered in the following section.

4. Emerging zoonotic risk of schistosomiasis: Causes, diagnosis and analysis

A consideration of past reports of schistosomiasis in animals in Africa would not be complete without an evaluation of potential risks of emerging zoonotic infections, including methods for researchers to determine the origin, transmission direction and causes of infections found both in humans and wildlife. In order to do so, scientists should be encouraged to employ the same up-to-date technology on animal populations as is used in humans, for consistency of results. Finally, research on zoonotic parasitic infections should embrace the use of a multidisciplinary tools in order to analyse their results and thus produce conclusions that can be used to inform other interested parties across different fields, from public health to conservation medicine and encompassing biogeography, molecular epidemiology and mathematical modeling (Daszak et al., 2004, Morens et al., 2004, Stephens et al., 1998, Wilcox and Gubler, 2005).

4.1 Hybridization of schistosomes: Risk of emerging zoonotic schistosomes

While it is beyond the scope of this chapter to review comprehensively the literature on hybridization of schistosomes, it is worth mentioning a few key examples of how interbreeding between human and non-human schistosome species has been reported as infections of novel hosts, and thus how these parasites might constitute risk of an emerging zoonotic disease, either from humans to wildlife or vice versa. Similarly, there are examples where hybridization may also protect against transmission of disease.

The two main instances of hybridization that involve so-called 'human' species of schistosome are those between *Schistosoma haematobium* and *S. bovis* and between *S. mansoni* and *S. rodhaini*. Natural hybrids between *S. haematobium* and *S. bovis* have been documented from children living in the Senegal River Basin (Huyse et al., 2009). In this example, the construction of the Diama Dam led to the creation of suitable habitat for the snail intermediate hosts of *S. mansoni*, *S. haematobium* and *S. bovis*, which spread rapidly through the region (De Clercq et al., 1999). Individuals co-infected with all three genotypes are relatively common; 4 out of 15 children infected with hybrids also excreted *S. mansoni* and *S. haematobium* eggs (Huyse et al., 2009). While to the authors' knowledge, accounts of these hybrids in cattle have yet to be reported from this region, given the presence of cattle schistosome hybrids in humans and the close phylogenetic relationships between these species (see Figure 1), searching for hybrids in bovine species should also be recommending in this setting, as well as other locations where known *S. haematobium/bovis* hybrids occur in humans (Coyne and Orr, 1998).

In contrast to the situation with *Schistosoma haematobium/bovis* hybrids, natural occurrence of hybridization between *S. mansoni* and *S. rodhaini* has thus far only been reported from snail intermediate hosts and rodents, and not mammals (Morgan et al., 2003, Steinauer et al., 2008a). In this case, the concern is that such infections could pass from rodent hosts into

humans; these natural hybrids from the Kisumu region of Kenya have similar cercarial emergence times as *S. mansoni*, thus putting humans more at risk of exposure than if *S. rodhaini*-like emergence behaviour were the dominant phenotype (Steinauer et al., 2008a).
There are also examples of hybridization involving the relatively rare *Schistosoma intercalatum/guineensis* species, both primarily infections of humans. These hybridize successfully with both *S. haematobium* and *S. bovis* in areas where their ranges and intermediate hosts overlap (Southgate et al., 1976, Tchuenté et al., 1997); *S. guineensis*, being transmitted by *Bulinus forskalii* snails, can come into contact with *S. bovis* in the snail host, as can *S. intercalatum* and *S. haematobium* in snails of the *Bulinus africanus* complex. All four may also come into contact in various definitive hosts, depending on susceptibility. It has actually been suggested that the process of hybridization is responsible for the limited distribution range of *S. intercalatum* and *S. guineensis*; given that males of *S. haematobium* and *S. bovis* are more reproductively successful, gene flow in the hybrids tends to be in the direction of the loss of *S. intercalatum/guineensis* genome and dominance of genetic material from *S. haematobium/bovis* (Tchuenté et al., 1997). In the case of hybrids with *S. bovis*, this might actually result in the reduction of exposure risk of schistosomiasis infection caused by human schistosomes, but at the same time it may increase the distribution and extent of animal species of the parasite. In both instances, a danger is that changes to the genome could result in enhanced pathology or virulence, either in humans or animals, which could then exacerbate the public health, veterinary and conservation burden of the hybrid infection.

4.2 Diagnosis, identification and analysis of zoonotic schistosomiasis infections and risk

The observation and identification of forms of schistosomiasis passing between humans and animals is often a non-trivial matter, given the wide variety of definitive host species at risk of infection as well as morphological similarities between different schistosome species across several life stages. This section will briefly outline some suggestions for new methods of diagnosis of infection for use in non-human settings, ways in which direction of transmission can be confirmed and also alternative, cross-disciplinary tools which should be employed by parasitological researchers in order to maximize the analyses which can be achieved from their data.
A crucial obstacle facing researchers in terms of the observation and diagnosis of schistosomiasis in non-human hosts is the difficulty in accessing samples from populations of wild animals. Given that primates and rodents are suspected to be the main animal groups at risk of infection with human schistosomes, and therefore the most likely reservoirs of infection (Nelson et al., 1962, Ouma and Fenwick, 1991), standardized protocols for sampling and data collection of these animal groups should be employed, to ensure consistency of results between surveys. Such protocols have been developed for primate parasitology in the field (Gillespie, 2006); however, for rodents, it might be prudent to follow methods established by field surveys in the literature, for example that of Hanelt et al. (2010) in their rodent surveys in Kisumu, Kenya. Another approach should also be to increase surveying effort of non-primate and non-rodent mammals which are known to be naturally susceptible to schistosomiasis infection, or which have never before been sampling extensively; for example, insectivore species are known from recent surveys to be susceptible and naturally infected with *Schistosoma mansoni* and *S. kisumuensis* (Hanelt et al., 2010). Given their constant exposure to water and abundance through water bodies, such as Lake Victoria, where schistosomiasis is highly endemic, it is also suggested that African otters should be targeted for parasitological surveys, as a high-risk group of mammals.

Once the target definitive host group has been identified, the next question involves the type of sample and the methods used for diagnosing infection. The traditional method is to observe eggs passed either in the stool, for gastro-intestinal species (such as *Schistosoma mansoni, S. rodhaini, S. intercalatum* and *S. guineensis*) or urine, for *S. haematobium*. In non-threatened species, trapping and dissection for observation of adult worms is also an option; similarly, for domestic livestock that are routinely slaughtered, surveys of abattoirs can be performed. While these methods are cheap, simple and relatively effective, they are not in line with current diagnostic efforts in human populations. For example, the CCA dipstick utilizes a tiny drop of urine, but since only feeding adult worms produce circulating cathodic antigen, is more indicative than eggs in stool of an active infection. This method has been tested on Ngamba Island's semi-captive chimpanzee population (Standley et al., 2011), and was shown to have greater sensitivity than any stool-based diagnostic (apart from PCR), and so may be especially useful in animals that are not efficient egg excretors.

Similarly, blood samples can be used to test for antibodies (IgG/M) against schistosome egg antigen enzyme-linked immunosorbent assay (SEA-ELISA), which is highly sensitive in diagnosis of humans (Stothard et al., 2009). This method has also been tested on Ngamba Island, showing over 90% prevalence in the chimpanzees (Standley et al., 2011); given that antibodies may persist in the bloodstream up to several years after the infection has been cleared, this method may be particularly effective in gauging exposure to *Schistosoma*, especially where host antibodies are sufficiently similar to human IgG/M to allow cross-specific binding, but is not accurate in measuring current infection status. In order to ensure that surveys of animals are comparable and consistent with on-going and parallel human studies, the inclusion of these new, field-reliable and highly sensitive rapid diagnostic tests should be incorporated into future sampling efforts (see Figure 4). It should be noted the SEA-ELISA test does not work on bovids as their IgG does not bind with the protein conjugate; a bovine IgG/M conjugate is needed.

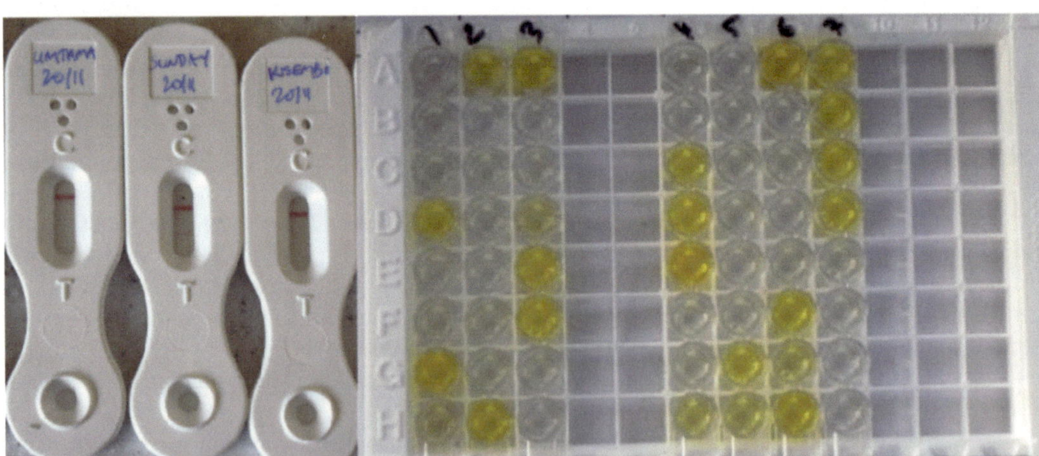

Fig. 4. Examples of the urine CCA lateral flow test (left) and SEA-ELISA serological diagnostic, both as used on chimpanzee urine and blood samples, respectively. In the CCA picture, a second pink line underneath the control band indicates a positive infection, as indicated with the central test. For the SEA-ELISA, a yellow test well indicates a sample positive for antibodies against schistosome egg antigen (photos taken by C. J. Standley).

One disadvantage with these rapid diagnostic tests is that they only diagnose schistosome infection to genus rather than species level. Morphology has traditionally been the first method for species identification; the shape, size, and spine location on schistosome eggs is often sufficient. Adult worms too have interspecies variations in body form and behaviour; cercarial identification is more difficult, but is aided by the type of intermediate snail host used and emergence behaviour. However, there have been observations of intraspecific variations in egg shape, perhaps due to host morphology; moreover, hybrids are difficult to detect through morphology alone. In these cases, the advent of molecular tools has revolutionized researchers' ability to confirm species identification (Webster et al., 2006), hybrids (Webster et al., 2007) and even the direction of transmission, in this setting as well as with other parasitic diseases (Graczyk et al., 2002, Standley et al., 2011). Moreover, monitoring changes in parasite genotype over time and comparing variation between human and animal populations can determine the source and maintenance of the infection (Nejsum et al., 2010). As such, when investigating purported cases of zoonotic transmission, it is recommended that conclusions are supported by these forms of additional evidence.

In addition to molecular tools, there are other methods that should be employed alongside traditional parasitological surveys for analyzing the zoonotic potential of parasitic diseases. For example, there is a growing movement to integrate spatial epidemiological data with human and animal population distribution information using geographical information systems (GIS), in order to evaluate high risk areas for the cross-over of infectious diseases (Eisen and Eisen, 2007). While geospatial models have been applied to schistosomiasis epidemiology in humans (Clements et al., 2010), and to human-animal schistosomiasis transmission in Asia (Ishikawa et al., 2006, Williams et al., 2002), it would be useful to integrate animals into these models within an African setting. These can also be informed by classic models of disease transmission, as developed by Anderson and May (1991), and used to gauge the risk of emergence of infection in particular areas, as well as evaluate the effect of control interventions.

5. Conclusions: Implications for public health initiatives and wildlife conservation management

As this chapter has demonstrated, species of the genus *Schistosoma* are widespread across the globe, causing infections in wildlife as well as in humans. In Africa, the public health burden of schistosomiasis, caused primarily by *S. mansoni*, *S. haematobium* and *S. intercalatum/guineensis*, is enormous (Hotez and Fenwick, 2009); less well recognized is the risk imparted on animal populations by these parasites. Human control interventions have been established across the Africa; usually coordinated at the national level and involving mass drug administration of praziquantel, such programmes have been effective at reducing the prevalence and intensity of schistosomiasis infection in a number of regions (Fenwick et al., 2009). However, it may be that in some settings, control will be confounded without a thorough understanding of the role animal reservoirs play in maintaining transmission; moreover, there are clear examples of how endangered non-human mammals, such as chimpanzees, will profit from a specific consideration of schistosomiasis as part of their conservation strategy. As such, human public health initiatives and wildlife monitoring groups should work synergistically together to produce disease control strategies that are beneficial to all animals, including humans, at risk of contracting diseases such as schistosomisias.

6. References

Alarcón De Noya, B., Pointier, J. P., Colmenares, C., Thèron, A., Balzan, C., Cesari, I. M., González, S. & Noya, O. (1997) Natural *Schistosoma mansoni* infection in wild rats from Guadeloupe: parasitological and immunological aspects. *Acta Tropica,* 68, 11-21.

Anderson, R. M. & May, R. M. (1991) Infectious Diseases of Humans, Oxford, Oxford University Press.

Appleton, C. & Henzi, S. (1993) Environmental correlates of gastrointestinal parasitism in montane and lowland baboons in Natal, South Africa. *International Journal of Primatology,* 14, 623-635.

Arafa, M. A. S. & Massoud, M. M. (1990) Natural *Schistosoma mansoni* infection in *Arvicanthis niloticus* in Ismailia, Egypt. *Journal of the Egyptian Society of Parasitology,* 20, 775-778.

Attwood, S. W., Fatih, F. A. & Upatham, E. S. (2008) DNA-sequence variation among *Schistosoma mekongi* populations and related taxa; Phylogeography and the current distribution of Asian schistosomiasis. *PLoS Neglected Tropical Diseases,* 2, e200.

Baidikul, V., Upatham, E. S., Kruatrachue, M., Viyanant, V., Vichasri, S., Lee, P. & Chantanawat, R. (1984) Study on *Schistosoma sinensium* in Fang district, Chiangmai province, Thailand. *Southeast Asian Journal of Tropical Medicine and Public Health,* 15, 141-147.

Bakuza, J. & Nkwengulila, G. (2009) Variation over time in parasite prevalence among free-ranging chimpanzees at Gombe National Park, Tanzania. *International Journal of Primatology,* 30, 43-53.

Bont, J. D., Aken, D. V., Vercruysse, J., Fransen, J., Southgate, V. R. & Rollinson, D. (1989) The effect of praziquantel on *Schistosoma nasale* infections in cattle. *Journal of Veterinary Pharmacology and Therapeutics,* 12, 455-458.

Bunnag, T., S., T., P., I., P., V. & S., I. (1983) *Schistosoma incognitum* and its zoonotic potential role in Phitsanulok and Phichit provinces, northern Thailand. *Southeast Asian Journal of Tropical Medicine and Public Health,* 14, 163-170.

Byram, J. E. & Von Lichtenberg, F. (1980) Experimental infection with *Schistosoma mekongi* in laboratory animals: parasitological and pathological findings. IN Bruce, J. I. & Sornmani, S. (Eds.) *The Mekong schistosome* Berkeley, Malacological Review.

Cheever, A. W., Kuntz, R. E., Moore, J. A. & Huang, T. C. (1976) Proliferative epithelial lesions of the urinary bladder in cynomolgus monkeys (*Macaca fascicularis*) Infected with *Schistosoma intercalatum*. *Cancer Research,* 36, 2928-2931.

Christensen, N. Ø., Mutani, A. & Frandsen, F. (1983) A review of the biology and transmission ecology of African bovine species of the genus *Schistosoma*. *Parasitology Research,* 69, 551-570.

Clements, A. C. A., Deville, M. A., Ndayishimiye, O., Brooker, S. & Fenwick, A. (2010) Spatial co-distribution of neglected tropical diseases in the East African Great Lakes region: revisiting the justification for integrated control. *Tropical Medicine & International Health,* 15, 198-207.

Coyne, J. A. & Orr, H. A. (1998) The evolutionary genetics of speciation. *Philosophical Transactions of the Royal Society of London Series B-Biological Sciences,* 353, 287-305.

Crosby, A. & Garnham, B. B. (2009) Experimental models of pulmonary vascular disease in schistosomiasis. *Experimental Models in Pulmonary Vascular Diseases,* 1, 39-41.

D'haenens, G. & Santele, A. (1955) A case of human infestation with *Schistosoma rodhaini* found in the outskirts of Elisabethville. *Annales de la Société Belge de Médecine Tropicale.,* 35, 497.

Daszak, P., Tabor, G. M., Kilpatrick, A. M., Epstein, J. O. N. & Plowright, R. (2004) Conservation Medicine and a New Agenda for Emerging Diseases. *Annals of the New York Academy of Sciences,* 1026, 1-11.

De Clercq, D., Vercruysse, J., Picquet, M., Shaw, D. J., Diop, M., Ly, A. & Gryseels, B. (1999) The epidemiology of a recent focus of mixed *Schistosoma haematobium* and *Schistosoma mansoni* infections around the 'Lac de Guiers' in the Senegal River Basin, Senegal. *Tropical Medicine & International Health,* 4, 544-550.

De Paoli, A. (1965) *Schistosoma haematobium* in the chimpanzee - a natural infection. *The American Journal of Tropical Medicine and Hygiene,* 14, 561-565.

Despres, L., Imbert-Establet, D., Combes, C. & Bonhomme, F. (1992) Molecular evidence linking hominid evolution to recent radiation of schistosomes (Platyhelminthes: Trematoda). *Molecular Phylogenetics and Evolution,* 1, 295-304.

Desprès, L., Imbert-Establet, D. & Monnerot, M. (1993) Molecular characterization of mitochondrial DNA provides evidence for the recent introduction of *Schistosoma mansoni* into America. *Molecular and Biochemical Parasitology,* 60, 221-229.

Duplantier, J. M. & Sène, M. (2000) Rodents as reservoir hosts in the transmission of *Schistosoma mansoni* in Richard-Toll, Senegal, West Africa. *Journal of Helminthology,* 74, 129-135.

Eisen, L. & Eisen, R. J. (2007) need for improved methods to collect and present spatial epidemiologic data for vectorborne diseases. *Emerging Infectious Diseases,* 13, 1816-1820.

Fenwick, A. (1969) Baboons as reservoirs hosts of *Schistosoma mansoni. Transactions of the Royal Society of Tropical Medicine and Hygiene,* 63, 557-567.

Fenwick, A., Webster, J. P., Bosque-Oliva, E., Blair, L., Fleming, F. M., Zhang, Y., Garba, A., Stothard, J. R., Gabrielli, A. F., Clements, A. C., Kabatereine, N. B., Toure, S., Dembele, R., Nyandindi, U., Mwansa, J. & Koukounari, A. (2009) The Schistosomiasis Control Initiative (SCI): rationale, development and implementation from 2002-2008. *Parasitology,* 136, 1719-1730.

Gear, J. H. S., Davis, D. H. S. & Pitchford, R. J. (1966) The susceptibility of rodents to schistosome infection, with special reference to *Schistosoma haematobium. Bulletin of the World Health Organization,* 35, 213-221.

Ghandour, A. M., Zahid, N. Z., Banaja, A. A., Kamal, K. B. & Bouq, A. I. (1995) Zoonotic intestinal parasites of hamadryan baboons *Papio hamadryas* in the western and northern regions of Saudi Arabia. *Journal of Tropical Medicine and Hygiene,* 98, 431-439.

Giboda, M., Ditrich, O. & Stěrba (1988) *Schistosoma margrebowiei* human patent zoonotic schistosomiasis imported from Zambia. *Bulletin de la Société de pathologie exotique et de ses filiales,* 81, 749-751.

Gillespie, T. (2006) noninvasive assessment of gastrointestinal parasite infections in free-ranging primates. *International Journal of Primatology,* 27, 1129-1143.

Gillespie, T. R. & Chapman, C. A. (2008) Forest fragmentation, the decline of an endangered primate, and changes in host-parasite interactions relative to an unfragmented forest. *American Journal of Primatology,* 70, 222-230.

Graczyk, T. K., Bosco-Nizeyi, J., Ssebide, B., Thompson, R. C., Read, C. & Cranfield, M. R. (2002) Anthropozoonotic *Giardia duodenalis* genotype (assemblage) a infections in habitats of free-ranging human-habituated gorillas, Uganda. *Journal of Parasitology,* 88, 905-9.

Haas, W., Granzer, M. & Brockelman, C. R. (1990) Finding and recognition of the bovine host by the cercariae *Schistosoma spindale. Parasitology Research,* 76, 343-350.

Hahn, N. E., Proulx, D., Muruthi, P. M., Alberts, S. & Altmann, J. (2003) Gastrointestinal parasites in free-ranging kenyan baboons (*Papio cynocephalus* and *P. anubis*). *International Journal of Primatology,* 24, 271-279.

Hanelt, B., Brant, S. V., Steinauer, M. L., Maina, G. M., Kinuthia, J. M., Agola, L. E., Mwangi, I. N., Mungai, B. N., Mutuku, M. W., Mkoji, G. M. & Loker, E. S. (2009) *Schistosoma kisumuensis* n. sp. (Digenea: Schistosomatidae) from murid rodents in the Lake Victoria Basin, Kenya and its phylogenetic position within the *S. haematobium* species group. *Parasitology,* 136, 987-1001.

Hanelt, B., Mwangi, I. N., Kinuthia, J. M., Maina, G. M., Agola, L. E., Mutuku, M. W., Steinauer, M. L., Agwanda, B. R., Kigo, L., Mungai, B. N., Loker, E. S. & Mkoji, G. M. (2010) Schistosomes of small mammals from the Lake Victoria Basin, Kenya: new species, familiar species, and implications for schistosomiasis control. *Parasitology,* 137, 1109-1118.

He, Y.-X., Salafsky, B. & Ramaswamy, K. (2001) Host-parasite relationships of *Schistosoma japonicum* in mammalian hosts. *Trends in Parasitology,* 17, 320-324.

Hotez, P. J., Bottazzi, M. E., Franco-Paredes, C., Ault, S. K. & Periago, M. R. (2008) The neglected tropical diseases of latin america and the caribbean: a review of disease burden and distribution and a roadmap for control and elimination. *PLoS Neglected Tropical Diseases,* 2, e300.

Hotez, P. J. & Fenwick, A. (2009) Schistosomiasis in Africa: An emerging tragedy in our new global health decade. *PLoS Neglected Tropical Diseases,* 3, e485.

Howells, M. E., Pruetz, J. & Gillespie, T. R. (2011) Patterns of gastro-intestinal parasites and commensals as an index of population and ecosystem health: the case of sympatric western chimpanzees (*Pan troglodytes verus*) and guinea baboons (*Papio hamadryas papio*) at Fongoli, Senegal. *American Journal of Primatology,* 73, 173-179.

Huyse, T., Webster, B. L., Geldof, S., Stothard, J. R., Diaw, O. T., Polman, K. & Rollinson, D. (2009) Bidirectional introgressive hybridization between a cattle and human schistosome species. *PLoS Pathogens,* 5, e1000571.

Imbert-Establet, D., Moné, H., Tchuenté, L. A. T. & Jourdane, J. (1997) Permissiveness of two African wild rodents, *Mastomys huberti* and *Arvicanthis niloticus*, to *Schistosoma intercalatum*: epidemiological consequences. *Parasitology Research,* 83, 569-573.

Ishikawa, H., Ohmae, H., Pangilinan, R., Redulla, A. & Matsuda, H. (2006) Modeling the dynamics and control of *Schistosoma japonicum* transmission on Bohol island, the Philippines. *Parasitology International,* 55, 23-29.

Karoum, K. O. & Amin, M. A. (1985) Domestic and wild animals naturally infected with *Schistosoma mansoni* in the Gezira Irrigated Scheme, Sudan. *Journal of Tropical Medicine and Hygiene,* 88, 83-89.

Kawashima, K., Katamine, D., Sakamoto, M., Shimada, M., Nojima, H. & Miyahara, M. (1978) Investigations on the role of wild rodents as reservoirs of human schistosomiasis in the Taveta area of Kenya, East Africa. *Japanese Journal of Tropical Medicine and Hygiene,* 6, 195-203.

Kuntz, R. E., Huang, T. C. & Moore, J. A. (1980) The capuchin monkey (*Cebus apella*) as an experimental host for *Schistosoma intercalatum*. *Proceedings of the Helminthological Society of Washington,* 47, 260-262.

Kuntz, R. E. & Malakatis, G. M. (1955a) Susceptibility studies in schistosomiasis. II. Susceptibility of wild mammals to infection by schistosoma mansoni in Egypt, with emphasis on rodents. *American Journal of Tropical Medicine and Hygiene,* 4, 75-89.

Kuntz, R. E. & Malakatis, G. M. (1955b) Susceptibility studies in schistosomiasis. IV. Susceptibility of wild mammals to infection by *Schistosoma haematobium* in Egypt, with emphasis on rodents. *The Journal of Parasitology,* 41, 467-475.

Kuntz, R. E., Mccullough, B., Huang, T. C. & Moore, J. A. (1978a) *Schistosoma intercalatum* Fisher, 1934 (Cameroon) infection in the patas monkey (*Erythrocebus patas* Schreber, 1775). *International Journal for Parasitology,* 8, 65-68.

Kuntz, R. E., Mccullough, B., Moore, J. A. & Huang, T.-C. (1978b) Experimental Infection with *Schistosoma intercalatum* (Fisher, 1934) in the Chimpanzee (*Pan troglodytes*) and the Gibbon (*Hylobates lar*). *The American Journal of Tropical Medicine and Hygiene,* 27, 632-634.

Lambert-Zazulak, P. I., Rutherford, P. & David, A. R. (2003) The International Ancient Egyptian Mummy Tissue Bank at the Manchester Museum as a Resource for the Palaeoepidemiological Study of Schistosomiasis. *World Archaeology,* 35, 223-240.

Legesse, M. & Erko, B. (2004) Zoonotic intestinal parasites in *Papio anubis* (baboon) and *Cercopithecus aethiops* (vervet) from four localities in Ethiopia. *Acta Tropica,* 90, 231-236.

Lockyer, A. E., Olson, P. D., Oslash, Stergaard, P., Rollinson, D., Johnston, D. A., Attwood, S. W., Southgate, V. R., Horak, P., Snyder, S. D., Le, T. H., Agatsuma, T., Mcmanus, D. P., Carmichael, A. C., Naem, S. & Littlewood, D. T. J. (2003) The phylogeny of the Schistosomatidae based on three genes with emphasis on the interrelationships of *Schistosoma* Weinland, 1858. *Parasitology,* 126, 203-224.

Loker, E. S. (1983) A comparative study of the life-histories of mammalian schistosomes. *Parasitology,* 87, 343-369.

Mango, A. M. (1971) The role of dogs as reservoirs in the transmission of *Schistosoma mansoni*. *East African Medical Journal,* 48, 298-306.

Mansour, N. S. (1973) *Schistosoma mansoni* and *Sch. haematobium* Found as a natural double infection in the Nile Rat, *Arvicanthis n. niloticus*, from a Human Endemic area in Egypt. *The Journal of Parasitology,* 59, 424.

Mcgrew, W. C., Tutin, C. E. G., Collins, D. A. & File, S. K. (1989) Intestinal parasites of sympatric *Pan troglodytes* and *Papio spp*. at two sites: Gombe (Tanzania) and Mt. Assirik (Senegal). *American Journal of Primatology,* 17, 147-155.

Modena, C. M., Lima, W. D. S. & Coelho, P. M. Z. (2008) Wild and domesticated animals as reservoirs of schistosomiasis mansoni in Brazil. *Acta Tropica,* 108, 242-244.

Morand, S., Krasnov, B. R., Poulin, R., Duplantier, J.-M. & Sene, M. (2006) Rodents as definitive hosts of *Schistosoma*, with special reference to *S. mansoni* transmission. In *Micromammals and Macroparasites.* Springer Japan.

Morens, D. M., Folkers, G. K. & Fauci, A. S. (2004) The challenge of emerging and re-emerging infectious diseases. *Nature,* 430, 242-249.

Morgan, J. A. T., Dejong, R. J., Lwambo, N. J. S., Mungai, B. N., Mkoji, G. M. & Loker, E. S. (2003) First report of a natural hybrid between *Schistosoma mansoni* and *S. rodhaini*. *Journal of Parasitology,* 89, 416-418.

Morgan, J. A. T., DeJong, R. J., Adeoye, G. O., Ansa, E. D. O., Barbosa, C. S., Brémond, P., Cesari, I. M., Charbonnel, N., Correa, L. R., Coulibaly, G., D'Andrea, P. S., De Souza, C. P., Doenhoff, M. J., File, S., Idris, M. A., Incani, N., Jarne, P., Karanja, D. M. S., Kazibwe, F., Kpikpi, J., Lwambo, N. J. S., Mabaye, A., Magalhaes, L. A., Makundi, A., Moné, H., Mouahid, G., Muchemi, G. M., Mungai, B. M., Séne, M., Southgate, V., Tcheum-Tchuenté, L. A., Théron, A., Yousif, F., Zanotti-Magalhaes, E. M., Mkoji, G. M. & Loker, E. S. (2005) Origin and diversification of the human parasite Schistosoma mansoni. Molecular Ecology, 14, 3889-3902.

Muller-Graf, C. D., Collins, D. A., Packer, C. & Woolhouse, M. E. (1997) *Schistosoma mansoni* infection in a natural population of olive baboons (*Papio cynocephalus anubis*) in Gombe Stream National Park, Tanzania. *Parasitology,* 115, 621-7.

Munene, E., Otsyula, M., Mbaabu, D. A. N., Mutahi, W. T., Muriuki, S. M. K. & Muchemi, G. M. (1998) Helminth and protozoan gastrointestinal tract parasites in captive and wild-trapped African non-human primates. *Veterinary Parasitology,* 78, 195-201.

Muriuki, S. M. K., Murugu, R. K., Munene, E., Karere, G. M. & Chai, D. C. (1998) Some gastro-intestinal parasites of zoonotic (public health) importance commonly observed in old world non-human primates in Kenya. *Acta Tropica,* 71, 73-82.

Murray, S., Stem, C., Boudreau, B. & Goodall, J. (2000) Intestinal parasites of baboons (*Papio cynocephalus anubis*) and chimpanzees (*Pan troglodytes*) in Gombe National Park. *Journal of Zoo and Wildlife Medicine,* 31, 176-178.

Ndifon, G. T., Betterton, C. & Rollinson, D. (1988) *Schistosoma curassoni* Brumpt, 1931 and *S. bovis* (Sonsino, 1876) in cattle in northern Nigeria. *Journal of Helminthology,* 62, 33-34.

Nejsum, P., Bertelsen, M. F., Betson, M., Stothard, J. R. & Murrell, K. D. (2010) Molecular evidence for sustained transmission of zoonotic *Ascaris suum* among zoo chimpanzees (*Pan troglodytes*). *Veterinary Parasitology,* 171, 273-276.

Nelson, G. S. (1960) Schistosome infections as zoonoses in Africa. *Transactions of the Royal Society of Tropical Medicine and Hygiene,* 54, 301-316.

Nelson, G. S. & Teesdale, C. (1965) *Schistosoma rodhaini* 'taken for a ride' by *S. mansoni* in baboons. *Transactions of the Royal Society of Tropical Medicine and Hygiene,* 59, 7.

Nelson, G. S., Teesdale, C. & Highton, R. B. (1962) The role of animals as reservoirs of bilharziasis in Africa. IN Wolstensholme, G. E. W. & O'connor, M. (Eds.) *Ciba Foundation symposium on bilharziasis held in commemoration of Theodor Maximilian Bilharz.* Boston.

Nutter, F. (1993) A comparison of gastrointestinal parasites in two communities of chimpanzees at Gombe National Park, Tanzania. MSc Thesis, Tufts University of Veterinary Medicine.

Ouma, J. H. & Fenwick, A. (1991) Animal reservoirs of schistosomiasis. IN Macpherson, C. N. L. & Craig, P. S. (Eds.) *Parasitic helminths and zoonoses in Africa.* London, Chapman and Hall.

Pagès, J.-R., Jourdane, J., Southgate, V. R., Tchuem Tchuenté, L.-A. & Combes, C. (2003) Reconnaissance de deux espèces jumelles au sein du taxon *Schistosoma intercalatum* Fisher, 1934, agent de la schistosomose humaine rectale en Afrique. Description de *Schistosoma guineensis* n.sp. IN Combes, C. & Jourdane, J. (Eds.) *Taxonomie, écologie et évolution des métazoaires parasites.* Perpignan, Presses Universitaires de Perpignan.

Petrášová, J., Modrý, D., Huffman, M., Mapua, M., Bobáková, L., Mazoch, V., Singh, J., Kaur, T. & Petrželková, K. (2010) Gastrointestinal parasites of indigenous and introduced primate species of Rubondo Island National Park, Tanzania. *International Journal of Primatology,* 31, 920-936.

Petrzelkova, K., Hasegawa, H., Moscovice, L., Kaur, T., Issa, M. & Huffman, M. (2006) Parasitic nematodes in the chimpanzee population on Rubondo Island, Tanzania. *International Journal of Primatology,* 27, 767-777.

Phillips-Conroy, J. E. (1986) Baboons, diet, and disease: food plant selection and schistosomiasis. IN Taub, D. M. & King, F. A. (Eds.) *Current Perspectives In Primates Social Dynamics.* New York, Van Nostrand Reinhold.

Pitchford, R. J. (1959a) Cattle schistosomiasis in man in the Eastern Transvaal. *Transactions of the Royal Society of Tropical Medicine and Hygiene,* 53, 285-90.

Pitchford, R. J. (1959b) Natural schistosome infections in South African rodents. *Transactions of the Royal Society of Tropical Medicine and Hygiene,* 53, 213.

Pitchford, R. J. (1977) A check list of definitive hosts exhibiting evidence of the genus *Schistosoma* Weinland, 1858 acquired naturally in Africa and the Middle East. *Journal of Helminthology,* 51, 229-251.

Pitchford, R. J. & Visser, P. S. (1962) The role of naturally infected wild rodents in the epidemiology of schistosomiasis in the Eastern Transvaal. *Transactions of the Royal Society of Tropical Medicine and Hygiene,* 56, 126-135.

Pitchford, R. J., Visser, P. S., Pienaar, U. D. V. & Young, E. (1974) Further observations on *Schistosoma mattheei* Veglia and Le Roux 1929 in the Kruger National Park. *Journal of the South African Veterinary Association,* 45, 211-218.

Ripert, C. (2003) Schistosomose dué á *Schistosoma intercalatum* et urbanisation en Afrique centrale. *Bulletin de la Société de pathologie exotique,* 96, 183-186.

Sandbach, F. R. (1976) The history of schistosomiasis research and policy for its control. *Medical History,* 20, 259–275.

Schwetz, J. (1954) On two schistosomes of wild rodents of the Belgian Congo: *Schistosoma rodhaini;* and *Schistosoma mansoni* var. *rodentorum* and ; and their relationship to *S. mansoni* of man. *Transactions of the Royal Society of Tropical Medicine and Hygiene,* 48, 89-92.

Schwetz, J. (1956) Role of wild rats and domestic rats (*Rattus rattus*) in schistosomiasis of man. *Transactions of the Royal Society of Tropical Medicine and Hygiene,* 50, 275-282.

Sinha, P. K. & Srivastava, H. D. (1960) Studies on *Schistosoma incognitum* Chandler, 1926. II. On the life history of the blood fluke. *The Journal of Parasitology,* 46, 629-641.

Sleeman, J. M., Meader, L. L., Mudakikwa, A. B., Foster, J. W. & Patton, S. (2009) Gastrointestinal parasites of mountain gorillas (*Gorilla gorilla beringei*) in the Parc National des Volcans, Rwanda. *Journal of Zoo and Wildlife Medicine,* 31, 322-328.

Southgate, V. R., Van Wijk, H. B. & Wright, C. A. (1976) Schistosomiasis at Loum, Cameroun; *Schistosoma haematobium, S. intercalatum* and their natural hybrid. *Parasitology Research,* 49, 145-159.

Standley, C. J., Adriko, M., Alinaitwe, M., Kazibwe, F., Kabatereine, N. B. & Stothard, J. R. (2009) Intestinal schistosomiasis and soil-transmitted helminthiasis in Ugandan schoolchildren: a rapid mapping assessment. *Geospatial Health,* 4, 39-53.

Standley, C.J., Kabatereine, N., Lange, C., Lwambo, N. & Stothard, J. R. (2010) Molecular epidemiology and phylogeography of *Schistosoma mansoni* around Lake Victoria. *Parasitology,* 137, 1937 - 1949.

Standley, C.J., Mugisha, L., Verweij, J., Adriko, M., Arinaitwe, M., Rowell, C., Atuhaire, A., Betson, M., Hobbs, E., Van Tulleken, C., Kane, R., Van Lieshout, L., Ajarova, L., Kabatereine, N. & Stothard, J. (2011) Confirmed infection with intestinal schistosomiasis in semi-captive wild born chimpanzees on Ngamba Island, Uganda. *Vector Borne and Zoonotic Diseases,* 11, 169-176.

Steinauer, M. L., Hanelt, B., Agola, L. E., Mkoji, G. M. & Loker, E. S. (2009) Genetic structure of *Schistosoma mansoni* in western Kenya: the effects of geography and host sharing. *International Journal for Parasitology,* 39, 1353-62.

Steinauer, M. L., Hanelt, B., Mwangi, I. N., Maina, G. M., Agola, L. E., Kinuthia, J. M., Mutuku, M. W., Mungai, B. N., Wilson, W. D., Mkoji, G. M. & Loker, E. S. (2008a) Introgressive hybridization of human and rodent schistosome parasites in western Kenya. *Molecular Ecology,* 17, 5062-5074.

Steinauer, M. L., Mwangi, I. N., Maina, G. M., Kinuthia, J. M., Mutuku, M. W., Agola, E. L., Mungai, B., Mkoji, G. M. & Loker, E. S. (2008b) Interactions between natural populations of human and rodent schistosomes in the Lake Victoria Region of Kenya: A molecular epidemiological approach. *PLoS Neglected Tropical Diseases,* 2, e222.

Steinmann, P., Keiser, J., Bos, R., Tanner, M. & Utzinger, J. R. (2006) Schistosomiasis and water resources development: systematic review, meta-analysis, and estimates of people at risk. *The Lancet Infectious Diseases,* 6, 411-425.

Stephens, D. S., Moxon, E. R., Adams, J., Altizer, S., Antonovics, J., Aral, S., Berkelman, R., Bond, E., Bull, J., Cauthen, G., Farley, M. M., Glasgow, A., Glasser, J. W., Katner, H. P., Kelley, S., Mittler, J., Nahmias, A. J., Nichol, S., Perrot, V., Pinner, R. W., Schrag, S., Small, P. & Thrall, P. H. (1998) Emerging and reemerging infectious diseases: A multidisciplinary perspective. *The American Journal of the Medical Sciences,* 315, 64-75.

Stirewalt, M. A., Kuntz, R. E. & Evans, A. S. (1951) The relative susceptibilities of the commonly-used laboratory mammals to infection by *Schistosoma Mansoni. The American Journal of Tropical Medicine and Hygiene,* s1-31, 57-82.

Stothard, J. R., Sousa-Figueiredo, J. C., Standley, C.J, Van Dam, G. J., Knopp, S., Utzinger, J., Ameri, H., Khamis, A. N., Khamis, I. S., Deelder, A. M., Mohammed, K. A. & Rollinson, D. (2009) An evaluation of urine-CCA strip test and fingerprick blood SEA-ELISA for detection of urinary schistosomiasis in schoolchildren in Zanzibar. *Acta Tropica,* 111, 64-70.

Sturrock, R. (2001) Schistosomiasis epidemiology and control: how did we get here and where should we go? *Memorias do Instituto Oswaldo Cruz,* 96, 17-27.

Tchuenté, L. A. T., Southgate, V. R., Njiokou, F., Njiné, T., Kouemeni, L. E. & Jourdane, J. (1997) The evolution of schistosomiasis at Loum, Cameroon: replacement of *Schistosoma intercalatum* by *S. haematobium* through introgressive hybridization. *Transactions of the Royal Society of Tropical Medicine and Hygiene,* 91, 664-665.

Theron, A. & Combes, C. (1995) Asynchrony of infection timing, habitat preference, and sympatric speciation of schistosome parasites. *Evolution,* 49, 372-375.

Vercruysse, J., Rollinson, D., Van Heerden, M. & Southgate, V. R. (2003) On the longevity of *Schistosoma curassoni. Journal of Helminthology,* 77, 89-90.

Vianna Martins, A. (1958) Non-human vertebrate hosts of *Schistosoma haematobium* and *Schistosoma mansoni. Bulletin of the World Health Organization,* 18, 931-944.

Webster, B., Tchuem Tchuenté, L. & Southgate, V. (2007) A single-strand conformation polymorphism (SSCP) approach for investigating genetic interactions of *Schistosoma haematobium* and *Schistosoma guineensis* in Loum, Cameroon. *Parasitology Research,* 100, 739-745.

Webster, B. L., Southgate, V. R. & Littlewood, D. T. J. (2006) A revision of the interrelationships of *Schistosoma* including the recently described *Schistosoma guineensis. International Journal for Parasitology,* 36, 947-955.

Weyher, A., Ross, C. & Semple, S. (2006) Gastrointestinal parasites in crop raiding and wild foraging *Papio anubis* in Nigeria. *International Journal of Primatology,* 27, 1519-1534.

Weyher, A. H., Phillips-Conroy, J. E., Fischer, K., Weil, G. J., Chansa, W. & Fischer, P. U. (2010) Molecular identification of *Schistosoma mattheei* from feces of Kinda (*Papio cynocephalus kindae*) and Grayfoot baboons (*Papio ursinus griseipes*) in Zambia. *Journal of Parasitology,* 96, 184-190.

Wilcox, B. & Gubler, D. (2005) Disease ecology and the global emergence of zoonotic pathogens. *Environmental Health and Preventive Medicine,* 10, 263-272.

Williams, G. M., Sleigh, A. C., Li, Y., Feng, Z., Davis, G. M., Chen, H., Ross, A. G. P., Bergquist, R. & McManus, D. P. (2002) Mathematical modelling of schistosomiasis japonica: comparison of control strategies in the People's Republic of China. *Acta Tropica,* 82, 253-262.

Wright, C. A., Southgate, V. R. & Knowles, R. J. (1978) What is *Schistosoma intercalatum* Fisher, 1934? *Transactions of the Royal Society of Tropical Medicine and Hygiene,* 66, 28-64.

Zahed, N. Z., Ghandour, A. M., Banaja, A. A., Banerjee, R. K. & Dehlawi, M. S. (1996) Hamadryas baboons *Papio hamadryas* as maintenance hosts of *Schistosoma mansoni* in Saudi Arabia. *Tropical Medicine & International Health,* 1, 449-455.

12

The Role of Wild Rodents in the Transmission of *Schistosoma mansoni* in Brazil

Rosana Gentile[1], Marisa S. Soares[2], Magali G. M. Barreto[2], Margareth M. L. Gonçalves[3] and Paulo S. D'Andrea[1]
[1]*Laboratório de Biologia e Parasitologia de Mamíferos Silvestres Reservatórios, Instituto Oswaldo Cruz, Fundação Oswaldo Cruz, Rio de Janeiro, RJ*
[2]*Laboratório de Avaliação e Promoção da Saúde Ambiental, Instituto Oswaldo Cruz, Fundação Oswaldo Cruz, Rio de Janeiro, RJ*
[3]*Laboratório de Helmintos Parasitos de Vertebrados, Instituo Oswaldo Cruz, Fundação Oswaldo Cruz, Rio de Janeiro, RJ*
Brasil

1. Introduction

The control of schistosomiasis still represents an important challenge for public health services around the world. Despite the success of schistosomiasis control programs in certain regions in reducing the prevalence and the intensity of infection, the global estimation of human cases has not changed. Schistosomiasis is an expanding, chronic parasitosis that affects about 200 million people in the world, and about 700 million people live in endemic areas (Who, 2010).

In Brazil, where this endemicity is caused only by *Schistosoma mansoni*, morbidity control has been favored by the use of Oxaminiquine and Praziquantel (Barbosa et al., 2008; Coura & Amaral, 2004; Lambertucci et al., 2000; TDR, 2005) and by an increase in sanitary sewer availability and medical assistance in the past few decades (Brasil, 2009). However, schistosomiasis still affects millions of people in Brazil (Katz & Peixoto, 2000). In 2010, there were diagnosed cases in 22 of the 27 federal units in Brazil, and the mortality between 1990 and 2008 oscillated around 500 deaths per year (Brasil, 2011a), which is more than the mortality observed for dengue and malaria during the same period (Brasil, 2011b). Despite considering schistosomiasis a rural endemicity in Brazil, there are frequent reports of the disease in urban areas in several localities (Barbosa et al., 2000; Barbosa et al., 2001; Graeff-Teixeira & Moraes, 1999; Guimarães & Neto, 2006; Guimarães et al., 1990; Guimarães et al., 1993; Kats et al., 1993; Mott et al., 1990; Soares et al., 1995). The greatest difficulty for schistosomiasis control is in transmission interruption because the occurrence of re-infection is frequent (Coura & Amaral, 2004), there are numerous favorable areas for the emergence and re-emergence of the parasistosis, and there is an evident expansion of the endemic areas (Brasil, 2010; Coura & Amaral, 2004; Graeff-Teixeira, 2004). This situation makes schistosomiasis a transmissible disease with a persistent profile in Brazil (Brasil, 2010).

Schistosomiasis transmission is favored under certain ecological, sociological, socio-economic, cultural, political and historical conditions existing in Brazil. Among them, we highlight the following: 1. Poverty and low economic development in many endemic areas (Katz & Peixoto, 2000); 2. Inadequate residential and environmental sanitation in rural and peri-urban areas (Barbosa et al., 1996; Silva, 1985); 3. Wide distribution of the mollusk intermediary hosts (Brasil, 2008); 4. Migrations, induced exodus and other permanent or transitory population movements (Coura & Amaral, 2004; Silva, 1985); 5. Absence of, scarcity of or inadequate health education programs (Schall et al., 2008); and 6. The complexity of the transmission processes with their multiple variables (Barbosa et al., 1996; Gazzinelli & Kloos, 2007; Martins Jr. & Barreto, 2003).

2. Small mammals naturally infected by *S. mansoni*

Schistosoma mansoni probably speciated from rodent schistosomas (*S. rodahini*) and is associated with the evolution of the first hominids (Després et al., 1992; Morgan et al., 2003; Morgan et al., 2005). Subsequently, *S. mansoni* became a parasite of wild rodents, and the presence of naturally infected wild rodents has become a complicating factor for control programs in endemic areas.

The presence of non-human definitive hosts increases the complexity of the epidemiologic situation of schistosomiasis in Brazil and constitutes one of the major problems for disease control because there is an overlap in the geographic distribution of the disease endemicity and the wild rodents potentially able to act as reservoirs.

In 1928, Cameron was the first to register a wild mammal naturally infected by *S. mansoni*: the African monkey introduced in the Antilles, *Cercopithecus sabaus*. Based on infection experiments carried out in rodents, he suggested the possibility of their participation in infection transmission, predicting complications in schistosomiasis control strategies. The first reports of naturally infected wild rodents were in the 1950s in Africa (Kuntz, 1952) and in Brazil (Amorim, 1953; Barbosa et al., 1953). At that time, Amorim (1953) emphasized the importance of animals with aquatic or semi-aquatic habits in the natural maintenance of *S. mansoni*. Among several wild and sinantropic rodent species found to be naturally parasitized in Brazil (*Oxymycterus* sp., *Necromys lasiurus, Akodon* spp., *Sooretamys* spp., *Calomys* spp., *Proechimys* sp., Cavia aperea, *Rattus rattus* and *Rattus norvegicus*), the species of the genera *Nectomys* and *Holochilus* are the most important and are generally considered wild reservoirs due to their semi-aquatic habits, wide geographic distribution and tolerance of human presence (Rey, 1993).

After those pioneering studies, several authors proposed investigating the participation of animals in the transmission cycle of mansonic schistosomiasis in the wild. Martins et al. (1955) evaluated schistosomiasis infection in *N. squamipes* in Belo Horizonte and Jabuticabas (MG) and found that they were naturally infected by *S. mansoni* with a prevalence of 26.1%. Rodrigues & Ferreira (1969) captured *N. squamipes* rodents naturally infected in São Paulo State, where they found new endemic human foci of the parasitosis. Bastos et al. (1984) captured *N. squamipes* in Maranhão State and reported that 70,6% of animals were parasitized. Silva & Andrade (1989) observed that *N. squamipes* had an important role in the maintenance of schistosomiasis in the rural area of Planalto (BA) because human prevalence was 3.26%, whereas rodent prevalence was 47%. Veiga-Borgeaud et al. (1986) found a high prevalence of *S. mansoni* in *H. brasiliensis* (currently *H. sciureus*) in swampy areas in Maranhão State. Picot (1992) confirmed the ability of the rodents *N. squamipes* and *H. brasiliensis* to eliminate viable eggs in feces in natural conditions.

Some other studies carried out in Africa and other countries of the Americas also investigated the importance of mammals as *S. mansoni* reservoirs. Borda & Rea (2006) observed *H. brasiliensis* (probably *H. vulpinus*) eliminating viable eggs in feces in Corrientes province, Argentina, and completing the transmission cycle in laboratory conditions. Sene et al. (1997) compared human and murine isolates of *S. mansoni* from Senegal in seven enzyme systems using isoeletric focusing. Rodent species studied were *Arvicanthis niloticus* and *Mastomys huberti*. They found no significant variation between human and rodent isolates. In the same region of Senegal, Duplantier & Sene (2000) investigated the importance of six rodent and one insectivore species as reservoir hosts of *S. mansoni*. Only *A. niloticus* and *M. huberti* were found infected with prevalence about 5%. They concluded that those rodents participate in the schistosomiasis transmission, but the human population is the main source of infection. Recently, Hanelt et al. (2010) examined the extent to which wild mammals acted as reservoirs of *S. mansoni* in Kenya. They found five murids and one shrew species infected with schistosomes (*S. manoni, S. bovi, S. rodhaini* and *S. kisumuensis*). The prevalence of *S. mansoni* in the reservoir populations was low (1.5%), however, the host could perpetuate snail infections and favor renewed transmission to humans.

In the 1980s, Théron, Pointier and Morand (Théron, 1984; Théron, 1985; Théron & Pointier, 1985; 1995; Morand et al., 1999) conducted the only study that incontestably demonstrated that in a wild focus, only the rodent *Rattus rattus* was responsible for schistosomiasis cycle maintenance, and in a semi-urban focus, both rodents and humans were equally responsible for the parasite cycle. Concerning the shedding pattern of cercariae, the same authors observed a late shedding pattern for wild focus mollusks, an early pattern for the urban focus, and a variable shedding pattern for the semi-urban focus. These results are in accordance with the epidemiologic context of each focus, as the late shedding patterns of cercariae relate to the crepuscular/nocturnal activity of rodents, confirming the adaptive value of the shedding patterns with the intermediary and definitive host populations involved in local transmission (Théron et al. 1992). The irrefutability of the conclusions is due to a unique characteristic of the study area: the occurrence of each species of the definitive hosts of *S. mansoni* (murine and human) separated in two distinct sub-areas and existing concomitantly in another one. This situation is very unusual and difficult to find.

The role of mammals in the schistosomiasis transmission was also investigated for *S. japonicum*, especially in China. He et al. (2001) studied the host-parasite relationships between *S. japonicum* and rodents, domesticated animals and simians and found that domesticated animals appeared to be the most important animal hosts in the transmission of *S. japonicum* infection, since they are very abundant. Rudge et al. (2009) compared the genetic differentiation of *S. japonicum* among habitat types and host species in China using microsatellite markers. They found strong genetic differences between habitat types, but little among host species, indicating high levels of parasite gene flow across species, what complicates the infection control. Lu et al. (2010) also investigated the role of small rodents and some domestic animals in the transmission of *S. japonicum* in six areas of China of different habitats over two years. The highest parasite prevalence was observed in rodents in a hilly region, whereas in marsh areas, bovines were considered as the main reservoirs.

3. The most important species of reservoir: Water-rats

The geographic distribution of the genera *Nectomys* in Brazil, which contains two species, is much wider than the distribution of mansonic schistosomiasis; nevertheless, they are

coincident in several regions. Studies of the participation of these rodents in schistosomiasis only mention *N. squamipes*, except for Bastos et al. (1982, 1984), who reported naturally infected *Nectomys squamipes amazonicus* (currently *Nectomys rattus* (Pelzen (1883)).
The water-rat *Nectomys squamipes* (Sigmodontinae) occurs in the Atlantic Forest, Rio São Francisco and Paraná Basins, and in small basins of Eastern Brazil below São Lourenço da Mata, Pernanbuco State, embracing the South, Southern and part of the Northeast regions (Fig. 1). *Nectomys rattus* occurs in the Paraná-Paraguai and Amazonic Basins and in small basins of Eastern Brazil from São Lourenço da Mata to the Amazon River (Fig. 1) (Bonvicino et al., 2008).

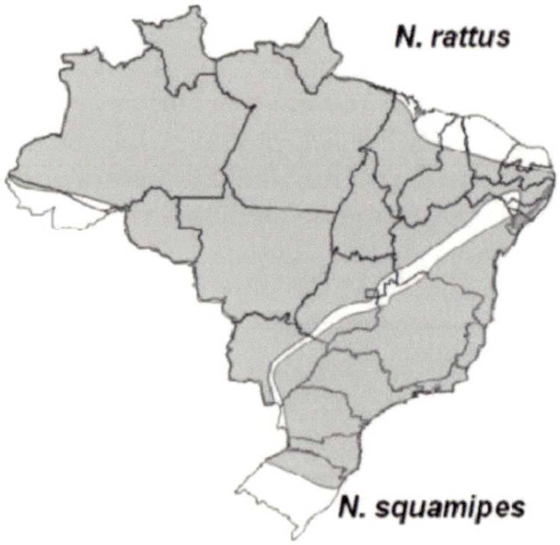

Fig. 1. Geographic distribution of the genera *Nectomys* in Brazil. Source: Bonvicino et al., 2008

N. squamipes is a semi-aquatic rodent, inhabiting streamside and swampy areas. It feeds primarily on insects, arthropods, snails and girinos found in the water and on fruits. Its activity is crepuscular and nocturnal (Fig. 2) (Ernest & Mares, 1986).
This species is undoubtedly the most important non-human, definitive host of *S. mansoni* in Brazil. The characteristics and studies that have proven its importance will be presented here along with the text.

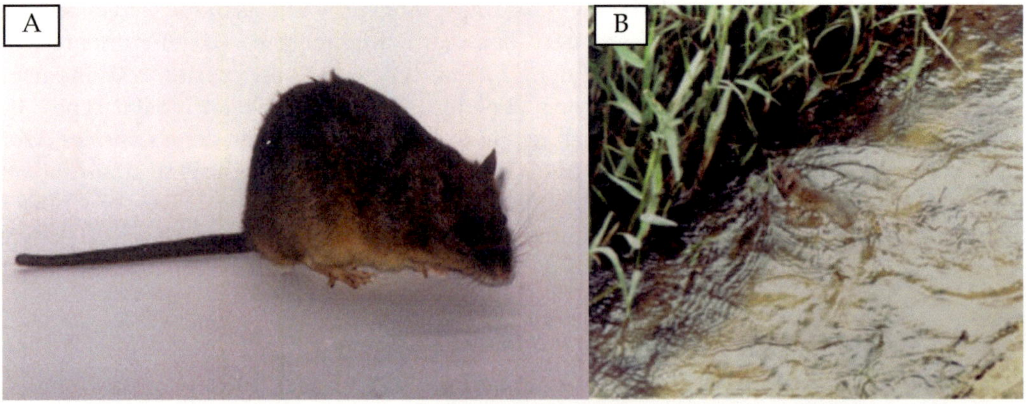

Fig. 2. *Nectomys squamipes*. A - Source: Cibele R. Bonvicino. B – Source: LABPMR

The genera *Holochilus* (Rodentia, Sigmodontinae) has four species occurring in Brazil: *H. brasiliensis, H. sciureus, H. chacaris* and *H. vulpinus* (Bonvicino et al., 2008). *H. sciureus* was formerly classified as *H. brasiliensis* (Wilson & Reeder, 2005). Only *H. sciureus* and *H. brasiliensis* occur in endemic areas of schistosomiasis in Brazil, the former occurring in the North region, part of the Northeast and north of the Middle-West, and the latter present from the Southeast to the South (Fig. 3).

These species live near streams and rivers or swampy and flooded areas. They are commonly found in humid fields, mostly in agricultural areas such as sugar cane, rice, corn and cotton plantations, and in vegetable gardens (Massoia, 1974; Ozanan, 1969). They are terrestrial and nocturnal, feeding on aquatic herbaceous vegetation and grass (Emmons & Feer, 1997). Outbreaks in population sizes called "ratadas" (Giovannoni et al., 1946) may occur, causing the species to become agricultural pests.

The potentiality of *Holochilus* sp. to act as wild reservoir of *S. mansoni* was demonstrated by their ability to eliminate viable eggs in feces in a natural environment (Dias et al., 1978) and by their ability to complete the parasite cycle without human presence in semi-natural conditions, using *Biomphalaria glabrata* as an intermediary host (Carvalho et al., 1976).

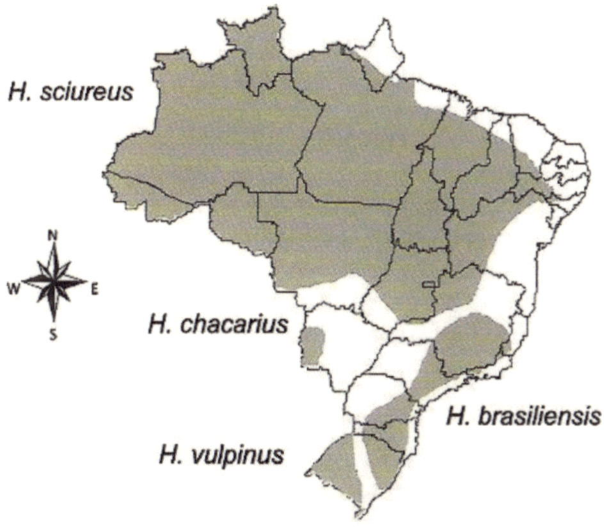

Fig. 3. Geographic distribution of the genera *Holochilus* in Brazil. Source: Bonvicino et al., 2008

4. Laboratory experiments: Water-rats as alternative experimental models for schistosomiasis studies

Several experimental studies have been carried out with the rodents *Nectomys* and *Holochilus* that proved that they can be considered alternative experimental models for studies of *S. mansoni* infection. They are highly susceptible to *S. mansoni* infections, easily handled and adapted to captivity conditions (D'Andrea et al., 1996). Here, we summarize the main results of the most relevant experimental studies on this theme.

Carvalho (1982) studied the pathology of schistosomiasis infection on *N. squamipes* and observed that most of the animals did not present with severe pathology and lesions due to the infection, suggesting a certain compatibility in the parasite-host relation.

Kawazoe & Pinto (1983) showed that the rodent *Holochilus brasiliensis* was able to eliminate viable eggs of *S. mansoni* in semi-natural conditions, but it was not able to complete the parasite transmission cycle if the intermediary host was *B. tenagophila*. However, they suggested that this rodent could have an important role in the eggs' dissemination in areas where the intermediary host was *B. glabrata*, even without the presence of parasitized humans.

Rodrigues-Silva (1988), Rodrigues-Silva et al. (1991) and Souza et al. (1992) evaluated the role of the rodents as natural hosts and as experimental models for schistosomiasis. They observed that naturally and experimentally infected animals presented tissue lesions in several organs similar to those found in mice. Based on these results, Rodrigues-Silva suggested that this rodent could be an alternative experimental model for schistosomiasis studies.

Rodrigues-Silva (1988) and Rodrigues-Silva et al. (1992) affirmed the importance of *N. squamipes* as a maintainer of the parasite cycle once the rodent proved to be a compatible or permissive host. This was demonstrated by the high infection duration and the elimination of viable, fertile and infective eggs for mollusks. *N. squamipes* is easily re-infected because the first infection facilitates the entrance of a new worm burden for the organism (Maldonado Jr. et al., 1994), assuring the elimination of viable eggs during the entire lifetime of the rodent (Costa-Silva, 2000).

Silva & Andrade (1989) studied naturally infected *N. squamipes* rodents and observed soft tissue lesions, and, despite the fact that the rodents exhibited a highly resistant immunopathology, the parasite seemed to suffer little interference with its oviposition and the number of egg eliminated.

Ribeiro et al. (1998) and Souza et al. (1992) showed that *N. squamipes* presented with a high rate of recovered worms even when infected with a low number of cercariaes, suggesting compatibility between *N. squamipes* and *S. mansoni*.

Picot (1992) showed that in semi-natural conditions, *N. squamipes* was able to close the transmission cycle of *S. mansoni* and to eliminate highly infectious, viable eggs.

Maldonado Jr. et al. (1994) evaluated the resistance of *S. mansoni* infection in *N. squamipes* by successive experimental infections, comparing the total number of worms recovered from re-infections with a control group. They concluded that previous infections did not reduce infectivity.

Ribeiro et al. (1998) evaluated the susceptibility of the rodents *N. squamipes* and *N. rattus* to *S. mansoni* infection, concluding that both species are highly susceptible to *S. mansoni* infection. *N. squamipes* presented 80% positivity after experimental infection and *N. rattus* presented 71%. They also demonstrated that the latter species was also able to complete the parasite cycle in laboratory conditions.

Costa-Silva (2000) observed that *N. squamipes* was susceptible to several *S. mansoni* strains, confirming its potential to act as a natural reservoir in some endemic areas and its utility as an experimental model for morphologic studies of *S. mansoni*.

Martinez et al. (2008) compared biological characteristics of four *S. mansoni* strains using *N. squamipes* as the experimental model. They concluded that this rodent was susceptible to different strains because the rodent did not present differences in biological parameters of infection when the different strains were compared.

5. A long term empiric study about the role of rodent reservoirs in Brazil

The first references of schistosomiasis in Sumidouro Municipality, Rio de Janeiro State, were related to studies carried out in 1959. S. Camargo (unpublished data) made the first

malacologic survey in 1962 in order to confirm the autochthony of the disease. By that time, the streams in the localities of Pamparrão, Porteira Verde and Boa Ventura were considered to be transmission foci due to the occurrence of infected snails (data recovered by Silva, 2004).
The first long-term study on schistosomiasis epidemiology in Sumidouro began in 1977 in the locality of Porteira Verde (Carvalho, 1982). The author observed that *S. mansoni* infection rates in *N. squamipes* were constant even after chemotherapy intervention in the human population and suggested that the rodent could be considered a potential natural reservoir of the disease in the region. The initial human *S. mansoni* prevalence varied between 11.2% and 17.4%. After treatment, it was reduced to 6.9% in the human population, whereas in the rodents, it was 48.2%.
Those findings on *N. squamipes* infection by *S. mansoni* in Sumidouro clearly showed the need to develop long-term studies to evaluate the role of this rodent in local transmission dynamics. With this goal in mind, a prospective survey on rodents and snails and a preliminary parasitological census in the human population were performed in 1990, thus creating the basis for the research on schistosomiasis in subsequent years. Below, we give a brief description of the project, with information on the methods, the main results and the conclusions on the schistosomiasis context in Sumidouro and, especially, on the role of rodents in the local transmission of *S. mansoni*.

5.1 Schistosomiasis context in Sumidouro

Sumidouro is a city of the State of Rio de Janeiro (22° 02 ' 59 " S, 42° 40 ' 29 " W), 179 km away from the state capital (Rio de Janeiro), which has a humid mesothermic climate (Fig. 4). Almost 63% of its 14920 inhabitants live in the rural area (IBGE 2010). In 2000, the Municipal HDI - (Human Development Index) was 0.712 (UNDP 2000). The work was carried out in five agricultural localities (Pamparrão, Porteira Verde, Encanto, Soledade and Volta), which had small portions of the Atlantic Forest on mountain summits and were cut by streams, small dams and irrigation ditches (Fig. 5).
In a new approach to schistosomiasis research in Brazil, different areas of scientific knowledge were adopted with an interdisciplinary perspective, an approach deemed more suitable for the situation than a multidisciplinary one, according to Almeida Filho (1997). This approach went beyond the domain of biomedical sciences, searching, for example, to understand cultural and behavioral factors that contribute to the complexity of the local schistosomiasis situation (Soares et al., 2002; Stotz et al., 2006). Thus, it was possible to understand the context of the role of rodents in the local cycle of the parasite and the situations that underlie the occurrence of schistosomiasis in the region. This was the only study with such characteristics carried out in Brazil on schistosomiasis.
Throughout the study period, the human population participated in a process that included questionnaires, interviews, focus groups, video sessions, debates, science fairs and coprology (Hoffman, Kato-Katz and other auxiliary methods, on average, 3 samples and 9 blades per person), serology (ELISA IgG and IgA; soluble extract of *S. mansoni* adults), clinical examination and treatment for all the diagnosed parasites. At the same time, the transmission foci were mapped according to the population density, dispersion and natural infection of the snail *Biomphalaria glabrata* by *S. mansoni* (Giovanelli et al., 2001). The serum samples were submitted to immunoenzymatic reactions using adult *S. mansoni* membrane soluble extract as antigen. One of the techniques used was western blotting to analyze the reactivity profile of anti-*S. mansoni* IgG antibodies. ELISAs were also carried out for anti-*S. mansoni* IgG, IgG1 and IgE.

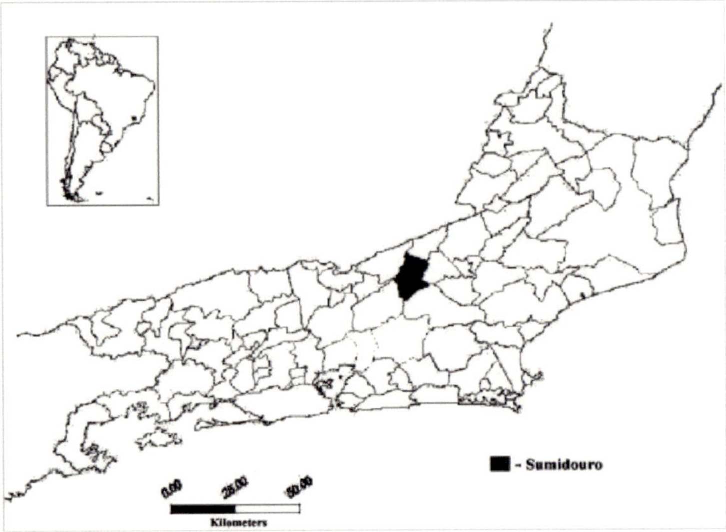

Fig. 4. Study area, indicating the Sumidouro Municipality in Rio de Janeiro State and in South America. Source: D'Andrea et. al., 2000.

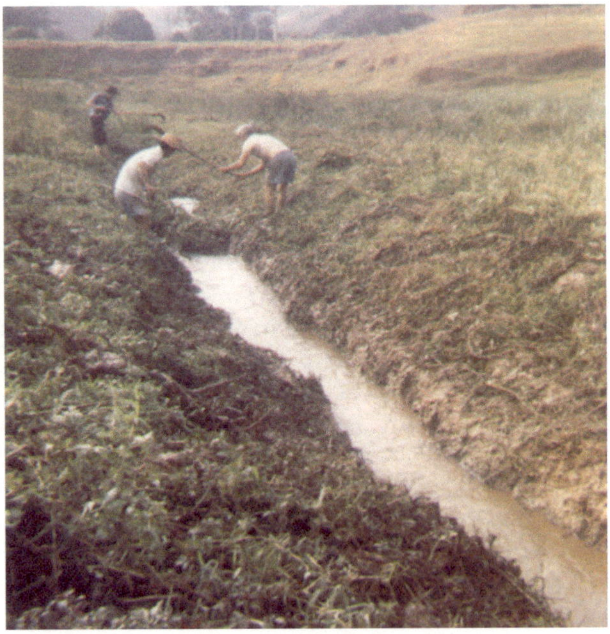

Fig. 5. Human activities in the study area.

These approaches disclosed bio-ecological, socio-ecological, socio-economic, historical, cultural and behavioral peculiarities that could not explain the persistence of transmission and the recurrence of high focal prevalences and hepatoesplenomegaly cases, despite all of the investments in controlling schistosomiasis in Sumidouro since the 1960s by several research groups and institutions. Amongst these peculiarities and beyond the relevance of the presence of the water-rat as a complicating factor for the control of schistosomiasis, the precariousness of the socio-ecologic and socio-economic conditions that put the populations under different environmental risks, including schistosomiasis, was notable.

The socio-ecologic precariousness was evidenced by the observation of the following conditions in the study territory: a) leisure, residential supply, farming, and other activities dependent on water contaminated by sewers *in natura* from almost all the houses; b) proliferation of snail vectors as a consequence of overflows due to alterations in the topography by deforestation and farming activities; c) perennial and occasional foci of *B. glabrata*, with high intensities of infection by *S. mansoni*, that occurred downstream, upstream and around residences, and water bodies visited daily by wild rodents of semi-aquatic habits during foraging activities; d) blockage of water bodies due to inadequate collection and disposal of garbage; e) scarcity of health water sources due to different types of environmental contamination and increasing deforestation around the springs; f) convergence of small water bodies and larger ones used by the population of other localities for residential supply, leisure, irrigation and other activities.

The socio-economic conditions contributed to the complexity of schistosomiasis control by exposing the population to psycho-social and chemical risks, given that irregularities and excesses in pesticide use were common in local agricultural production, with strong consequences for human and environmental health. The historical approach of schistosomiasis in Sumidouro showed the following: a) since the 1960s, there were cases of severe collateral effects from medicine, failures of sanitation, as well as environmental and material injuries after the use of moluscicides for snail control; b) in addition to these low quality of life, poverty, lack of good life quality perspectives, alcoholism and other factors that stimulate pessimism and inaction turned part of the communities against the diagnosis and treatment of schistosomiasis, as well as against the methodologies of sanitation and snail control suggested by the public powers and by the researchers; c) these refusals increased the limitations of coprological diagnosis that contributed to uncertainty in the real number of infected people; d) these facts demand the adoption of a wide range of measures, such as methodologies to understand the needs of the population and to make people understand schistosomiasis transmission and the serological techniques used for diagnosis (Gonçalves et al., 2005; Soares et al. 2002).

In this complex context, schistosomiasis transmission to the human population occurred in home backyards and for other reasons (occupational, recreational and occasional), with high ratios of non-treatment due to migration, refusal or medical precaution and with a high prevalence in specific groups (men and farm workers).

To simplify the comprehension of key aspects of the relevance of rodents' participation in schistosomiasis transmission in Sumidouro, the next section will describe each phase of the study concerning *N squamipes*.

5.2 Eco-epidemiologic monitoring - The rodent as a focus transmission biological indicator – Pamparrão and Encanto localities

Long-term monitoring of the ecology and parasitology of the water-rat *Nectomys squamipes*, together with an epidemiologic study of the human population, was carried out in two localities in Sumidouro Municipality, at different times: in Pamparrão from 1991 to 1996, and in Encanto from 2001 to 2006. In both localities, a capture-mark-recapture study of small mammals was conducted. Trappings were conducted along streamsides, which is the habitat of the rodent (Fig. 6). Stool and serologic diagnostics were performed on the rodents. Human populations were also diagnosed and treated. With this design, we obtained results that have enabled us to raise the small mammal fauna of the area (D'Andrea et al., 1999), understand the pattern of population dynamics of the water-rat (Bonecker et al., 2009; D'Andrea et al. 2007; Gentile et al. 2000) and its habitat use (Gentile & Fernandez 1999), understand aspects of the relationship between *S. mansoni* and *N. squamipes* (D'Andrea et al. 2000; Gentile et al., 2006), and adapt procedures and techniques to local particularities.

In Pamparrão, which is a low endemicity area, the population dynamic study of the water-rat showed that it reproduced throughout the year, predominantly during the rainy periods. The population size also increased during and after rainy periods and was related to survival rather than population outbreaks (Fig. 6) (Gentile et al., 2000).

The habitat preference study showed that *N. squamipes* preferred areas of dense herbaceous vegetation near the ground as well as courses and water bodies (Gentile & Fernandez 1999). In the parasitological survey, the high prevalence and parasitic burden confirmed that *N. squamipes* was highly susceptible to infection by *S. mansoni*. Three factors were related to the level of infection of the rodent: human sewage contamination in the home range of the rodents, local snail abundance and the movement pattern of rodents between transmission sites. The *S. mansoni* infection rates in snails was generally very low throughout the study area, except for some isolated sites where concentrated infected specimens were found with infection rates ranging from 10 to 25%. The level of *S. mansoni* infection in rodents increased with the proximity to human habitations, which was also related to the level of infection in humans. There was no correlation between population size and the *S. mansoni* infection rates in the rodents (Fig. 7).

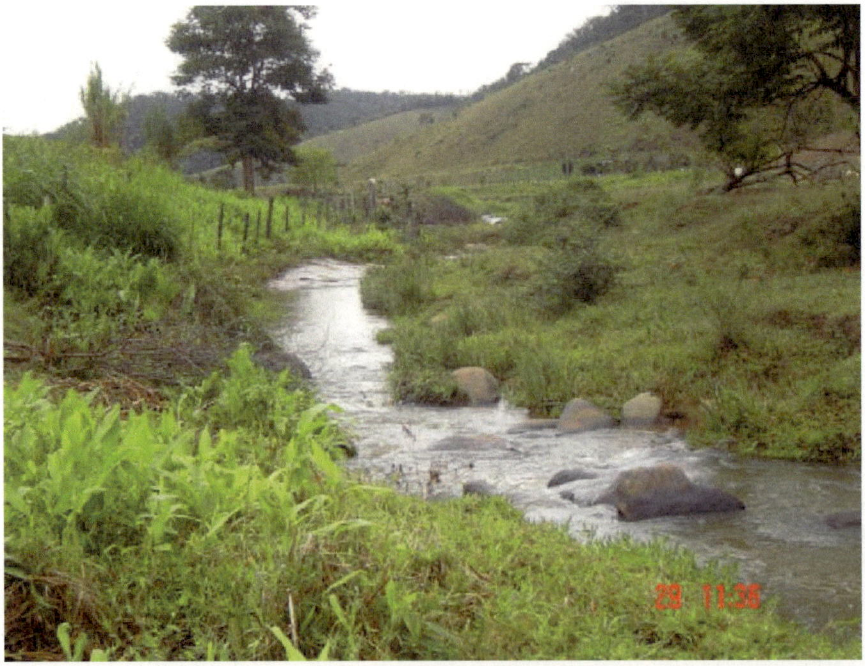

Fig. 6. A general view of a transect capture site of the water-rats. Source: LABPMR.

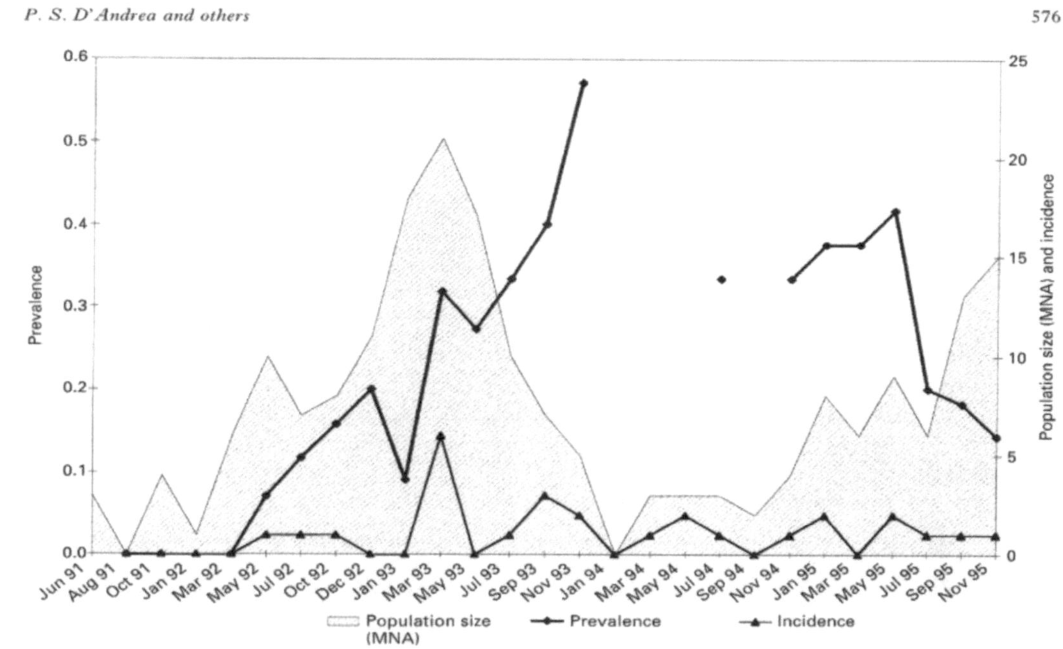

Fig. 7. Population parameters of the *Nectomys squamipes* in Pamparrão, Sumidouro, Rio de Janeiro State, Brazil. Source: D'Andrea et al., 2000.

The population of the parasite did not regulate the host population and did not affect the longevity of the animals. Parasitism did not affect the survival of the rodents, who continued to eliminate viable eggs of the parasite throughout their lifecycle, as shown in the laboratory. In general, the infection did not seem to reduce the fitness (survival rates, reproduction and movement) of the rodents. The presence of infected animals in locations removed from areas contaminated by human feces and the observation of rodent movement suggested that the rodent is capable of carrying *S. mansoni* to non-transmission sites and may introduce the parasite into new areas, creating new foci and complicating disease control (D'Andrea et al., 2000).

In the Encanto locality, where schistosomiasis present at a medium endemicity, another phase of the study was conducted over four years to evaluate the effects of chemotherapy treatment in the infected human population on the rate of rodent infection and to compare diagnostic methods. During this phase, we also studied the population dynamics of the rodent *N. squamipes*, the infection rate of schistosomiasis on the water-rat populations and its change over time, and different methods for *S. mansoni* diagnosis (Bonecker et al., 2009; Gentile et al., 2006).

The population dynamics of *N. squamipes* were in accordance with other studies and with the Pamparrão study, where the reproduction of the animals occurred throughout the year but primarily during rainy periods, a trend that is related to the close association of this rodent to resources found in water (Ernest & Mares, 1986; Gentile et al., 2000). These animals reproduce opportunistically so that reproduction is triggered by resource availability according to rainfall pattern (Gentile et al., 2000), resulting in rapid population increases with higher survivorship a few months after the rainy periods, and young individuals are primarily observed in those periods (Fig. 8). The rodents showed no potential for outbreaks or for becoming agricultural pests (Bonecker et al., 2008).

There was a positive correlation between the prevalence rates estimated by the two methods of diagnosis; however, the coprological method underestimated the rate of *S. mansoni* infection in rodents at about 35%, mainly when prevalence was low. The two methods showed the same trends over time. Therefore, diagnosis by the serological method was more appropriate for assessing rates of *S. mansoni* infection in rodents, especially when the intensity of infection was low (Gentile et al., 2006).

The abundance of *N. squamipes* was related to rainfall, which, in turn, had a direct influence on the rates of *S. mansoni* transmission in rodents. *S. mansoni* prevalence was negatively correlated with rainfall at a delay of four months, and the highest prevalence rates were observed during periods of lower abundance in the rodent population, which occurred at the end of the dry season. The incidence of the parasite in the rodent population did not show a seasonal pattern. Serologic conversion was observed in five animals monitored over time. There was no difference regarding the sex of the infected and uninfected animals (Gentile et al., 2006).

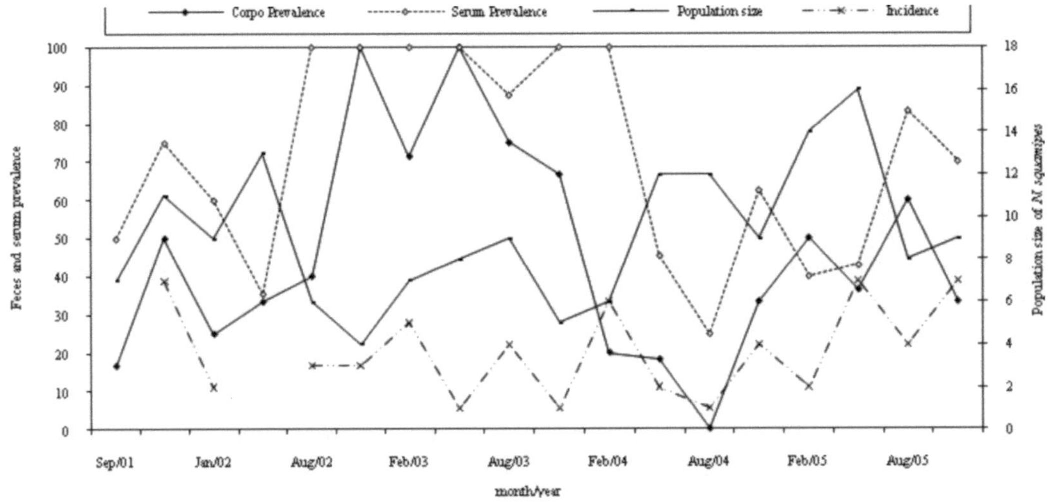

Fig. 8. Prevalences and incidences of *Schistosoma mansoni* in *Nectomys squamipes* and rodent population sizes over four years at Encanto, Sumidouro, Rio de Janeiro State, Brazil. Source: Gentile et al., 2006.

Despite the low rodent infection rate at 18 months after the chemotherapy in the human population, this treatment did not interrupt the rodent infection, as after one year, there was a resurgence in the rodent infection rate, whereas the human population prevalence was considerably reduced (from 19.3% to 4.8%). The high incidence and the serologic conversions observed in the last year of the study corroborated these data and indicated a continuous process of *S. mansoni* transmission in the area, despite the chemotherapy in the human population (Gentile et al., 2006).

5.3 The *S. mansoni* – water-rat interaction

In an another phase of the study, aspects of the parasite interaction between *S. mansoni* and *N. squamipes* were evaluated. In this study, the collected animals were examined for *S.*

mansoni and other helminth species. The abundance and intensity of *S. mansoni* in the population of *N. squamipes* were determined, as well as the degree of aggregation and the interaction with other helminths.

The distribution of *S. mansoni* in the population of *N. squamipes* was highly aggregated, and 50% of the worms were concentrated in 4.2% of the host population. Considering only the infected rodents, 11.4% of them harbored half the population of parasites (D'Andrea et al., 2000). Spatial heterogeneity and low infection rates in snails explain the patchy distribution, which restricts the foci of transmission to only a few areas.

The prevalence of *S. mansoni* on the water-rats was 34.5%, the intensity was 48.3 individuals and the abundance was 16.7. These high intensity and abundance values reflect the high susceptibility of the rodent to the parasite and the high transmissibility of the parasite in the region. In the *N. squamipes* population, *S. mansoni* was the dominant species of the helminth community. There was no antagonistic or synergistic interaction between *S. mansoni* and the other helminth species (Maldonado Jr. et al., 2006).

5.4 On a regional scale

Cross-sectional studies were conducted in other localities during the same time as the study in Encanto. In Pamparrão and Soledade, areas of low and high endemicity, respectively, animals were captured and necropsied. In Volta, an area with no human cases of schistosomiasis, a mark-recapture study of the rodents was carried out. The *S. mansoni* diagnosis was made by serological and parasitological methods and necropsy to compare the techniques and refine the diagnosis for areas of low endemicity.

At this step of the study, we observed different patterns regarding the participation of the water-rat in the *S. mansoni* transmission dynamics in each location. In Volta, the rodents were able to maintain the *S. mansoni* infection even without infected humans, at least over a short period of time. In Pamparrão, the low rodent population size and the absence of rodent infection over two years did not eliminate infection transmission, as human prevalence was 13.4%. In Soledade, a high endemic area, we observed infected rodents far from human habitations, and the human and rodent transmission cycles did not seem to be affecting each other. (Gentile et al., 2006).

Regarding the comparison of diagnostic methods, the similarity in the reactive serology profile between individuals diagnosed coprology/necropsy negative and those diagnosed coprology/necropsy positive demonstrates that serology detects recent infection, including the false negatives in coprology, because antibodies can be found after five days of infection in laboratory experiments with *N. squamipes* (Peralta et al., 2009). The low titers of antibodies in most of these samples corroborates this hypothesis.

5.5 A natural experiment on the time of activity of the water-rat

D'Andrea et al. (2002) conducted two field experiments in the location of Pamparrão with the following objectives: 1) Determine the activity pattern of *N. squamipes* and its use of the aquatic environment; and 2) Prove the occurrence of late transmission of *S. mansoni* cercariae to *N. squamipes* in natural conditions using sentinel animals. These experiments showed the occurrence of infection of *N. squamipes* by cercariae in natural conditions in daylight and twilight hours with no significant differences, demonstrated by the recovery of worms used in rodent sentinels. The observation of the occurrence of infections in rodents during their natural time of activity (at dusk) raised the possibility of an adaptative process of *S. mansoni* to different definitive hosts (D'Andrea et al., 2002). The emission peak during the day would be more related to human infection, as this is the time of greatest activity for the local people and of increased contact with contaminated water bodies, and the crepuscular peak could be related to infection in rodents, as they have twilight/nocturnal activity (Fig. 9 and Table 1) (D'Andrea et al., 2002).

	Diurnal (10 a.m. – 2 p.m.)		Crepuscular / Nocturnal (5 p.m. – 9 p.m.)	
	July	November	July	November
Number of water-rats exposed	8	6(3[a])	8	6
Number of water-rats infected	5	3	4	4
Total of adult worms recovered	14	8	8	5
Total of worms pairs recovered	3	1	3	1

Table 1. Exposure of water-rats (born in captivity) to early and late *Schisotosoma mansoni* infection and worm recoveries. [a] Water-rats died during the experiment. Source: D'Andrea et al., 2002.

Previous studies have attempted to show differences between rodents and human *S. mansoni* strains through the following factors: external morphology of adult worms (Machado-Silva et al., 1994), pathogenicity in mice (Bastos et al., 1984, Silva & Andrade 1989), compatibility with snails (Bastos et al., 1984; Dias et al., 1978), sensitivity to drugs

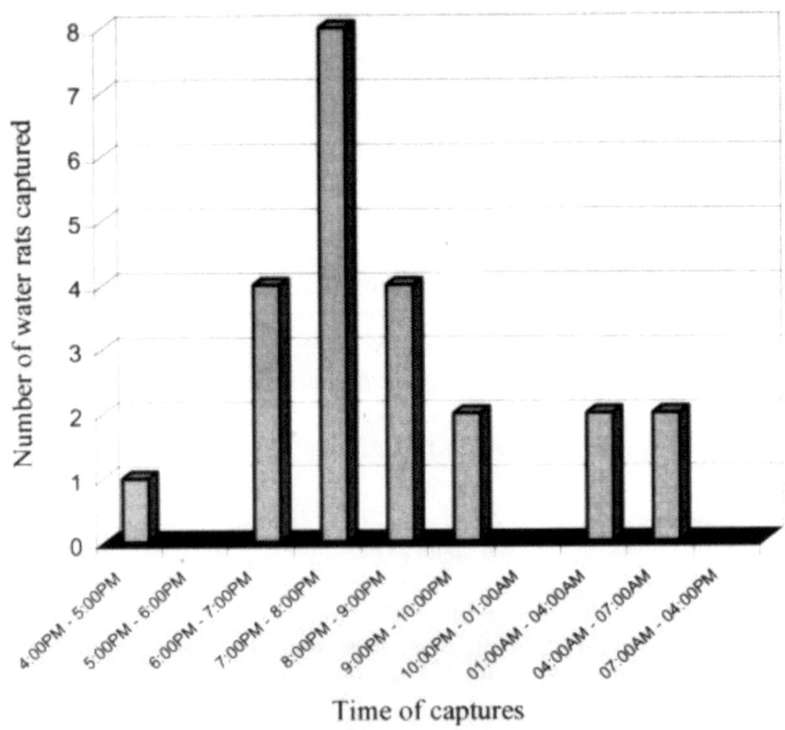

Fig. 9. Daily activity pattern of the water-rat *Nectomys squamipes*. Source: D'Andrea et al., 2002.

(Souza et al. 1992) and iso-enzyme patterns (Oliveira, 1996). These biological differences, coupled with the existence of two different patterns of cercariae emission (diurnal and crepuscular / nocturnal), led to the hypothesis that there could be differences at the molecular level between the human and rodent strains and between different geographical regions (Gentile & Oliveira, 2008). Several studies had previously shown intra-specific *S. mansoni* differences in enzymes (Fletcher et al., 1981; Navarro et al., 1992), molecular mitochondrial DNA (Blair et al., 1999; Després et al., 1991; Després et al., 1993; Le et al . 2000; Pena et al., 1995) and total DNA (Barral et al., 1993; Barral et al., 1996; Neto et al., 1993; Simpson et al., 1995; Sire et al., 1999).

6. Conclusions

The information obtained in these studies provides a more realistic and innovative support to the schistosomiasis control program in Sumidouro by contributing to the knowledge of the epidemiological complexity in the study area and, in particular, by elucidating the role of wild rodents in the local transmission of this disease. It is important to note that despite not having ideal conditions, as achieved in the work of Théron & Pointier (1995), the information obtained by this empirical long-term study carried out in Sumidouro, as well as the results of the laboratory experiments, allows for the establishment of a set of criteria for characterizing *N. squamipes* as a host-reservoir of *S. mansoni*:

1. High susceptibility to infection: The species proved to be extremely susceptible to contracting the infection, even in areas of low endemicity.
2. Ability to complete the parasite cycle: The water-rat eliminates viable eggs of *S. mansoni* in its stool, and because of its semi-aquatic habit, these eggs are very likely to hatch, allowing the infection of intermediate hosts and the completion of the cycle of the parasite.
3. The rodent is not affected by the infection, allowing transmission of the parasite throughout its life - the data show that natural infection with *S. mansoni* does not affect survival, reproduction or mobility, and, in general, the infection causes no reduction in the fitness of infected individuals or interference with population dynamics.
4. The infection is chronic and persistent over the life time of the animal - data from experimental infections show mild disease with no change in the survival of the animal and, under natural conditions, show that the disease is cumulative, that there is no immunization or self-healing, and that the elimination of viable eggs of the parasite is persistent throughout the life of the animal.
5. Overlap of areas of *S. mansoni* distribution and reservoir distribution - there is overlap between the geographic and ecological distribution of *N. squamipes* and schistosomiasis in Brazil.
6. The reservoir must make the link between the wild and domestic environment - the water-rat is an abundant rodent and totally adapted to degraded natural areas and rural areas, which occur frequently in the surroundings of domicile areas and small crops, thereby increasing transmission to human populations.
7. The reservoir must maintain the infection in the absence of man - experiments in controlled conditions (semi-natural) and evidence from this study suggest that possibility.
8. The possibility of adaptation of *S. mansoni* to *N. squamipes* with an independent parasitic cycle - chronobiological differences between rodents and humans

concerning their activity time and exposure to water courses and experimental evidence of two peaks in cercariae emission (one during the day and another at twilight), with the possibility of late infection in rodents, suggest adaptation process of a *S. mansoni* strain to the water-rat.

Observing these criteria in the studied localities, the importance of the water-rats as wild reservoirs of *S. mansoni* in Sumidouro was demonstrated, despite transmission power of different degrees in each area, even on a small regional scale. It was clear that, independent of other reasons for the complexity of the situation, the presence of these rodents must always be taken into account in schistosomiasis control programs, as its participation in transmission increases this complexity. Thus, the main impact of the results was the perception that the solution to the problem of schistosomiasis in Sumidouro must be determined through an approach based both on the needs of the ecosystem and of the human population. This approach must emphasize the presence of the rodent and its participation in the transmission of the parasite to humans, in addition to considering historical, social, economical, anthropological and other peculiarities of the situation. From both social and scientific perspectives, this will represent a favorable conclusion to this long-term study.

This approach must be able to alter schistosomiasis transmission control by dealing with the complexity of the situation, which means considering ethical aspects and other aspects that cannot be mathematically modeled, stimulating the participation of the population of Sumidouro to search for solutions to its problems, and training teachers, doctors, health and environmental agents, and other local professionals for interventions in the local context. To make the establishment of more adequate environmental health public policies possible, this approach must also supply the municipal sectors of health, environment, education and sanitation with qualified and up-to-date technical procedures. In principle, the Ecosystem Approach to Health (OPAS, 2009; Waltner Toews et al., 2008,) fits these objectives.

The Ecosystem Approach to Health, already proposed to deal with schistosomiasis and other parasitic and infectious diseases (Augusto et al., 2005; PAHO, 2009; Waltner-Toews, 2004), is a process of participative management in the health/environment interface that is designed to construct information, foresee changes (as for example, an epidemic), and carry through choices that involve the judgment of values, interests and uncertainties. This approach is adaptive because it is based on methodological pluralism and on a protocol of basic lines fed back by a collective appreciation of the problem. Therefore, it can indicate paths for management strategies and public policies that are adequate to social/ecological systems like those we observed in Sumidouro. The investment in an Ecosystem Approach to Health would certainly answer the desires of our research group in effectively contributing to the improvement of the quality of life of the people in that city.

7. Acknowledgements

We would like to thank several people who contributed to this study, especially Arnaldo Maldonado Jr., José Roberto Machado e Silva, Rosângela Rodrigues e Silva, Sócrates F. C. Neto, José M. Peralta, Juberlan S. Garcia, José W. F. da Costa, Cláudia H. Almeida, Carlos E.V. Grelle, Fabiano F. Fernandes, Alexandre Giovanelli, Regina M.O. Figueiredo, Elaine M. Martinez, Simone T. Bonecker, Luciana G. Portugal, Cibele R. Bonvicino, M. Gusmão, T. Figueiredo, R. P. Igreja, A. C. Santana, M. T. Paulino, W. Abreu, I. Pimenta, W. Valim and all the people of LABPMR and LAPSA in FIOCRUZ from 1990 to 2006 for helping with the field and laboratory work. We also thank the Municipal Secretary of Agriculture and Environment in Sumidouro, S. S. Serafim, for providing many operational facilities and a field base; the people of Encanto, Pamparrão, Volta and Soledade in Sumidouro, who allowed us to carry out the field work on their properties and participated in the schistosomiasis inquiry; and the Municipal Government, the Office of Education and Culture and the Office of Health and Social Promotion in Sumidouro, Rio de Janeiro, for extensive operational support. We would like to make a special acknowledgement to Dr. Luis Rey, who was responsible for the original conception of this study and its viability. This study was supported by Fundação Oswaldo Cruz (IOC), CNPq, FAPERJ, PAPES - FIOCRUZ and the Sumidouro Municipal Government.

8. References

Almeida-Filho, N. (1997). Transdisciplinaridade e saúde coletiva. *Ciência e Saúde Coletiva*, Vol. 2, No1/2, pp. 5-20.

Amorim, J.P. (1953). Infestação experimental e natural de murídeos pelo *Schistosoma mansoni* (nota prévia). *Revista Brasileira de Malariologia e Doenças Tropicais*, Vol.5, pp. 219-222.

Augusto, L. G.S.; Carneiro, R.M. & Martins, P.H. (2005). *Abordagem ecossistêmica em saúde: Ensaios para o controle de dengue*, 382pp., Ed. Universitária da UFPE, Recife, Brasil.

Barbosa, F.S.; Dobbin, J.E. Jr. & Coelho, M.V. (1953). Infestação natural de *Rattus rattus frugivorus* por *Schistosoma mansoni* em Pernambuco. *Publicação Avulso do Instituto Aggeu Magalhães*, Vol. 2, pp. 42-43.

Barbosa, C. S.; Pieri, O. S.; Silva, C. B. & Barbosa, F. S. (2000). Ecoepidemiologia da esquistossomose urbana na ilha de Itamaracá, Pernambuco. *Revista de Saúde Pública*, Vol.34, pp. 337-341.

Barbosa, C.S.; Coutinho, A.L.; Montenegro, S.M.L.; Abath, F.; Guida, U.; Spinelli, V. (2001). Epidemia de esquistossomose aguda na praia de Porto de Galinhas, Pernambuco. *Cadernos de Saúde Pública*, Vol.17, pp. 725-728.

Barbosa, C. S. ; Favre, T. C. ; Amaral ; Pieri, O. S. (2008). Epidemiologia e Controle da Esquistossomose Mansonica. In: *Schistosoma Mansoni e Esquistossomose : Uma Visão Multidisciplinar vol 1*, O. Carvalho & H. Lenzi, (Eds.), 965-1008, Editora Fiocruz, Rio de Janeiro, Brasil.

Barbosa, C. S.; Silva, C. B.; Barbosa, F. S. (1996). Esquistossomose: Reprodução e Expansão da Endemia no Estado de Pernambuco no Brasil. *Revista de Saúde Pública*, Vol.30, No.6, pp. 609-616.

Barral, V.; Morand, S.; Pointier, J.P. & Theron, A. (1996). Distribution of schistosome genetic diversity within naturally infected *Rattus rattus* detected by RAPD markers. *Parasitology*, Vol.113, pp. 511-517.

Barral, V.; This, P.; Imbert-Establet, D.; Combes, C. & Delseny, M. (1993). Genetic variability and evolution of the *Schistosoma* genome analysed by using random amplified polymorphic DNA markers. *Molecular and Biochemical Parasitology*, Vol.59, pp. 211-221.

Bastos, O.C.; Sadigurky, M.; Nascimento, M.D.S.B.; Brazil, R.P. & Holanda, J.C. (1984). *Holochilus brasiliensis nanus* Thomas, 1897. Sugestão de modelo experimental para filariose, leishimaniose e esquistossomose. *Revista do Instituto de Medicina Tropical São Paulo*, Vo.26, pp. 307-315.

Bastos, O.C.; Silva, A.M.A.; Souza, E.P.; Lemos-Neto, R.C. & Piedrabuena, A.E. (1982). Ocorrências de linhagens humana e silvestre de *Schistosoma mansoni*, na pré-amazônia. 1° Estudo em molusco. *Revista de Saúde Pública*, Vo.16, pp. 292-298.

Blair, D.; Le, T.H.; Despres, L. & Mcmanus, D.P. (1999). Mitochondrial genes of *Schistosoma mansoni*. *Parasitology*, Vol.119, pp. 303-313.

Bonecker, S.T.; Portugal, L.G.; Costa-Neto, S.F. & Gentile, R. (2009). A long term study of small mammal populations in a Brazilian agricultural landscape. *Mammalian Biology*, Vol.74, pp. 467-477.

Bonvicino, C.R.; Oliveira, J.A. & D'andrea, P.S. (2008). *Guia dos roedores do Brasil, com chaves para gêneros baseadas em caracteres externos*, Centro Pan-Anamericano de Febre Aftosa - OPAS/OMS, 120pp, Rio de Janeiro, Brasil.

Borda, C.E. & Rea, M.J.F. (2006). Intermediate and definitive hosts of *Schistosoma mansoni* in Corrientes province, Argentina. *Memórias do Instituto Oswaldo Cruz*, Vol.101, No.I, pp. 233-234.

Brasil. (2008). *Vigilância e controle de moluscos de importância epidemiológica: diretrizes técnicas; programa de vigilância e controle da esquistossomose (PCE)*, ilus.(Série A. Normas e manuais técnicos), Ministério da Saúde. Secretaria de Vigilância em Saúde. Departamento de Vigilância Epidemiológica,178 pp, Brasília, Brasil.

Brasil. (2010). *Doenças infecciosas e parasitárias: guia de bolso*, 8. ed. Ver, Série B. Textos Básicos de Saúde, Ministério da Saúde. Secretaria de Vigilância em Saúde. Departamento de Vigilância Epidemiológica, 448 pp., Brasília, Brasil.

Brasil (2011a). Óbitos por Esquistossomose. Brasil, Grandes Regiões e Unidades Federadas 1990-2009. In: *Portal Saúde*, Accessed in 06/09/2011, Available from: http://portal.saude.gov.br/portal/arquivos/pdf/obitos_1990_ 2008.

Brasil (2011b). Glossário de Doenças. In: Portal Saúde, Acccessed in 06/09/2011, Available from:
http://portal.saude.gov.br/portal/saude/Gestor/area.cfm?id_area=1498

Cameron, T.W.M. (1928). A new definitive host for *Schistosoma mansoni*. *Journal of Helminthology*, Vol.6, pp. 219-222.

Carvalho, D.M. (1982). *Sobre a importância de Nectomys squamipes na epidemiologia da esquistossomose mansônica no município de Sumidouro, MSc Dissertation*, Fundação Oswaldo Cruz, 87pp., Rio de Janeiro, Brasil.

Carvalho, O.S.; Andrade, R.M. & Cortês, M.I.N. (1976). Ciclo vital de *Schistosoma mansoni* através do *Holochilus brasiliensis* (Desmarest, 1818), em ambiente semi-natural (Trematoda: Schistosomatidae; Rodentia: Cricetidae). *Revista da Sociedade Brasileira de Medicina Tropical*, Vol.10, pp. 235-247.

Costa-Silva, M. (2000). *Suscetibilidade experimental de Nectomys squamipes (Rodentia: Sigmodontinae) a cepas de Schistosoma mansoni (Trematoda: Schistosomatidade): Estudo morfológico de vermes adultos machos e fêmeas por microscopia de luz, MSc Dissertation*, Universidade do Estado do Rio de Janeiro, 56pp., Rio de Janeiro, Brasil.

Coura, J.R. & Amaral, R.S. (2004). Epidemiological and Control Aspects of Schistosomiasis in Brazilian Endemic Areas *Memórias do Instituto Oswaldo Cruz*, Vol. 99, No.Suppl. I, pp. 13-19, 2004

D'Andrea, P.S.; Fernandes, F.A.; Cerqueira, R. & Rey, L. (2002). Experimental evidence and ecological perspectives for the adaptation of *Schistosoma mansoni* Sambon, 1907 (Digenea: Schistosomatidae) to a wild host, the water-rat, *Nectomys squamipes*

Brants, 1827 (Rodentia: Sigmodontinae). *Memórias do Instituto Oswaldo Cruz*, Vol.97, No.1, pp. 11-14.

D'Andrea, P.S.; Gentile, R.; Cerqueira, R.; Grelle, C.E.V.; Horta, C. & Rey, L. (1999). Ecology of small mammals in a Brazilian rural area. *Revista Brasilera de Zoologia*, Vol.16, No.3, pp. 611-620.

D'Andrea, P.S.; Gentile, R.; Maroja, L.S.; Fernandez, F.A.; Coura, R.S. & Cerqueira, R. (2007). Small mammal populations of an agroecosystem in the Atlantic Forest domain, southeastern of Brazil. *Brazil Journal of Biology*, Vo.67, No.1, pp. 179-186.

D'Andrea, P.S.; Horta, C.; Cerqueira, R. & Rey, L. (1996). Breeding of the water-rat (*Nectomys squamipes*) in the laboratory. *Laboratory Animals*, Vo.30, pp. 369-376.

D'Andrea, P.S.; Maroja, L.S.; Gentile, R.; Cerqueira, R.; Maldonado Jr., A. & Rey, L. (2000). The parasitism of *Schistosoma mansoni* (Digenea-Trematoda) in a naturally infected population of water-rats, *Nectomys squamipes* (Rodentia-Sigmodontinae) in Brazil. *Parasitology*, Vo.120, pp. 573-582.

Despres, L.; Imbert-Establet, D. & Monnerot, M. (1993). Molecular characterization of mitochondrial DNA provides evidence for the recent introduction of *Schistosoma mansoni* into America. *Molecular and Biochemical Parasitology*, Vo.60, pp. 221-229.

Després, L.; Imbert-Establet, D.; Combes, C. & Bonhomme, E. (1992). Molecular evidence linking hominid evolution to recent radiation of *Schistosome* (Platyhelminths: Trematoda). *Molecular Phylogeny and Evolution*, Vo.4:, pp. 295-304.

Despres, L.; Imbert-Establet, D.; Combes, C.; Bonhomme, F. & Monnerot, M. (1991). Isolation and polymorphism in mitochondrial DNA from *Schistosoma mansoni*. *Molecular and Biochemical Parasitology*, Vo.47, pp. 139-141.

Dias, L.C.S.; Pires, F.A. & Pinto, A.C.W. (1978). Parasitological and ecological aspects of schistosomiasis mansoni in the valley of Paraiba do Sul river (São Paulo, Brazil). 1. Natural infection of small mammals with *Schistosoma mansoni*. *Transactions of Royal Society of Tropical Medicine. Hygiene*, Vol.72, pp. 496-500.

Duplantier, J.M. & Sène, M. (2000). Rodents as reservoir hosts in the transmission of Schistosoma mansoni in Richard-Toll, Senegal, West Africa. *Journal of Helminthology*, Vol.74, pp. 129-135.

Emmons, L.H. & Feer, F. (1997). *Neotropical Rainforest Mammals: A field Guide*, University of Chicago Press, 307pp., Chicago, USA.

Ernest, K.A. & Mares, M.A. (1986). Ecology of *Nectomys squamipes*, the Neotropical Water-rat, in central Brazil: home range, habitat selection, reproduction and behaviour. *Journal of Zoology*, Vol.210, pp. 599-612.

Fletcher, M.; Loverde, P.T. & Woodruff, D.S. (1981). Genetic variation in *Schistosoma mansoni* enzyme polymorphisms in populations from Africa, Southwest Asia, South America and West Indies. *American Journal of Tropical Medicine Hygiene*, Vol.30, pp. 406-421.

Gazzinelli, A & Kloos, H. (2007). The use of spatial tools in the study of *Schistosoma mansoni* and its intermediate host snails in Brazil: a brief review. *Geospatial Health*, Vol.2, No.1, pp.51-58

Gentile, R. & Fernandez, F.A.S. (1999). Influence of habitat structure on a streamside small mammal community in a Brazilian rural area. *Mammalia*, Vol.63, pp. 29-40.

Gentile, R.; Costa-Neto, S.F.; Gonçalves, M.M.L.; Bonecker, S.T.; Fernandes, F.A.; Garcia, J.S.; Barreto, M.G.M.; Soares, M.S.; D'andrea, P.S.; Peralta, J.M. & Rey, L. (2006). An ecological field study of the water-rat *Nectomys squamipes* as a wild reservoir

indicator of *Schistosoma mansoni* transmission in an endemic area. *Memórias do Instituto Oswaldo*, Vo.101, No.I, pp. 111-117.
Gentile, R.; D'andrea, P.S.; Cerqueira, R. & Maroja, L.S. (2000). Population dynamics and reproduction of marsupials and rodents in a Brazilian rural area: a five-year study. *Study Neotropical Fauna & Environment*, Vol.35, pp. 1-9.
Gentile., R. & Oliveira. G. (2008). Brazilian studies on the genetics of *Schistosoma mansoni*. *Acta Tropica*, Vol.108, No.2-3, pp. 175–178.
Giovanelli, A.; Soares, M.S.; D'andrea, P.S.; Gonçalves, M.M.L. & Rey, L. (2001). Abundância e infecção do molusco *Biomphalaria glabrata* pelo *Schistosoma mansoni* no Estado do Rio de Janeiro, Brasil. *Memórias do Instituto Oswaldo Cruz*, Vol.35, pp. 523-530.
Giovannoni, M.; Vellozo, L.G.C. & Kubiak, G.V.L. (1946). Sobre as "ratadas" do primeiro planalto paranaense. *Arquivos de Biologia e Tecnologia*, Vo.1, pp. 185-195.
Gonçalves, M.M.L.; Barreto, M.G.M. & Maldonado Jr., A. (2005). Fatores sócio-culturais e éticos relacionados com os processos de diagnóstico da esquistossomose mansônica em área de baixa endemicidade. *Cadernos de Saúde Pública*, Vol.21, No.1, pp. 92-100.
Graeff-Teixeira, C. (2004). The initial epidemiological studies in the low endemicity schistosomiasis area in Esteio, Rio Grande do Sul, the southernmost Brazilian state, 1997 to 2000. *Memorias do Instituto Oswaldo Cruz*, Vol.99, No.S, pp. 73–78.
Graeff-Teixeira, C. & Moraes, C. (1999). Identification of a transmission focus of *Schistosoma mansoni* in the southermost Brazilian state, Rio Grande do Sul. *Memórias do Instituto Oswaldo Cruz*, Vol.94, pp. 9-10.
Guimarães, C.T.; Souza, C.P.; Carvalho, O.S. & Katz, N. (1993). Sobre um foco urbano de esquistossomose em área metropolitana da região sudeste do Brasil. *Revista de Saúde Pública*, Vol.27, pp. 210-213.
Guimarães, C.T.; Souza, C.P.; Soares, D.M.; Araújo, N. & Schuster, L.M.R. (1990). Occurrence of moluscs in aquaria of ornamental fishes in Belo Horizonte, Minas Gerais, Brasil. *Memórias do Instituto Oswaldo Cruz*, Vol.85, pp. 127-129.
Guimarães, I.C.S. & Neto, J. T. (2006). Transmissão urbana de esquistossomose em crianças de um bairro de Salvador, Bahia. *Revista da Sociedade Brasileira de Medicina Tropical*, Vol.39, pp.451-455.
Hanelt, B.; Mwangi, L.N.; Kinuthia, J.M; Maina, G.M.; Agola, L.E.; Mutuku, M.W.; Steinauer, M.L.; Agwanda, B.R.; Kigo, L.; Mungai, B.N.; Loker, E.S. & Mkoji, G.M. (2010). Schistosomes of small mammals from the Lake Victoria Basin, Kenya: new species, familiar species, and implications for schistosomiasis control. *Parasitology*, Vol.137, pp. 1109-118.
He, Y.X.; Salafsky, B. & Ramaswamy, K. (2001). Host-parasite relationships of Schistosoma japonicum in mammalian hosts. Trends in Parasitology, Vol 17, pp.320-324.
Instituto Brasileiro de Geografia e Estatística. (2010). Sumidouro RJ - População 2010, In: *IBGE Cidades@*, Access in 04/23/2011, Available from: http://www.ibge.gov.br/cidadesat/topwindow.htm
Katz, N.; Guimarães, C.T.; Souza, C.P.; Santos, O.C. (1993). Sobre um foco urbano de esquistossomose em área metropolitana da região sudeste do Brasil. *Revista Saúde Pública (São Paulo)*, Vol.27, pp. 210-213.
Katz, N.; Peixoto, S. U. (2000). Análise crítica da estimativa do número de portadores de esquistossomose mansoni no Brasil. *Revista da Sociedade Brasileira de Medicina Tropical*, Vol.33, No.3, pp. 303-308.

Kawazoe, U. & Pinto, A.C.M. (1983). Importância epidemiológica de alguns animais silvestres na esquistossomose mansônica. *Revista de Saúde Pública*, Vol.17, pp. 345-366.

Kuntz, R.E. (1952). Natural infection of an Egyptian gerbil with *Schistosoma mansoni*. *Proceedings of the Helminthological Society of Washington*, Vol.19, pp. 123-124.

Lambertucci, J.R.; Serufo, J.K.; Lara, R.G.; Rayes, A.A.M.; Teixeira, R.; Nobre, V. & Antunes, C.M.F. (2000). *Schistosoma mansoni*: assessment of morbidity before and after control. Acta Tropica, Vol.77, pp. 101–109

Le, T.H.; Blair, D. & Mcmanus, D.P. (2000). Mitochondrial DNA sequences of human schistosomes: the current status. *International Journal for Parasitology*, Vol.30, pp. 283-290.

Lu, D.B.; Wang, T.P.; Rudge, J.W.; Donnelly, C.A.; Fang, G.R. & Webster, J.P. (2010). Contrasting reservoirs for Schistosoma japonicum between marshland and hilly regions in Anhui, China - a two-year longitudinal parasitological survey. *Parasitology*, Vol 137, pp. 99-110.

Machado-Silva, J.R.; Galvão, C.; Presgrave, O.A.; F.; Rey, L. & Gomes, D.C. (1994). Host induced morphological changes of *Schistosoma mansoni* Sambon, 1907 male worms. *Memórias do Instituto Oswaldo Cruz*, Vol.89, pp. 411-416.

Maldonado Jr., A.; Gentile, R.; Fernandes, C.M.; D'andrea, P.S.; Lanfredi, R.M. & Rey, L. (2006). Helminth communities of *Nectomys squamipes* (Rodentia: Sigmodontine) naturally infected by the exotic trematode *Schistosoma mansoni* in southeastern Brazil. *Journal of Helminthology*, Vol.80, pp. 369-375.

Maldonado Jr., A.; Machado E Silva, J.R.; Rodrigues E Silva, R.; Lenzi, H.L. & Rey, L. (1994). Evaluation of the resistance to *Schistosoma mansoni* infection in *Nectomys squamipes* (Rodentia: Cricetidae), a natural host of infection in Brazil. *Revista do Instituto de Medicina Tropical de São Paulo*, Vol.36, pp. 193-198.

Martinez, E.M.; Costa-Silva, M.; Neves, R.H.; Oliveira, R.M.F. & Machado-Silva, J.R. (2008). Biological implications of the phenotypic plasticity in the *Schistosoma mansoni-Nectomys squamipes* model. *Revista do Instituto de Medicina tropical de São Paulo*, Vol.50, No.4, pp. 229-232.

Martins, A.V.; Martins, G. & Brito, R.S. (1955). Reservatórios silvestres do *Schistosoma mansoni* no estado de Minas Gerais. *Revista Brasileira de Malariologia e Doenças Tropicais*, Vol.7, pp. 259-265.

Martins Jr., D.F. & Barreto, M.L.. (2003). Aspectos macroepidemiológicos da esquistossomose mansônica: análise da relação da irrigação no perfil espacial da endemia no Estado da Bahia, Brasil. *Cadernos de Saúde Pública*, Vol.19, No.2, pp. 383-393.

Massoia, E. (1974). Ataques graves de *Holochilus* y otros roedores a cultivos de cana de azúcar. *Instituto Nacional de Tecnología Agropecuaria*, Vol.321, No.24, pp. 1-12.

Morand, S.; Pointier, J.P. & Théron, A. (1999). Population biology of Schistosoma mansoni in the black rat: host regulation and basic transmission rate. *International Journal for Parasitology*, Vol.29, pp. 673-684.

Morgan, J.A.T.; Dejong, R.J.; Adoye, G.O.; Ansa, E.D.O.; Barbosa, C.S.; Brémond, P.; Cesari, I.M.; Charbonnel, N.; Corrêa, L.R.; Coulibaly, G.; D'andrea, P.S.; Souza, C.P.; Doenhoff, M.J.; File, S.; Idris, M.A.; Incani, N.; Jarne, F.; Karanja, D.M.S.; Kazibwe, F.; Kpikpi, J.; Lwambo, N.J.S.; Mabaye, A.; Magalhães, L.A.; Makundi, A.; Moné, H.; Mouahid, G.; Muchemi, G.M.; Mungai, B.N.; Séne, M.; Southgate, V.; Tchuenté, L.A.T.; Théron, A.; Yousif, F.; Zanotti-Magalhães, E.M.; Mkoji, G.M. & Loker, E.S.

(2005). Origin and diversification of the human parasite *Schistosoma mansoni*. *Molecular Ecology*, Vol.14, pp. 3889-3902.

Morgan, J.A.T.; Dejong, R.J.; Kazibwe, F.; Mkoji, G.M. & Locker, E.S. (2003). A newly - identified lineage of *Schistosoma*. *International Journal for Parasitology*, Vol.33, pp. 977-985.

Mott, K.E.; Desjeux, P.; Moncayo, A.; Ranque, P. & De Raadt, P. (1990). Parasitic diseases and urban development. *Bulletin of the World Health Organization*, Vol.68, pp. 691-698.

Navarro, M.C.; Cesari, I.M. & Incani, R.N. (1992). Isoenzyme studies in one Brazilian and two Venezuelan strains of *Schistosoma mansoni*. *Comparative Biochemistry and Physiology - Part B: Biochemistry & Molecular Biology*, Vol.102, pp. 471-474.

Neto, E.D.; Souza, C.P.; Rollinson, D.; Katz, N.; Pena, S.D.J. & Simpson, A.J.G. (1993). The random amplification of polymorphic DNA allows the identification of strains and species of schistosome. *Molecular and Biochemical Parasitology*, Vol.57, pp. 83-88.

Oliveira, R.M.F. (1996). *Características parasitológicas e perfil enzimáticos deamostras de Schistosoma mansoni Sambon, 1907, MSc Dissertation*, Instituto Oswaldo Cruz, FIOCRUZ, 170pp., Rio de Janeiro, Brasil.

OPAS - Organização Pan-Americana da Saúde (2009). *Enfoques ecossistêmicos em saúde – perspectivas para sua adoção no Brasil e países da América Latina*, Organização Pan-Americana da Saúde, 44 pp., Brasília, Brasil.

Ozanan, C.C.A.F. (1969). Notas sobre o rato de cana, "*Holochilus sciureus*" Wagner, na região do Cariri, Ceará. *Revista Brasileira de Biologia*, Vol.29, No.4, pp. 567-570.

Pan-American Health Organization (PAHO). (2009). *Enfoques ecossistêmicos em saúde – perspectivas para sua adoção no Brasil e países da América Latina,* Organização Pan-Americana da Saúde, 44pp., Brasília, Brasil.

Pena, H.B.; De Souza, C.P.; Simpson, A.J. & Pena, S.D. (1995). Intracellular promiscuity in *Schistosoma mansoni*: nuclear transcribed DNA sequences are part of a mitochondrial minisatellite region. *Proceedings of the National Academy Sciences of the United States America*, Vol.92, pp. 915-919.

Peralta, R.H.S.; Melo, D.G.S.; Gonçalves, M.M.L.; D'andrea, P.S.; Rey, L.; Machado-Silva, J.R. & Peralta, J.M. (2009). Serological Studies in *Nectomys Squamipes* demonstrate the low sensitivity of coprological exams for the diagnosis of schistosomiasis. *The Journal of Parasitology*, Vol.95, pp. 764-766.

Picot, H. (1992). *Holochilus brasiliensis* and *Nectomys squamipes* (Rodentia, Cricetidae) natural hosts of *Schistosoma mansoni*. *Memórias do Instituto Oswaldo Cruz*, Vol.87, pp. 255-260.

Programa das Nações Unidas para o Desenvolvimento (2010). Índice de Desenvolvimento Humano - Municipal,1991-2000 - Todos os municípios do Brasil, In: *IDH-PNUD*, Accessed in 04/23/2011, Available from: http://www.pnud.org.br/atlas/ranking/IDH-M%2091%2000%20Ranking%20decrescente%20(pelos%20dados %20de%202000).htm

Rey, L. (1993). Non-human vertebrate hosts of *Schistosoma mansoni* and schistosomiasis transmission in Brazil. *Research and Review in Parasitology*, Vol.53, pp. 13-25.

Ribeiro, A.C.; Maldonado Jr, A.; D'andrea, P.S.; Vieira, G.O. & Rey, L. (1998). Susceptibility of *Nectomys rattus* (Pelsen, 1883) to experimental infection with *Schistosoma mansoni* (Sambon, 1907): a potencial reservoir in Brazil. *Memórias do Instituto Oswaldo Cruz*, Vol.93, No.I, pp. 295-299.

Rodrigues, D.C. & Ferreira, C.S. (1969). Primeiro encontro de roedores (*Nectomys squamipes)* naturalmente infestado pelo *Schistosoma mansoni,* no Estado de São Paulo, Brasil. *Revista do Instituto de Medicina Tropical. São Paulo,* Vol.11, pp. 306-308.

Rodrigues-Silva, R. (1988). *Nectomys squamipes e Akodon arviculoides (Rodentia: Cricetae) como hospedeiro naturais do Schistosoma mansoni em Sumidouro (RJ – Brasil). Emprego do Nectomys como modelo alternativo no estudo da esquistossomose mansoni, MSc Dissertation,* Fundação Oswaldo Cruz, 147pp., Rio de Janeiro, Brasil.

Rodrigues-Silva, R.; Machado E Silva, J.R.; Faerstein, N.F.; Lenzi, H.L. & Rey, L. (1992). Natural infection of wild rodents by *Schistosoma mansoni.* Parasitological aspects. *Memórias do Instituto Oswaldo Cruz,* Vol.87, pp. 271-276.

Rodrigues-Silva, R.; Machado E Silva, J.R.; Oliveira, R.M.F.; Maldonado Jr, A. & Rey, L. (1991). Roedores silvestres como modelos experimentais da esquistossomose mansônica: *Akodon arviculoides* (Rodentia: Cricetidae). *Revista do Instituto de Medicina Tropical de São Paulo,* Vol.33, No.4, pp. 257-261.

Rudge, J.W.; Lu, D.B.; Fang, G.R.; Wang, T.P.; Basanez, M.G. & Webster, J.P. (2009). Parasite genetic differentiation by habitat type and host species: molecular epidemiology of Schistosoma japonicum in hilly and marshland áreas of Anhui Province, China. *Molecular Ecology,* Vol.18, No.10, pp. 2134-2147.

Schall, V.T., Massara, C.L & Diniz, M.C.P. (2008). Educação em Saúde no Controle da Esquistossomose: uma visão multidisciplinar, In: *Schistosoma mansoni & Esquistossomose,* O.S. Carvalho, P.M.Z. Coelho & H.L. Lenzi. (Eds.), 1029-1079, Editora Fiocruz, Rio de Janeiro, Brasil.

Sene, M.; Bremond, P.; Herve, J.P.; Southgate, V.R.; Sellin, B.; Marchand, B. & Duplantier, J.M. (1997). Comparison of human and murine isolates of *Schistosoma mansoni* from Richard-Toll, Senegal, by isoeletric focusing. *Journal of Helminthology,* Vol.71, pp. 175-181.

Silva, L.J. (1985). Crescimento urbano e doença- A esquistossomose no município de São Paulo (Brasil). *Revista de Saúde Pública de São Paulo,* Vol.19, pp. 1-7.

Silva, M.D. 2004. Memória da Esquistossomose no Município de Sumidouro, RJ, Brasil. *Monografia do Programa de Vocação Científica.* Escola Politécnica de Saúde Joaquim Venâncio, Fiocruz, 54p.

Silva, T.M. & Andrade, Z.A. (1989). Infecção natural de roedores silvestres pelo *Schistosoma mansoni. Memórias do Instituto Oswaldo Cruz,* Vol.84, pp. 227-235.

Simpson, A.J.; Dias, N.E.; Vidigal, T.H.; Pena. H.B.; Carvalho, O.S. & Pena, S.D. (1995). DNA polymorphism of schistosomes and their snail hosts. *Memórias do Instituto Oswaldo Cruz,* Vol.90, pp. 211-213.

Sire, C.; Durand, P.; Pointier, J.P. & Theron, A. (1999). Genetic diversity and recruitment pattern of *Schistosoma mansoni* in a *Biomphalaria glabrata* snail population: a field study using random-amplified polymorphic DNA markers. *Journal Parasitology,* Vol.85, pp. 436-441.

Soares, S.M.; Barreto, M.G.M.; Silva, C.L.P.A.C.; Pereira, J.B.; Moza, P.; Rey, L.; Calçado, M.S.; Lustoza, A. & Maspero, R. (1995). Schistosomiasis in a low prevalence area: Incomplete urbanization increasing risk of infection in Paracambi, RJ, Brazil. *Memórias do Instituto Oswaldo Cruz,* Vol.90, pp. 451-458.

Soares, M.S., Roque, O.C. & Barbosa, C.S. (2002). Relato Preliminar de Reflexões sobre Prevenção de Impasses no Enfrentamento de Doenças Transmissíveis de Origem Socioambiental. *Informe Epidemiológico do SUS, Brasilia,* Vol.11, No.3, pp. 167-176..

Souza, V.A.M.; Silva, R.R.; Maldonado Jr, A.; Machado E Silva, J.R. & Rey, L. (1992). *Nectomys squamipes* (Rodentia - Cricetidae) as an experimental model for schistosomiasis mansoni. *Memórias do Instituto Oswaldo Cruz*, Vol.87, pp. 277-280.

Stotz, E.N.; Barreto, M.G.M. & Soares, M.S. (2006). Aprendizagem de pesquisadores científicos com agricultores: reflexões sobre uma prática em Sumidouro (RJ), Brasil. *Moçambras*, Vol.1, pp. 19/01.

TDR/SWG/07 (2005). Report of the Scientific Working Group meeting on Schistosomiasis. Geneva, 14–16 november 2005, Geneva, Switzerland, In: *World Health Organization*, Accessed in 06/09/2011, Available from: www.who. int/tdr.

Théron, A & Pointier, J.P. (1985). Recherche des facteurs susceptibles démpécher la réalisation du cycle de *Schistosoma mansoni* dans les mares de la Grand Terre de Guadeloupe. *Annales de Parasitologie Humaine et Comparée*, Vol.60, pp. 155-164.

Théron, A. & Pointier, J.P. (1995). Ecology, dynamics, genetics and divergence of trematode populations in heterogeneous environments: The model of *Schistosoma mansoni* in the insular focus of Guadeloupe. *Research and Reviews in Parasitology*, Vol.55, pp. 49-64.

Théron, A. (1984). Early and late shedding patterns of *Schistosoma mansoni* cercarie: ecological significance in transmission to human and murine hosts. *Journal Parasitology*, Vol.70, pp. 652-655.

Théron, A. (1985). Polymorphisme du rhythme d'émision des cercaries de *Schistosoma mansoni* et ses relations avec l'écologie de la transmission du parasite. *Vie et Milleu*, Vol.35, pp. 23-31.

Théron, A.; Pointer, J.P.; Morand, S.; Imbert-Establlet, D. & Borel, G. (1992). Long-term dynamics of natural populations of *Schistosoma mansoni* among *Rattus rattus* in patchy environment. *Parasitology*, Vol.104, pp. 291-298.

Veiga-Borgeaud, T.; Neto, R.C.L.; Peter, F. & Bastos, O.C. (1986). Constatações sobre a importância dos roedores silvestres (*Holochilus brasiliensis nanus* Thomas, 1897) na epidemiologia da esquistossomose mansônica própria da pré-Amazônia, Maranhão-Brasil. *Cadernos de Pesquisa, São Luis*, Vol.2, pp. 86-99.

Waltner-Toews, D. (2004). *Ecosystem Sustainability and Health: A Practical Approach*, Cambridge University Press, Cambridge, UK.

Waltner-Toews, D.; Kay, J.J. & Lister, N.M.E. (2008). *The ecosystem approach: complexity, uncertainty, and managing for sustainability*, Columbia University Press, 383pp., New York, USA.

Wilson, D.E. & Reeder, D.M. (2005). *Mammal Species of the World. A taxonomic and Geographic Reference,* The John Hopkins University Press, 2142pp., Baltimore, USA.

World Health Organization (2010). Schistosomiaisis - A major public health, In: *Programs and Projects*, Accessed in 02/25/2010, Available from: http://www.who.int/schistosomiaisis/en/

13

A Study of Schistosomiasis Prevalence and Risk of Snail Presence Spatial Distributions Using Geo-Statistical Tools

Ricardo J.P.S. Guimarães[1], Fernanda R. Fonseca[1], Luciano V. Dutra[1], Corina C. Freitas[1], Guilherme C. Oliveira[2] and Omar S. Carvalho[2]
[1]*Instituto Nacional de Pesquisas Espaciais/INPE*
[2]*Centro de Pesquisas René Rachou/FIOCRUZ, MG*
Brasil

1. Introduction

Schistosomiasis mansoni is an endemic disease, typical of developing countries. In Brazil, schistosomiasis is caused by the etiological agent *Schistosoma mansoni*, whose intermediate hosts are species of mollusc of the *Biomphalaria* genus.

It is a fact, accepted by almost all the researchers, that *S. mansoni* was introduced in Brazil by the African slavery trade during the sixteenth century (Almeida Machado, 1982).

It was in the northeast of Brazil that the sugar cane found fertile and favourable soil, especially in the coastal plains with their hot and humid climate, where today the states of Pernambuco and Bahia are located. The scarce manpower, obtained from the native Indian, did not meet demand and it was more profitable to import slave labour from Africa. From the mid-sixteenth century (1551-1575) until mid-nineteenth century (1851-1860) about four million slaves arrived in Brazil. This migration started in the main African regions of the west, the east, southwest and Mozambique. Although many regions of Africa supplied slave labour to Brazil, the majority originated from the Congo and Angola. The Portuguese colonization of Angola in the early sixteenth century, enabled the migration of more than two thirds of Africans, from the ports of Luanda, Benguela and Cabinda. During the sixteenth and early seventeenth centuries, there was a large influx of Africans from the ports of the Bay of Benin (region of Ghana/Nigeria). The Brazilian port of Salvador and Recife received most of the slaves (Klein, 2002), originated from endemic regions of both *S. mansoni* and *S. haematobium* infections. However, the absence of an intermediate host for *S. haematobium* in Brazil was a limiting factor which minimized the later problem in the country (Camargo, 1980).

The wetlands used for planting sugar cane almost always follow the rivers' banks and streams and the presence of molluscs of the *Biomphalaria* genus, susceptible to *S. mansoni*, provided the ideal environmental conditions for the schistosomiasis introduction into the country (Camargo, 1980).

The endemic area has remained unchanged for several years, probably due to the shortage at that time of roads and transportation, hampering the population movement (Camargo, 1980).

With the entrance of other countries into the sugar trade, sugar production in the northeast of Brazil declined in the early eighteenth century, leading to a decline in demand for slave labour. At that time the gold and diamond rush initiated in the state of Minas Gerais began and thus, with the urgent need of workers for the mines, the first great migratory flow to the gold and diamonds mines brought the slave labour from the northeast to Minas Gerais. It is estimated that one fifth of the population at that time moved to Minas Gerais (Prado Junior, 1986), using the "ways of São Francisco" (Rey, 1956) as the main access route. It is probable that schistosomiasis also came along with these early migrants.

Nowadays, Minas Gerais has 853 municipalities and schistosomiasis is present in 518 of them. According to official data, approximately 12 million people are at risk of disease (SES, 2006).

1.1 Schistosomiasis prevalence

Pirajá Silva made the first report about the *S. mansoni* presence in Brazil in 1908. This researcher noted the presence of parasite eggs in faeces of a patient treated at the Medical School of Bahia (Silva, 1908).

Teixeira (1919) observed the first cases in the city of Belo Horizonte, Minas Gerais. On that occasion the eggs of *S. mansoni* were found in the faeces of 49 patients (0.5%) from 9,995 people considered "of all ages and conditions". Among those infected, 36 (73.5%) were children under the age of 15.

Martins (1938) worked in the cities of Montes Claros, Salinas, Jequitinhonha, Espinosa, Brejo das Almas, Rio Pardo, Fortaleza and Tremedal. Using the sedimentation method, 348 people of different ages were examined, with 100 (28.7%) having a positive stool examination for *S. mansoni*.

Versiani et al. (1945) examined 2,352 schoolchildren of both sexes, aged 7 to 15 in the city of Belo Horizonte. The screening method was used for sedimentation. 294 (12.5%) excreted eggs of *S. mansoni* in their stools.

Pellon and Teixeira (1950) published the most comprehensive Helminthological School Survey ever conducted in Brazil. 440,786 schoolchildren were examined, covering eleven states: Maranhão, Piauí, Ceará, Rio Grande do Norte, Paraíba, Pernambuco, Alagoas, Sergipe, Bahia, Espírito Santo and Minas Gerais. The screening method used was qualitative (Lutz , 1917). The survey revealed that 44,478 people had schistosomiasis mansoni, resulting in a prevalence of 10.09%. In the state of Minas Gerais, in thirteen physiographic zones, 7,991 people were diagnosed with schistosomiasis, yielding a prevalence of 4.92%.

Pellon and Teixeira (1953) presented a new survey conducted in five other states (Goiás, Mato Grosso, Paraná, Rio de Janeiro and Santa Catarina), supposedly non-endemic areas for schistosomiasis. The Lutz method diagnosed 145 (0.08%) cases of schistosomiasis, after examining 174,206 people. Other surveys are described in Pellegrino et al. (1975) and Katz et al. (1978).

The Ministry of Health in the northeast of Brazil implemented the Special Programme for Schistosomiasis Control (PECE) in Brazil in 1976, covering the states of Alagoas, Ceará, Paraíba, Pernambuco, Rio Grande do Norte and Sergipe. Due to the diversity of methodologies used in the diagnosis, the results became difficult to evaluate, however, it is admitted that PECE has been effective in reducing the disease morbidity (Almeida Machado, 1982; Lima e Costa et al., 1996).

In 1980 PECE became a routine programme named the Schistosomiasis Control Programme (PCE) and was extended to the states of Bahia and Minas Gerais (Massara, 2005). The PCE started in 1983 with management and execution by the Superintendent of Public Health Campaigns (SUCAM) of the Ministry of Health in five municipalities in the north and northeast. Since 1990 these responsibilities were transferred to the National Health Foundation (FUNASA) and in 1993 the Municipal Health Agents started implementation of activities of the PCE (Lima e Costa et al., 1996).

The evaluation and monitoring of activities of the PCE, done manually until 1996, is now performed by computer with the creation of Localities System (SISLOC) and the Schistosomiasis Control Programme System (SISPCE) (Guimarães, 2010).

Between 1988 and 2004, the PCE identified low prevalence (less than 5.0%) in 24.5% of the municipalities studied and average prevalence (between 5% and 15%) in 35.0%. High prevalence (greater than 15.0%) was found in 40.5% of the studied municipalities (SES, 2006).

Carvalho et al. (1987, 1988, 1989, 1994, 1997, 1998a), Katz & Carvalho (1983), Campos & Briques (1988), Kloss et al. (2004), Gazzinelli et al. (2006), Enk et al. (2008, 2009), Massara et al. (2008) and Tibiriça (2008) also published results of schistomiasis prevalence studies in Minas Gerais state.

Finally, Drummond et al. (2010) reported that the PCE examined 2,643,564 stool samples in the period of 2003-2007 and obtained 141,284 positives for *S. mansoni* in Minas Gerais.

1.2 Molluscs of the *Biomphalaria* genus

So far in Brazil, eleven species and one subspecies of *Biomphalaria* genus molluscs have been described: *B. glabrata* (Say, 1818), *B. tenagophila* (Orbigny, 1835), *B. straminea* (Dunker, 1848), *B. peregrina* (Orbigny, 1835), *B. schrammi* (Crosse, 1864), *B. kuhniana* (Clessin, 1883), *B. intermedia* (Paraense & Deslandes, 1962), *B. amazonica* (Paraense, 1966), *B. oligoza* (Paraense, 1974), *B. occidentalis* (Paraense, 1981), *B. cousini* (Paraense, 1966) and *B. tenagophila guaibensis* (Paraense, 1984). Among these, only the first three are naturally found infected with *S. mansoni*. Another three species, *B. amazonica*, *B. peregrina* and *B. cousini*, were experimentally infected, being considered as potential hosts of this trematode (Corrêa & Paraense, 1971; Paraense & Correa, 1973; Caldeira et al., 2010).

Seven species have been reported as having a presence in Minas Gerais state. Based on work by Souza et al. (2001) and supplemented with information obtained from the Laboratory of Helminthology and Medical Malacology, René Rachou Research Center, Oswaldo Cruz Foundation (LHMM-CPqRR/Fiocruz) and the Regional Health Management of Juiz de Fora (GRS-JF), 484 of the 853 municipalities of the state were surveyed and molluscs were found in 345 of them with the following distribution: *B. glabrata* (216 municipalities), *B. straminea* (160), *B. tenagophila* (86), *B. peregrina* (80), *B. schrammi* (28), *B. intermedia* (21) and *B. occidentalis* (05). The three host species have been found in 35 counties simultaneously.

Observations on the biology and understanding of the molluscs' population structure of the *Biomphalaria* genus are important, especially for studying the epidemiology and prevention of schistosomiasis (Kawazoe, 1975).

The presence of the Planorbidae family of molluscs is acknowledged since the Jurassic period, reported in the United States and Europe and occupying large tracts of land between latitudes 70° N and 40° S. The altitude does not influence the survival of the molluscs, since they are observed from sea level to 3,000 metres of altitude in the Rocky Mountains, or Lake Titicaca, 4,280 metres (Baker, 1945).

The study of the habitat of these molluscs, as well as their behaviour in relation to the climate, results in valuable information when the goal is disease transmission control. They are commonly found in small water collections, both natural (streams, creeks, ponds, swamps) and artificial (irrigation ditches, small dams), wind speed less than 30 cm/s and a vegetation necessary for their nourishment and protection of eggs under aquatic foliage.

In most habitats the presence of microflora and organic matter, little turbidity, good sunshine, pH between 6 and 8, NaCl content below 3 by 1000 and average temperature between 20 and 25 degrees C is observed. However, molluscs can tolerate wide variations in physical, chemical and biological characteristics of their environments and some specimens may migrate slowly against the current occupying other breeding sites upstream of the original colonies (WHO, 1957; Paraense, 1972,;Rey, 2001).

Biomphalaria molluscs developed a wide repertoire of survival mechanisms. In the rainy season, mainly due to flooding, the mollusc population decreases. The repopulation and breeding occurs mostly in the late dry season, when the number of areas with standing water (lentic) increases. In dry regions, drying reduces the number of individuals in each rainy season and the population is re-established from the few survivors.

The desiccation resistance is a physiological adaptation of *Biomphalaria* molluscs who enter a state of dormancy, reducing the need for and water loss. Another adaptation of molluscs is the acceleration of development during the rainy season to ensure the production of new individuals and thus the colony can withstand the next dry season. (Paraense, 1955, 1972; Grisolia & Freitas, 1985; Juberg et al., 1987).

The mollusc's reproductive mechanism has a fundamental role in the species' perpetuation. Because they are hermaphrodites, there is both self and cross-fertilization. The egg is wrapped in elastic capsules, gelatinous, tough and transparent. The average number of eggs per egg capsule is 20 and can reach a hundred.

Under favourable conditions, molluscs opt for cross-fertilization, however, under unfavourable conditions, a few individuals can use the mechanism of self-fertilization, initiating a new population (founder effect). The molluscs are highly prolific; a single individual is capable of generating at the end of three months, nearly 10 million descendants (Barbosa, 1970; Paraense, 1972; Thomas, 1995).

Excluding fortuitous factors, survival of molluscs will not exceed one year. Its persistence in an outbreak stems from the multiplication rate, which depends on several ecological factors influencing fertility, laying and egg viability (Paraense, 1972; Baptista & Juberg, 1993).

Of the three host species of *S. mansoni*, *B. glabrata* is the most important, due to its extensive geographic distribution, high rates of infection and efficiency in eliminating cercariae and consequently the agent spreading. Moreover, its distribution in Brazil is almost always associated with schistosomiasis occurrence (Lutz, 1917). The species was found in the municipality of Esteio located in the metropolitan region of Porto Alegre, RS (Carvalho et al., 1998b).

Biomphalaria tenagophila has epidemiological importance in the south of Brazil, being responsible for outbreaks in São Paulo. In the state of Minas Gerais it is responsible for maintaining the focus on Itajubá city (Katz & Carvalho, 1983).

B. straminea has the widest distribution among the three species, being found in almost all river basins. However it has greater epidemiological importance in the northeast of Brazil, where, in some areas, it is solely responsible for the foci maintenance with high disease prevalence. This species has been epidemiologically linked to the occurrence of cases of schistosomiasis in Paracatu in Minas Gerais (Carvalho et al., 1988).

Working in non-endemic regions in Minas Gerais (Carvalho et al., 1994, 1997, 1998a), located in the west of the state, two districts were found with *B. glabrata* (Araxá and Sacramento), 20 with *B. straminea* (Bonfinópolis de Minas, Cachoeira Dourada, Cascalho Rico, Centralina, Conceição das Alagoas, Douradoquara, Grupiara, Ipiaçu, Ituiutaba, João Pinheiro, Lagamar, Lagoa Grande, Monte Alegre de Minas, Paracatu, Sacramento, Santa Vitória, Uberaba, Uberlândia, Unaí and Vazante) and 4 with *B. tenagophila* (Agua Comprida, Patos de Minas, Uberaba and Uberlândia).

The schistosomiasis distribution in Minas Gerais is not regular. The disease is endemic in the northern (including parts of Médio São Francisco and Itacambira), eastern and central areas (Alto Jequitinhonha, Metalúrgica, Oeste e Alto São Francisco). The highest infection rates are found in the northeast and east of the state which encompasses the areas of Mucuri, Rio Doce and Zona da Mata (Pellon & Teixeira, 1950; Katz et al., 1978; Carvalho et al., 1987; Lambertucci et al., 1987). In endemic areas, large concentrations of these molluscs, together with other risk factors, favour the existence of cities with a high prevalence of schistosomiasis.

1.3 Schistosomiasis and geoprocessing

Schistosomiasis is a parasitosis determined in space and time by environmental and behavioural factors of residents in endemic areas. Its distribution in the state of Minas Gerais is not regular, since areas of high prevalence are close to non-endemic regions. Thus, despite advances in knowledge in the field of schistosomiasis, the disease remains a major public health problem in the country, requiring larger investments in preventive measures such as sanitation and health education, as well as in studies that allow for disease control through geoprocessing methodologies (Amaral et al., 2006; Guimarães et al., 2009).

Another aspect of this problem is the increasing occurrence of repeated little outbreaks of acute schistosomiasis related to rural tourism, especially in Minas Gerais. This phenomenon involves the middle and upper class sections of the population who have first time contact with the disease during leisure activities practicing rural tourism in nearby endemic areas (Enk et al., 2003; Massara et al., 2008; Enk et al., 2010).

Under these circumstances geoprocessing can be applied to characterize, to better understand the interconnection of these factors and to provide a more complete picture of disease transmission. Computational resources, such as Geographic Information System (GIS), allow for complex analysis of a large amount of information and to display the results of this analysis in graphical maps. Data generated by the GIS have an important role in the study of schistosomiasis, especially in relation to the interaction of disease with environmental conditions (Guimarães et al., 2006).

The use of GIS for the study of schistosomiasis in Brazil was also done in several states: Bahia (Bavia et al., 1999, 2001); Minas Gerais (Brooker et al., 2006; Fonseca et al., 2007a; Fonseca, 2009; Freitas et al., 2006; Gazzinelli et al., 2006; Guimarães et al., 2006, 2008, 2009, 2010a, 2010b; Guimarães, 2010; Martins, 2008; Martins-Bedê et al., 2009, 2010; Carvalho et al., 2010; Tibiriça et al., 2011); Pernambuco (Barbosa et al., 2004; Araújo et al., 2007; Galvão et al., 2010).

This work has two main objectives: the first is to estimate the probability of occurrence of each mollusc species (*B. glabrata, B. tenagophila, B. straminea*) in the state of Minas Gerais, Brazil, and to determine which of these species is more related to the prevalence of the disease; the second is to estimate the prevalence of schistosomiasis for the entire state of Minas Gerais, using the estimated probability of snail existence, besides socio-economic and environmental variables.

2. Materials and methods

This study was carried out in the Minas Gerais state, Brazil. Minas Gerais is 586,520.368 km^2 in size and is located in the west of the southeastern region of Brazil, which also contains the states of São Paulo, Rio de Janeiro and Espírito Santo. It borders with Bahia and Goiás (north), Mato Grosso do Sul (far west), the states of São Paulo and Rio de Janeiro (south) and the state of Espírito Santo (east). It also shares a short boundary with the Brazilian Federal District. It is situated between 14°13'58" and 22°54'00" S latitude and between 39°51'32" and 51°02'35" W longitude.

Minas Gerais is one of the 26 states of Brazil, of which it is the second most populous, the third richest and the fourth largest in area. The landscape of the state is marked by mountains, valleys and large areas of fertile lands presenting altitudes between 198.88 to 1573.18 metres.

According to the IBGE (2010), there were 19,597,330 people residing in the state. The last census revealed the following numbers: urbanization (85.3%), population growth between 2000-2010 (1.1%), men (49.2%), women (50.8%).

Ethnic groups found in Minas Gerais include: Caucasian (45.39%), Multiracial (44.28%), African (9.22%), Asian (0.95%) and Amerindian people (0.16%) (IBGE 2010).

The population was divided into: 0-4 (6.52%), 5-14 (15.91%), 15-19 (8.77%), 20-39 (32.91%), 40-59 (24.1%) and above 60 (11.79%) years of age (IBGE, 2010).

The Human Development Index (HDI) of Minas Gerais was 0.800, with variations between 0.568 (Angelândia) and 0.841 (Poços de Caldas) (SNIU, 2000).

On average, 66.36% of households have access to the main water supply, of which the worst municipality has 3.91% and the best has 99.26%. Also, on average about 49.2% of households have a bathroom or toilet and general sewage network, being that the worst and the best municipality have 0% and 97.5%, respectively (SNIU, 2000).

Minas Gerais is composed of 853 municipalities. Of these, 523 have active transmission of schistosomiasis and a population of 10,870,063 living in endemic areas (Drummond et al., 2010). In 440 municipalities, the Schistosomiasis Control Programme has been implemented. It includes health education activities that emphasize the importance of schistosomiasis, stool examinations, treatment of positive cases and a sanitation programme has been implanted in some areas with the help of local communities interested in the control of the disease and willing to work as a team (Drummond et al., 2006).

The Figure 1 shows the localization of all municipalities of Minas Gerais and the endemic region.

2.1 Materials

The following data were used to achieve the objectives:

2.1.1 Schistosomiasis prevalence data

Schistosomiasis prevalence values (*Pv*) were obtained from the Brazilian Schistosomiasis Control Programme (PCE) through the annual reports of the Secretary of Public Health Surveillance (SVS) and the Secretary of Health in the State of Minas Gerais (SESMG).

The PCE in Minas Gerais began in 1986 and since 2000 it has been under the coordination of the SESMG in collaboration with Municipal Health Systems. The aim of the PCE is to prevent the occurrence of the hepatosplenic form and to prevent the transmission in focus areas (SESMG, 2006). The Kato Katz technique is the methodology used to determine prevalence, examining one slide per person.

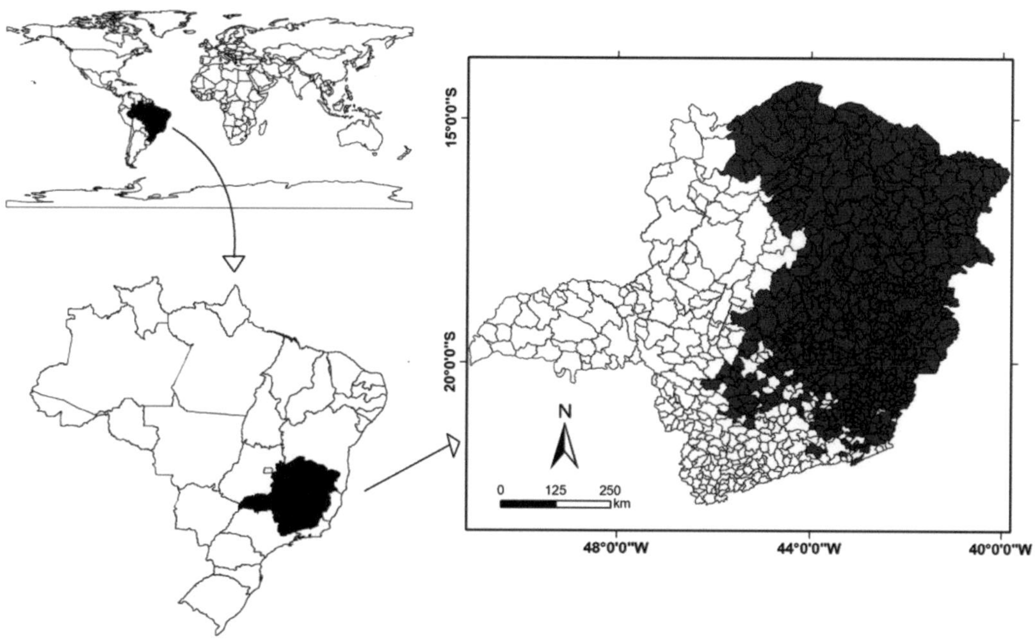

Fig. 1. Spatial localization of Minas Gerais in Brazil and the endemic region in highlight.

Among the 853 municipalities of Minas Gerais state, only 255 municipalities presented information on disease prevalence. The disease is considered non-endemic in the west, northwest and south of the state, and endemic in the northern, eastern and central areas. The largest infection rates are found in the northeastern and eastern areas of the state (Pellon & Teixeira, 1950; Katz et al., 1978; Carvalho et al., 1987). The spatial distribution of the schistosomiasis prevalence is presented in Figure 2a.

2.1.2 Intermediate hosts' data

Data on the distribution of *Biomphalaria* molluscs were provided by the Laboratory of Helminthiasis and Medical Malacology of the René Rachou Research Center (CPqRR/Fiocruz-MG). Molluscs were collected in breeding places from different municipalities in Minas Gerais at different periods, using scoops and tweezers, and then packed to be transported to the laboratory (Souza & Lima, 1990). Specific identification was performed according to the morphology of the shells, reproductive system and renal ridge of the molluscs (Deslandes, 1951; Paraense & Deslandes, 1955a, 1955b, 1959; Paraense, 1975, 1981), and more recently by low stringency polymerase chain reaction and restriction fragment length polymorphism (Vidigal et al., 2000).

Among the 853 municipalities of Minas Gerais state, 194 municipalities did not present any of the three species (*B. glabrata, B. tenagophila* and *B. straminea*), 216 municipalities presented information of the *B. glabrata*, 86 of *B. tenagophila*, 160 of *B. straminea*, 60 municipalities found *B. glabrata* and *B. tenagophila*, 101 reported the presence of *B. glabrata* and *B. straminea*, 44 had *B. tenagophila* and *B. straminea*, and 35 municipalities presented information of the three *Biomphalaria* species.

The spatial distribution of the *Biomphalaria* species data are presented in Figure 2b.

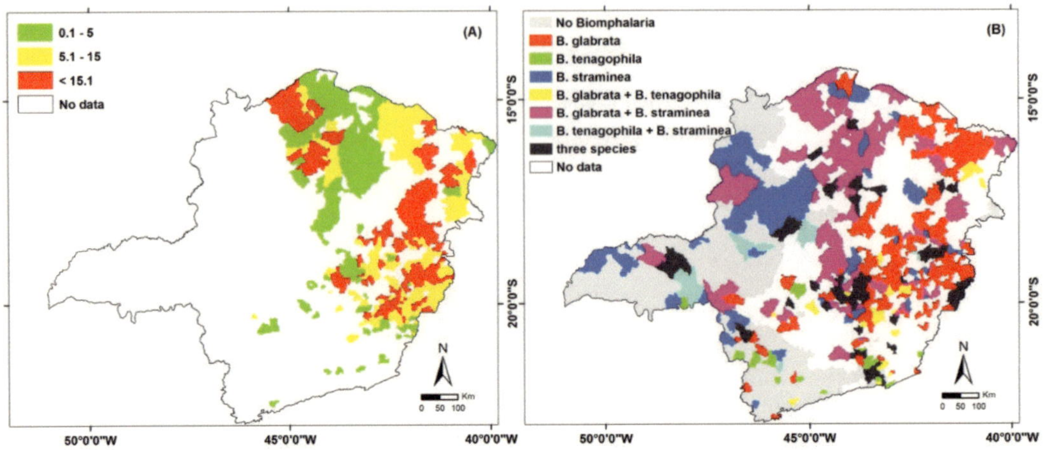

Fig. 2. (a) Distribution of the schistosomiasis prevalence and (b) distribution of the Biomphalaria species in Minas Gerais state, Brazil.

2.1.4 Environmental data

Environmental data were derived from Moderate Resolution Imaging Spectroradiometer (MODIS) and from the Shuttle Radar Topography Mission (SRTM) sensor. Nine variables of MODIS sensor were used, collected in two seasons, summer (from 17/Jan/2002 to 01/Feb/2002 period) and winter (from 28/Jul/2002 to 12/Aug/2002 period) and two in February of 2000 from the SRTM. MODIS product comprises the Blue, Red, Near Infrared (*NIR*) and the Middle Infrared (*MIR*) bands, the Normalized Difference Vegetation Index (*NDVI*) and the Enhanced Vegetation Index (*EVI*) and the derived indexes of the mixture model: vegetation (*Veg*), soil (*Soil*) and shadow (*Shad*).

The variables from SRTM sensor are: the digital elevation model (*DEM*) and the declivity (*DEC*), derived of DEM.

The Linear Spectral Mixture Model (LSMM) is an image processing algorithm that generates the fraction images with the proportion of each component (vegetation, soil and shade) inside the pixel, which is estimated by minimizing the sum of square of the errors. In this work the so called vegetation, soil and shade fraction images were generated using the MODIS data and the estimated values for the spectral reflectance components were also used as an input to the model (Guimarães et al., 2010b).

Some indices related to the water presence and quantification as defined in Fonseca et al. (2007b) were also used in the work. The median of the water accumulation (*WA*) was used to measure the amount of water that may exist in the municipality. Based on the declivity and water accumulation data, the mobility of water (*MW*) in the same seasons was calculated.

The meteorological variables consisted of total precipitation (*PC*) and the minimum (*TN*) and maximum (*TX*) temperature average for summer and winter seasons, which were obtained from the Center for Weather Forecast and Climate Studies (CPTEC), in the same date of MODIS images. With the attempt of characterizing the disease using aspects related to the climate, the day temperature difference (*dT*) variable was developed in the present work: in the summer and winter seasons. That variable was used and proposed by the authors Malone et al. (1994) and Bavia et al. (2001), and is associated with the difference among the maximum and minimum temperature, in the winter and summer seasons.

2.1.5 Socioeconomic data

Three socioeconomic variables, obtained by the Foundation João Pinheiro (FJP) in 2004, were used in the work: the index of need in health (*INH*), the economical index (*IE*) and the Factor of Allocation of Financial Resources for Attention to Health (*FA*).

Eighteen socioeconomic variables supplied by the Brazilian National System of Urban Indicators (SNIU) were also used, and they included data of human development index (*HDI*), of longevity (*HDIL*), income (*HDII*) and education (*HDIE*) for the years 1991 and 2000. Three variables with information of water quality from 2000 were also included referring to the percentage of domiciles with access to the general net of water supply (*WaterNet*), with access to the water through wells or nascents (*WaterWellNasc*) and with other access forms to water (*WaterOther*). Eight more variables from 2000 were included regarding the sanitary conditions of the municipalities being studied, which are: the percentage of domiciles with a bathroom connected to rivers or lakes (*SanRiverLake*), connected to a ditch (*SanDitch*), to rudimentary sewage (*SanSewageR*), to septic sewage (*SanSewageS*), to a general net (*SanNet*), to other sewerage type (*SanOther*), with a bathroom or sanitarium (*WithSan*) and without a bathroom or sanitarium (*WithoutSan*).

2.2 Methods

To achieve the first objective, two approaches have been considered: indicator kriging and logistic regression. The logistic regressions were based on the information of the snail species (*B. glabrata, B. tenagophila* and *B. straminea*), as well as environmental variables; indicator kriging methodology uses only the snail distribution information. The second objective was achieved by applying multiple regressions methodology.

2.2.1 Indicator kriging

Geostatistical methods, such as indicator kriging, may be defined as a technique of statistical inference, which allows the estimation of values and the uncertainties associated with the attribute during the spatialization of a sample property (Felgueiras et al., 1999). It is a nonlinear estimator, which is applied on a sample set of the attribute whose values are modified according to a nonlinear transformation. According to Felgueiras (1999), the indicator kriging is considered non-parametric because it does not use any kind of distribution of a priori probability for a random variable. Instead, it enables the construction of a discretized approximation of the cumulative distribution function of the random variable.

The indicator kriging was performed in each of the 15 river basins: Buranhém, Doce, Grande, Itabapoana, Itanhém, Itapemirim, Jequitinhonha, Jucuruçu, Mucuri, Paraíba do Sul, Paranaíba, Pardo, Piracicaba/Jaguari, São Francisco and, São Mateus.

The classes used for this study were defined as: B. glabrata, B. tenagophila, B. straminea, B. glabrata + B. tenagophila, B. glabrata + B. straminea, B. tenagophila + B. straminea, B. glabrata + B. tenagophila + B. straminea, and without Biomphalaria.

The class without *Biomphalaria* includes information about the non-occurrence of *Biomphalaria* species or information about non-transmitter species in Brazil, such as *B. peregrina, B. schrammi, B. intermedia, B. occidentalis* etc.

The mollusc attributes (class of species and localization) were distributed along the drainage network of 15 river basins, according to the methodology used by Guimarães et al. (2009).

Variogram models were fitted for each class (*Biomphalaria* species), in each basin, through exploratory analysis, using the geostatistical procedures. These procedures involved the creation of experimental semivariograms and fitting them to mathematical theoretical models. After model fitting, indicator kriging procedures were applied to obtain an approximation of the conditional distribution function of the random variables. Based on the estimated function, maps of mollusc spatial distributions along with the corresponding uncertainties for the entire basin were built.

2.2.2 Logistic regression

The logistic regression was applied in this work with the purpose of predicting the existence probability of *Biomphalaria* species in Minas Gerais state, Brazil, and after to diagnose which of the three species (*B. glabrata, B. tenagophila* and *B. straminea*) have a greater influence on the risk of schistosomiasis in Minas Gerais state.

The logistic regression is used to predict the dependent variable and this variable should be qualitative. The dependent variable possesses two answers (0 or 1). In this work, the dependent variables are *B. glabrata* (*BG*), *B. tenagophila* (*BT*) and *B. straminea* (*BS*) species. So using logistic regression, the *BG* species variable receives the value '0' for the municipalities where they do not exist and the value '1' where they do exist. The *BT* species variable receives the value '0' for the municipalities where they do not exist and the value '1' where they do exist. Finally, the *BS* species variable receives the value '0' for the municipalities where they do not exist and the value '1' where they do exist.

Therefore, this work had as dependent variables the *B. glabrata, B. tenagophila* and *B. straminea* species and the socioeconomic and environmental variables mentioned above were considered as explanatory variables.

The variable selection for the logistic regression models was performed in steps:

1. data collection and variables preparation: transformations were tested in the explanatory variable, such as quadratic, inverse, logarithm and square root, with the purpose of normalizing the explanatory variables,
2. reduction of the number of explanatory variables: all variables whose correlations with the dependent variable were not significant at 5% level, and explanatory variables with correlation higher than 0.8 with another explanatory variable were discarded,
3. production of logistic regression models: all possible regressions were generated with the remaining variables,
4. selection of the best model: goodness-of-fit and ROC curve were analyzed.

2.2.3 Multiple regression

The prevalence data has been generated on a municipality level, therefore all the input variables were integrated inside the municipalities' boundaries, using GIS systems and exported to a standard spreadsheet for the statistical analysis and modelling.

A logarithmic transformation was made to the dependent variable (prevalence, denoted by Pv) to increase the correlation with independent variables.

Multicollinearity effects among the independent variables were detected. The variables selection technique was used in order to choose a set of variables that better explain the dependent variable. It was done by the R^2 criterion, using all possible regression procedures (Neter et al., 1996). This selection technique consists of the identification of a subset with few variables and a coefficient of determination R^2 sufficiently closed to that when all variables are used in the model. Interaction effects were also included in the model.

The dependent variable was randomly divided into two sets: one with 123 cases for variables selection and model definition, and another with 132 cases for model validation.

The multiple linear regressions were employed based on two approaches: the global model, where a linear regression model was established to estimate the disease throughout the state (Guimarães et al., 2006, 2008), and the regional model (Guimarães et al., 2010b) where a regression model was generated to estimate the disease in each region determined by the SKATER algorithm (Assunção et al., 2006).

The purpose of regionalization is to divide Minas Gerais state into four regions where selected variables are considered uniform in those regions. Thereby, it is possible to obtain better models to estimate the schistosomiasis prevalence.

The regionalization consisted of two steps. In the first step, homogeneous and contiguous regions were determined from the Minas Gerais state, using the following variables: calcareous areas, percentage of water in the city, *Biomphalaria* species, index of need for health, digital elevation model, vegetation (obtained by the mixture model), accumulated rainfall and average temperature. The second step consisted of fitting different linear regression models for each region.

The obtained models were then used to build the risk map for all municipalities of the Minas Gerais state.

3. Results and discussion

All the variables previously mentioned were generated and transferred to a database using the software TerraView/TerraLib (http://www.dpi.inpe.br/geoschisto/).

3.1 Indicator kriging

Indicator kriging was used to make inferences about the presence of the species of *Biomphalaria*. As described in section 2.2.1, eight classes are the results of the methodology. The result was a map of the species' distribution and a map of the uncertainties associated with the classification. Figure 3a shows the associated classes to the *Biomphalaria* species, with a maximum level of uncertainty of 0.78. The map of uncertainties (Figure 3b) showed that the higher uncertainties have been concentrated along class transition areas. As a

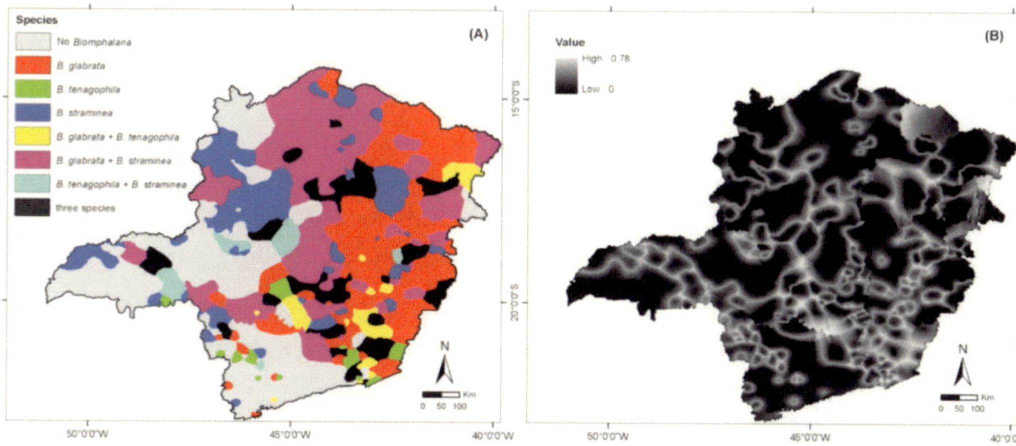

Fig. 3. (a) Estimated *Biomphalaria* species distribution with a maximum level of uncertainties of ≤ 0.78; (b) Uncertainties associated with the classification.

consequence, regions where several classes may occur, more transitions have been found and, therefore, higher uncertainties.

3.2 Logistic regression

Unlike indicator kriging, logistic regression estimates the occurrence probability for each species separately. Variables that represent vegetation, temperature, precipitation and topography, were found in the logistic regression models, giving an indication of important conditions for the mollusc's development.

The first model generated by logistic regression, for *B. glabrata* species, has five variables and is presented in Equations 1 and 2.

$$\hat{\text{Prob}}_{BG} = \frac{\exp^{Xb}}{1+\exp^{Xb}} = \frac{G}{1+G} \quad (1)$$

where $\hat{\text{Prob}}_{BG}$ is the estimated probability of existence of the *B. glabrata* species in Minas Gerais state, *b* are estimated parameters, *X* are the explanatory variables and *G* is given by Equation 2.

$$G = \exp(1.837 - 0.003(DEM) + 11.173(NDVI_W) - 0.121(PC_W) + 0.015(PC_S) - 0.390(TN_W)) \quad (2)$$

where *DEM* is the digital elevation model, $NDVI_W$ is the winter normalized vegetation index, PC_W is the mean winter precipitation and TN_W is the winter minimum temperature.

It is observed that the *DEM* variable possesses an inverse relationship with the presence of the *B. glabrata* species; in other words, the lower the digital elevation model, the larger is the presence of *B. glabrata*. The PC_W and TN_W (winter minimum temperature) variables also presented an inverse relationship with the presence of the *B. glabrata* species. It is noticed that the larger the vegetation index (*NDVI*) and precipitation in summer, the larger is the presence of the *B. glabrata* species. This can be explained by the natural conditions of the habitat of the mollusc that lives close to vegetation and water, in search of protection against solar radiation and high temperatures.

The second model generated by logistic regression, for *B. tenagophila* species, has four variables and it is presented in Equations 3 and 4

$$\hat{\text{Prob}}_{BT} = \frac{\exp^{Xb}}{1+\exp^{Xb}} = \frac{T}{1+T} \quad (3)$$

where $\hat{\text{Prob}}_{BT}$ is the probability estimated of the existence of the *B. tenagophila* species in Minas Gerais state, b are parameters estimated, X are the explanatory variables and *T* is presented in Equation 4.

$$T = \exp(21.887 - 0.003(DEM) - 0.041(Shad_S) - 23.723(MIR_W) - 0.543(TX_S)) \quad (4)$$

According to Equations 3 and 4, an indirect relationship in all the variables can be noticed. This coincides with the ideal conditions for the snail's development, as the topography of low elevated defined by *DEM*, the water concentration or low topographical variation that

can be associated to the $Shad_S$ variable, the humidity of the plants defined by the MIR_W and the maximum temperature average for summer seasons associated to the TX_S variable.
Equations 5 and 6 present the model generated by logistic regression for *B. straminea* species and five variables

$$\hat{Prob}_{BS} = \frac{\exp^{Xb}}{1+\exp^{Xb}} = \frac{S}{1+S} \tag{5}$$

where $\hat{Prob}_{BS}$ is the probability estimated of the existence of the *B. straminea* species in Minas Gerais state, b are parameters estimated, X are the explanatory variables and S is presented in Equation 6

$$\begin{aligned} S = \exp(0.351 - 0.081(SanRiverLake) + 0.020(WithoutSan) \\ - 0.002(DEM) - 0.076(PC_W) + 0.013(PC_S)) \end{aligned} \tag{6}$$

Equations 5 and 6 emphasize that environmental and socioeconomic aspects contribute to the presence of the *B. straminea* species. It is observed that the smaller the *SanRiverLake*, *DEM* and PC_W variables, the larger is the presence of *B. straminea*, while the *WithoutSan* and PC_S variables possess a direct relationship.
The models selected, for each one of the snail species, were analyzed to verify if they presented a good adjustment, through Receiver Operating Characteristic (ROC) or ROC curve. ROC curve is a measure that confronts mistakes with successes and successes with mistakes. The larger the area below the curve, the better is the model adjustment.
The result of ROC curve of the models selected for each one of the snail species is presented in Figure 4.
Based on Figure 4, sensitivity and specificity are statistical measures of the performance used for the logistic regression test. Sensitivity measures the proportion of actual positives which are correctly identified (the percentage of municipalities where the *Biomphalaria* species exist and are identified as *Biomphalaria*), and specificity measures the proportion of negatives which are correctly identified (the percentage of municipalities where the *Biomphalaria* species exist and are not identified as *Biomphalaria*). According to the Figure 4 it

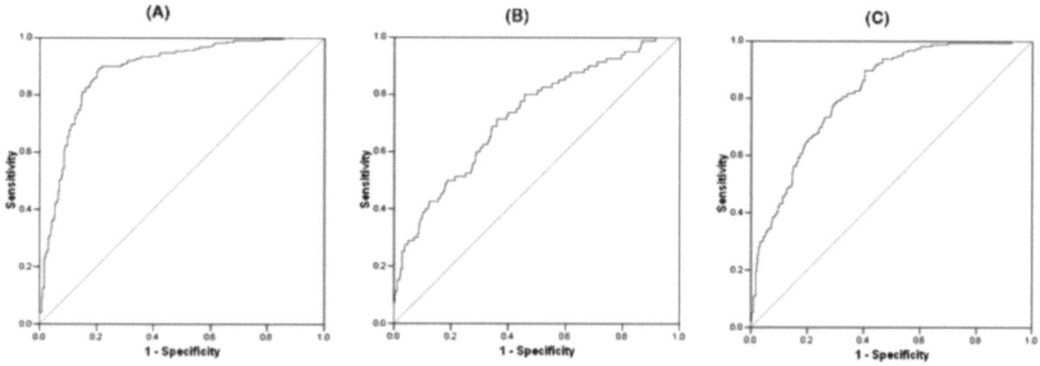

Fig. 4. ROC curve of the models selected for each one of the *Biomphalaria* species: (a) ROC curve of the *B. glabrata* species, (b) ROC curve of the *B. tenagophila* species, (c) ROC curve of the *B. straminea* species.

is observed that the model of the *B. glabrata* species presented the best adjustment, with 98% of area below the ROC curve. The *B. tenagophila* and *B. straminea* species obtained 73% and 82%, respectively. Based on the models selected, the probabilities of presence of *Biomphalaria* species were estimated for the whole Minas Gerais state.

Figure 5 presents the probability of the presence of *B. glabrata* (Figure 5a), *B. tenagophila* (Figure 5c) and *B. straminea* (Figure 5e) species using logistic regression. Additionally, Figure 5 shows the estimated presence of *B. glabrata* (Figure 5b), *B. tenagophila* (Figure 5d) and *B. straminea* (Figure 5f) species using indicator kriging which is obtained from section 3.1 results by merging the probabilities of the joint classes.

The estimative of the presence of each species was correlated with the historical data of schistosomiasis prevalence (*Pv*), with the intention of determining which of the *Biomphalaria* species is more related with the disease prevalence (Table 1). The values in highlights (*) are the estimates of the species that possess significant correlation on a 95% confidence level ($p<0.05$).

Estimated species	Logistic regression	Kriging
B. glabrata	0.18*	0.15*
B. tenagophila	0.07	-0.05
B. straminea	-0.04	-0.10

Table 1. Correlation of the estimative of *Biomphalaria* species with the historical data of schistosomiasis prevalence.

Based on Table 1, *B. glabrata* is the species of *Biomphalaria* that has more correlation with the disease prevalence. This result is confirmed by the study of Lutz (1917), which affirms the distribution of *B. glabrata* is more associated to the occurrence of the schistosomiasis in Brazil.

3.3 Multiple regression

The purpose of this section is to use the *Biomphalaria* presence probabilities, as estimated by logistic regressions, as explanatory variables together with the environmental variables.

The analysis of the correlation matrix showed that some variables had non-significative correlations with the prevalence of schistosomiasis (*Pv*) at a 95% confidence level and some variables were highly correlated among themselves, indicating that the model could be further simplified. Variable selection was performed by the R^2 criterion using all possible regressions (Neter et al., 1996).

3.3.1 Global model

The four variables selected were: probability estimated of *B. glabrata* using logistic regression (LR_G), winter precipitation (PC_W), summer minimum temperature (TN_S) and human development index (HDI_{91}) for the year 1991.

The final model, with $R^2 = 0.28$, was

$$\hat{Pv} = e^{(-4.22+1.76LR_G+0.03PC_W+0.35TN_S-3.28HDI_{91})} - 1 \quad (7)$$

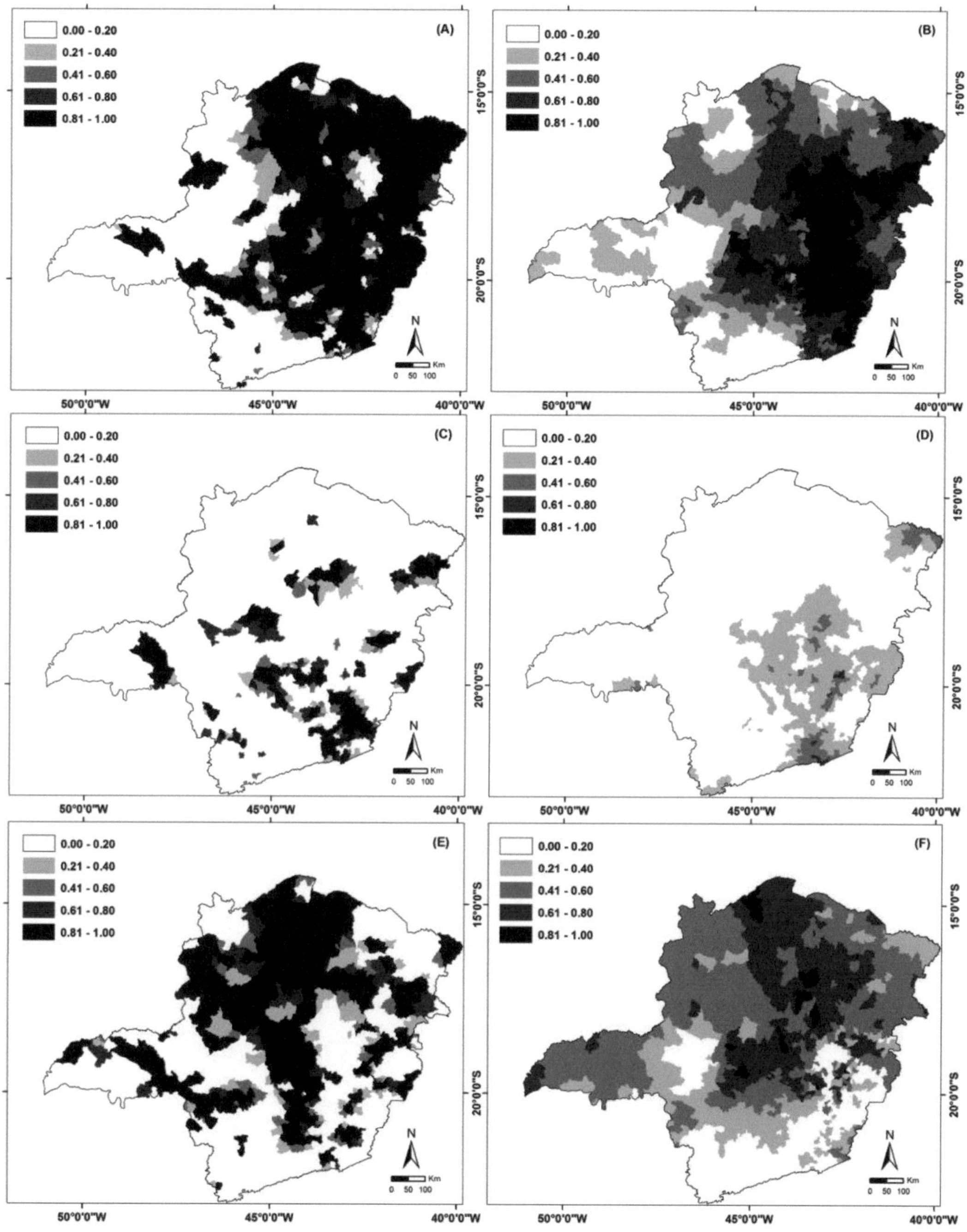

Fig. 5. Probability estimated of *B. glabrata* (a), *B. tenagophila* (c) and *B. straminea* (e) using logistic regression; and the estimate of *B. glabrata* (b), *B. tenagophila* (d) and *B. straminea* (f) using indicator kriging.

Figure 6a shows the estimated *Pv* for all municipalities in the Minas Gerais state using the estimated regression equation (7). Figure 6b presents the plot of the residuals, resulting from the difference between observed (Figure 2a) and estimated *Pv* from 255 municipalities. In Figure 6b, dark colours (red and blue) represent overestimated values, light colours (red and blue) underestimated ones, and in white are the municipalities where the estimated prevalence differs very little from the true values.

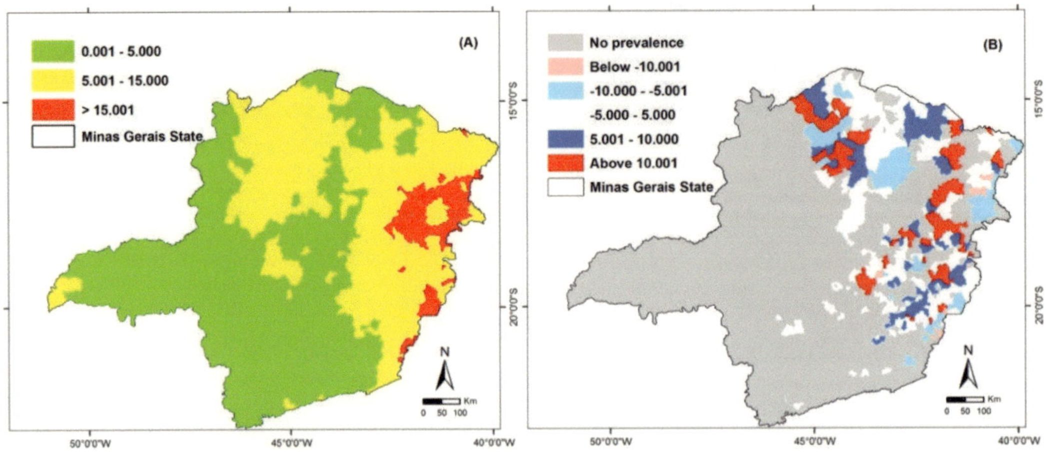

Fig. 6. (a) Global model - prevalence (%) 0.001–5.000 (green), 5.001–15.000 (yellow) and above 15.001 (red); (b) Residuals models.

The precipitation, minimum temperature and estimate of *B. glabrata* were positively correlated with *Pv*. The human development index was negatively correlated with *Pv*. This is consistent with the adequate environmental conditions for the transmission of schistosomiasis. The transmission depends on the presence of *B. glabrata*, places with temperature above 15°C, hydric collections and low economic status.

The result of this model has the same variables (precipitation, temperature and HDI) obtained by Guimarães et al. (2006). The difference is that the variable obtained by Guimarães et al. (2006) related to the type of vegetation (forest, savannah and caatinga) and in this study to the presence of the *B. glabrata*. However, this variable (presence of the *B. glabrata*) had already been obtained by Guimarães et al. (2010b) using indicator kriging.

3.3.2 Regional model

The state of Minas Gerais was divided into four regions using the Skater algorithm. The result of the regionalization is shown in Figure 7a. Regression models were developed for each of the four regions with the same 255 variables used in the global model and the same selection procedure (123 cases for variables selection and model definition, and another with 132 cases for model validation). Different numbers of variables were selected in each region to determine the best regression model.

The final models generated for each region and their R^2 were

$$\hat{Pv}_1 = e^{(8.29+13.14LR_T-0.12DEC-10.95NDVI_S-0.16C)} - 1 \Rightarrow R^2 = 0.91 \quad (8)$$

$$\hat{Pv}_2 = e^{(-6.86+4.08NDVI_W+1.31TN_S-0.57TN_W-0.36TX_W)} - 1 \Rightarrow R^2 = 0.45 \quad (9)$$

$$\hat{Pv}_3 = e^{(11.44-0.002DEM+0.47TN_S-0.64TX_S+1.79NHI)} - 1 \Rightarrow R^2 = 0.35 \quad (10)$$

$$\hat{Pv}_4 = e^{(-8.54+0.003DEM+0.24TX_W+3.64HDIE_{00}+0.03C)} - 1 \Rightarrow R^2 = 0.51 \quad (11)$$

where: LR_T (probability estimated of *B. tenagophila* using logistic regression), *DEC* (slope from SRTM), $NDVI_S$ (summer normalized difference vegetation index), *C* (percentage of housing with bathroom or toilet connected to a ditch), $NDVI_W$ (winter normalized difference vegetation index), TN_S (summer minimum temperature), TN_W (winter minimum temperature), TX_W (winter maximum temperature), *DEM* (digital elevation model from SRTM), TX_S (summer maximum temperature), *NHI* (need of health index), $HDIE_{00}$ (HDI education for the year of 2000).

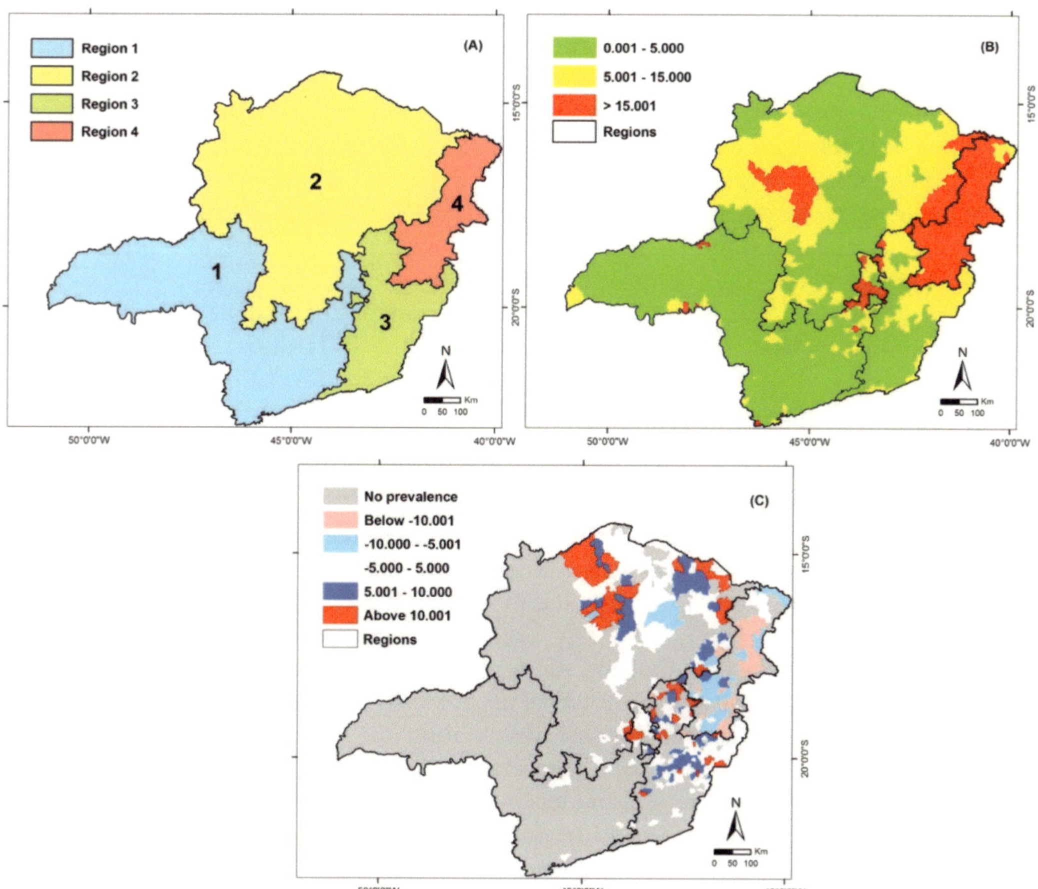

Fig. 7. (a) Regionalization; (b) Regional models - prevalence (%) 0.001–5.000 (green), 5.001–15.000 (yellow) and above 15.001 (red); (c) Residuals.

Figure 7b shows the estimated values of *Pv* for the whole state of Minas Gerais using equations (8, 9, 10 and 11). In addition, Figure 7c shows the residuals from 255 municipalities. In this figure, gray represents "no prevalence", dark colours represent overestimated values, light colours represent the underestimated values and in the white municipalities with good estimates.

The regional model for Region 1 (R_1) reflects the effect of sanitation (housing with bathroom or toilet connected to a ditch), topography (*DEC*), vegetation ($NDVI_S$) and the influence of molluscs (*B. tenagophila*). Region 1 achieved a R^2 value of 0.91. The result obtained by Guimarães (2010) suggested it would be interesting to do a detailed study in the Sul Meso region, which is part of Region 1, to determine the prevalence and the transmitter of schistosomiasis.

The model for Region 2 (R_2) shows the effect of vegetation ($NDVI_w$) and temperature. The same relationship between temperature and vegetation was also obtained by Bavia et al. (2001) in Bahia state and Guimarães et al. (2006, 2010b) in Minas Gerais state. The R^2 found for this model was 0.45.

The models for Regions 3 and 4 (R_3 and R_4) show that *Pv* was associated with topography (*DEM*), weather (temperature) and socioeconomic effects. Among the regional models, Region 3 had the lowest R^2 (0.35). Region 4 had R^2 of 0.51. The variables obtained in Regions 3 and 4 were the same variables found by Guimarães et al. (2010b) also in the same regions.

In all models (global and regional) the presence of *Biomphalaria*, socioeconomic effects, vegetation index and temperature were the most important variables. These characteristics are the same as environmental conditions for the presence and development of molluscs (infection of the intermediate host) and sanitation (water contamination - presence of *S. mansoni* cercariae) obtained by Guimarães et al. (2010b).

Bavia et al. (2001), in Bahia, showed that the distribution of schistosomiasis is related to the vegetation index and temperature using data from NOAA/AVHRR.

4. Conclusion and further work

The use of GIS, remote sensing, geostatistical and statistical techniques together proved to be quite suitable for the study of schistosomiasis.

This study explored the relationship between the schistosomiasis prevalence and the existing snail species in Minas Gerais state, Brazil (*B. glabrata, B. tenagophila, B.straminea*). The results showed that the snail species that has more correlation with the disease prevalence is *B. glabrata*.

The generated results showed that logistic regression or indicator kriging are consistent tools and the obtained map can be used as an auxiliary tool to formulate proper public health strategies and to guide fieldwork, considering the places with higher occurrence probability for occurrence of the most important species. Although not shown here, it is interesting to notice that among the models generated for regression logistic for the three *Biomphalaria* species, there was coincidence in the selection of variables. Variables that represent the vegetation, temperature, precipitation and topography were presented in the models, giving an indication of the important conditions for the mollusc's development.

Most of the selected explanatory variables in the global and regional models were related to environmental conditions for the presence and development of the mollusc, even as to the transmission of schistosomiasis.

The results of the regression models show that regionalization improves the estimation of the schistosomiasis prevalence in Minas Gerais state. Based on this model, a schistosomiasis risk map was built for Minas Gerais using an interpolator. Martins-Bedê et al. (2009) and Guimarães et al. (2010b) also obtained a better model with the use of regionalization.

To conclude, this study can contribute significantly to the choice of actions by the health decision makers, allowing them, on the one hand to narrow the set of municipalities in the state of Minas Gerais for which treatment and sanitation should be a priority, and on the other hand, to focus on preventive measures in the municipalities where transmission can occur.

The use of GPS is recommended for field surveys to obtain the coordinates of the foci of *Biomphalaria*. Thus the results can be compared to the logistic regression and the accuracy of predictive models can also be improved.

The methodology used in this study can be utilized to control and to take preventive measures to prevent schistosomiasis transmission in the areas with occurrence of the disease.

5. Acknowledgment

Sandra C Drummond (Secretary of Health in the state of Minas Gerais) and CNPq (grants #300679/2011-4, 384571/2010-7, 302966/2009-9, 308253/2008-6).

6. References

Almeida Machado P (1982). The Brazilian Program for Schistosomiasis Control. *Am J Trop Med Hyg*, Vol. 31, No. 1, pp. 76-86, 0002-9637.

Amaral RS, Tauil PL, Lima DD, Engels D (2006). An analysis of the impact of the Schistosomiasis Control Programme in Brazil. *Mem Inst Oswaldo Cruz*, Vol. 101, No. Suppl. I, pp. 79-85, 0074-0276.

Araújo KCGM, Resendes APC, Souza-Santos R, Silveira Júnior JC, Barbosa CS (2007). Análise espacial dos focos de *Biomphalaria glabrata* e de casos humanos de esquistossomose mansônica em Porto de Galinhas, Pernambuco, Brasil, no ano 2000. *Cadernos de Saúde Pública*, Vol. 23, No. 2, pp. 409-417, 0102-311X.

Assunção RM, Neves MC, Camara G, Freitas CC (2006). Efficient regionalization techniques for socio-economic geographical units using minimum spanning trees. *International Journal of Geographical Information Science*, Vol. 20, No. 7, pp. 797-811, 1365-8816.

Baker FC (1945). *The molluscan family Planorbidae* University of Illinois, Illinois.

Baptista DF, Jurberg P (1993). Factors conditioning the habitat and the density of *Biomphalaria tenagophila* (Orbigny, 1835) in an isolated schistosomiasis focus in Rio de Janeiro city. *Mem Inst Oswaldo Cruz*, Vol. 88, No. 3, pp. 457-464, 0074-0276.

Barbosa CS, Araújo KC, Antunes L, Favre T, Pieri OS (2004). Spatial distribution of schistosomiasis foci on Itamaracá Island, Pernambuco, Brazil. *Mem Inst Oswaldo Cruz*, Vol. 99, No. Suppl. I, pp. 79-83, 0074-0276.

Barbosa FS (1970). Epidemiologia. In: *Esquistossomose mansoni,* A. S. Cunha, pp. (31-60), Editora da U.S.P., São Paulo.

Bavia ME, Hale L, Malone JB, Braud DH, Shane SM (1999). Geographic information systems and the enviromental risk of schistosomiasis in Bahia, Brazil. *Am J Trop Med Hyg*, Vol. 60, No. 4, pp. 566-572, 1476-1645.

Bavia ME, Malone JB, Hale L, Dantas A, Marroni L, Reis R (2001). Use of thermal and vegetation index data from earth observing satellites to evaluate the risk of schistosomiasis in Bahia, Brazil. *Acta Trop*, Vol. 79, No. 1, pp. 79-85, 0001-706X.

Brooker S, Alexander N, Geiger S, Moyeed RA, Stander J, Fleming F, Hotez PJ, Correa-Oliveira R, Bethony J (2006). Contrasting patterns in the small-scale heterogeneity of human helminth infections in urban and rural environments in Brazil. *Int. J. Parasitol.*, Vol. 36, No. 10-11, pp. 1143-1151, 0020-7519.

Caldeira RL, Teodoro TM, Gomes MFB, Carvalho OS (2010). Preliminary studies investigating the occurrence of *Biomphalaria cousini* in Brazil. *Mem Inst Oswaldo Cruz*, Vol. 105, No. 4, pp. 485-487, 0074-0276.

Camargo S (1980). Impacto do desenvolvimento na expansão da esquistossomose. *Rev Inst Med Trop São Paulo*, Vol. 22, No. Supl. 4, pp. 117-119.

Campos R, Briques W (1988). *Levantamento multicêntricode parasitoses intestinais no Brasil. Os resultados finais.* Rhodia, São Paulo.

Carvalho OS, Rocha RS, Massara CL, Katz N (1987). Expansão da esquistossomose mansoni em Minas Gerais. *Mem Inst Oswaldo Cruz*, Vol. 82, No. Suppl. IV, pp. 295-298, 0074-0276.

Carvalho OS, Rocha RS, Massara CL, Katz N (1988). Primeiros casos autóctones de esquistossomose mansonica em região do noroeste do Estado de Minas Gerais (Brasil). *Rev Saúde Públ S Paulo*, Vol. 22, No. 3, pp. 237-239, 1518-8787.

Carvalho OS, Massara CL, Rocha RS, Katz N (1989). Esquistossomose Mansoni no Sudoeste do Estado de Minas Gerais (Brasil). *Rev Saude Publica*, Vol. 23, No. 4, pp. 341-344, 1518-8787.

Carvalho OS, Massara CL, Silveira Neto HV, Alvarenga AG, Vidigal THDA, Chaves A, Katz N (1994). Schistosomiasis mansoni in the region of Triângulo Mineiro - State of Minas Gerais (Brasil). *Mem Inst Oswaldo Cruz*, Vol. 89, No. 4, pp. 509-512, 0074-0276.

Carvalho OS, Massara CL, Silveira Neto HV, Guerra HL, Caldeira RL, Mendonça CLF, Vidigal THDA, Chaves A, Katz N (1997). Re-evaluation of schistosomiasis mansoni in Minas Gerais, Brazil. II. Alto Paranaiba Mesoregion. *Mem Inst Oswaldo Cruz*, Vol. 92, No. 2, pp. 141-142, 0074-0276.

Carvalho OS, Massara CL, Guerra HL, Campos YR, Caldeira RL, Chaves A, Katz N (1998a). Re-evaluation of schistosomiasis mansoni in Minas Gerais - Brazil. III. "Noroeste de Minas" mesoregion. *Rev Inst Med Trop São Paulo*, Vol. 40, No. 5, pp. 277-279, 1678-9946.

Carvalho OS, Nunes IM, Caldeira RL (1998b). First report of *Biomphalaria glabrata* in the state of Rio Grande do Sul, Brazil *Mem Inst Oswaldo Cruz*, Vol. 93, No. 1, pp. 39-40, 0074-0276.

Carvalho OS, Scholte RGC, Guimarães RJPS, Freitas CC, Drummond SC, Amaral RS, Dutra LV, Oliveira G, Massara CL, Enk MJ (2010). The Estrada Real project and endemic diseases: the case of schistosomiasis, geoprocessing and tourism. *Mem Inst Oswaldo Cruz*, Vol. 105, No. 4, pp. 532-536, 0074-0276.

Correa LR, Paraense WL (1971). Susceptibility of *Biomphalaria amazonica* to infection with two strains of *Schistosoma mansoni*. *Rev Inst Med Trop São Paulo,* Vol. 13, No. 6, pp. 387-390, 0036-4665.

Deslandes N (1951). Técnica de dissecção e exame de planorbídeos. *Rev Serv Espec Saúde Pública,* Vol. 4, No. 2, pp. 371-382,

Drummond SC, Silva LCS, Amaral RS, Sousa-Pereira SR, Antunes CMF, Lambertucci JR (2006). Morbidity of schistosomiasis in the state of Minas Gerais, Brazil. *Mem Inst Oswaldo Cruz,* Vol. 101, No. Suppl. I, pp. 37-44, 0074-0276.

Drummond SC, Pereira SRS, Silva LCS, Antunes CMF, Lambertucci JR (2010). Schistosomiasis Control Program in the state of Minas Gerais in Brazil. *Mem Inst Oswaldo Cruz,* Vol. 105, No. 4, pp. 519-523, 0074-0276.

Enk MJ, Amorim A, Schall VT (2003). Acute schistosomiasis outbreak in the metropolitan area of Belo Horizonte, Minas Gerais: Alert about the risk of unnoticed transmission increased by growing rural tourism. *Mem Inst Oswaldo Cruz,* Vol. 98, No. pp. 745-750, 0074-0276.

Enk MJ, Lima ACL, Drummond SC, Schall VT, Coelho PMZ (2008). The effect of the number of stool samples on the observed prevalence and the infection intensity with *Schistosoma mansoni* among a population in an area of low transmission. *Acta Trop,* Vol. 108, No. 2-3, pp. 222-228, 0001-706X.

Enk MJ, Massara CL, Guimarães RJPS (2009). *Distribuição espacial da esquistossomose na localidade de Pedra Preta, município de Montes Claros, Minas Gerais - Brasil,* 45 Congresso da Sociedade Brasileira de Medicina Tropical Comunicações, ed. SBMT, Uberaba: SBMT, Recife, pp 508.

Enk MJ, Amaral GL, Costa e Silva MF, Silveira-Lemos D, Teixeira-Carvalho A, Martins-Filho OA, Correa-Oliveira R, Gazinnelli G, Coelho PMZ, Massara CL (2010). Rural tourism: a risk factor for schistosomiasis transmission in Brazil. *Mem Inst Oswaldo Cruz,* Vol. 105, No. 4, pp. 537-540, 0074-0276.

Felgueiras CA (1999). *Modelagem Ambiental com Tratamento de Incertezas em Sistemas de Informação Geográfica: O Paradigma Geoestatístico por Indicação,* Computação Aplicada, PhD Thesis, Instituto Nacional de Pesquisas Espaciais, São José dos Campos, pp 212. Retrieved from
< http://www.dpi.inpe.br/teses/carlos/>

Fonseca FR, Freitas CC, Dutra LV, Martins FT, Guimarães RJPS, Scholte RGC, Amaral RS, Drummond SC, Moura ACM, Rocha L, Carvalho OS (2007a). *Desenvolvimento de um modelo de regressão linear para a predição da prevalência de esquistossomose no Estado de Minas Gerais.* XIII Simpósio Brasileiro de Sensoriamento Remoto, INPE, Florianópolis-SC, pp. 2573-2580. Retrieved from
<http://www.dpi.inpe.br/geoschisto/publicacoes/Fonseca_Regressao.pdf>

Fonseca FR, Saraiva TS, Freitas CC, Dutra LV, Monteiro AMV, Rennó CD, Martins FT, Guimarães RJPS, Moura ACM, Scholte RGC, Amaral RS, Drummond SC, Carvalho OS (2007b). *Desenvolvimento de um índice hidrológico para aplicação em estudos de distribuição da prevalência de esquistossomose em Minas Gerais.* XIII Simpósio Brasileiro de Sensoriamento Remoto, INPE, Florianópolis-SC, pp. 2589-2595. Retrieved from
< http://www.dpi.inpe.br/geoschisto/publicacoes/Fonseca_IHidrologico.pdf>

Fonseca FR (2009). *Modelagem espacial da esquistossomose mansoni no estado de Minas Gerais, utilizando a conectividade de redes via estradas e rios*. Sensoriamento Remoto, MSc Thesis, Instituto Nacional de Pesquisas Espaciais, São José dos Campos, pp. 94. Retrieved from < http://www.dpi.inpe.br/geoschisto/publicacoes/Fonseca_dissertacao.pdf>

Freitas CC, Guimarães RJPS, Dutra LV, Martins FT, Gouvea EJC, Santos RAT, Moura ACM, Drummond SC, Carvalho OS (2006). *Remote Sensing and Geographic Information Systems for the Study of Schistosomiasis in the State of Minas Gerais, Brazil*, Geoscience and Remote Sensing Symposium. IGARSS 2006. IEEE International Conference on, pp 2436-2439.

Galvão AF, Favre TC, Guimarães RJPS, Pereira APB, Zani LC, Felipe KT, Domingues ALC, Carvalho OS, Barbosa CS, Pieri OS (2010). Spatial distribution of *Schistosoma mansoni* infection before and after chemotherapy with two praziquantel doses in a community of Pernambuco, Brazil. *Mem Inst Oswaldo Cruz*, Vol. 105, No. 4, pp. 555-562, 0074-0276.

Gazzinelli A, LoVerde PT, Haddad JPA, Pereira WR, Bethony J, Correa-Oliveira R, Kloos H (2006). The spatial distribution of *Schistosoma mansoni* infection before and after chemotherapy in the Jequitinhonha Valley in Brazil. *Mem Inst Oswaldo Cruz*, Vol. 101, No. Suppl. I, pp. 63-71, 0074-0276.

Grisolia MLM, Freitas JR (1985). Características físicas e químicas do habitat da *Biomphalaria tenagophila* (Mollusca, Planorbidae). *Mem Inst Oswaldo Cruz*, Vol. 80, No. 2, pp. 237-244, 0074-0276.

Guimarães RJPS, Freitas CC, Dutra LV, Moura ACM, Amaral RS, Drummond SC, Guerra M, Scholte RGC, Freitas CR, Carvalho OS (2006). Analysis and estimative of schistosomiasis prevalence for Minas Gerais state, Brazil, using multiple regression with social and environmental spatial data. *Mem Inst Oswaldo Cruz*, Vol. 101, No. Suppl. I, pp. 91-96, 0074-0276.

Guimarães RJPS, Freitas CC, Dutra LV, Moura ACM, Amaral RS, Drummond SC, Scholte RGC, Carvalho OS (2008). Schistosomiasis risk estimation in Minas Gerais state, Brazil, using environmental data and GIS techniques. *Acta Trop*, Vol. 108, No. 2-3, pp. 234-241, 0001-706X.

Guimarães RJPS, Freitas CC, Dutra LV, Felgueiras CA, Moura ACM, Amaral RS, Drummond SC, Scholte RGC, Oliveira GC, Carvalho OS (2009). Spatial distribution of *Biomphalaria* mollusks at São Francisco River Basin, Minas Gerais, Brazil, using geostatistical procedures. *Acta Trop*, Vol. 109, No. 3, pp. 181-186, 0001-706X.

Guimarães RJPS (2010). *Ferramentas de geoprocessamento para o estudo e controle da esquistossomose no Estado de Minas Gerais*. Biomedicina, PhD Thesis, Santa Casa de Belo Horizonte, Minas Gerais, pp. 226. Retrieved from < http://www.dpi.inpe.br/geoschisto/publicacoes/Tese_Ricardo.pdf>

Guimarães RJPS, Freitas CC, Dutra LV, Scholte RGC, Amaral RS, Drummond SC, Shimabukuro YE, Oliveira GC, Carvalho OS (2010a). Evaluation of a linear spectral mixture model and vegetation indices (NDVI and EVI) in a study of schistosomiasis mansoni and *Biomphalaria glabrata* distribution in the state of Minas Gerais, Brazil. *Mem Inst Oswaldo Cruz*, Vol. 105, No. 4, pp. 512-518, 0074-0276.

Guimarães RJPS, Freitas CC, Dutra LV, Scholte RGC, Martins-Bedê FT, Fonseca FR, Amaral RS, Drummond SC, Felgueiras CA, Oliveira GC, Carvalho OS (2010b). A geoprocessing approach for studying and controlling schistosomiasis in the state of Minas Gerais, Brazil. *Mem Inst Oswaldo Cruz*, Vol. 105, No. 4, pp. 524-531, 0074-0276.

IBGE (2010). (04/11/2010). Sinopse do Censo Demográfico 2010, In: *Instituto Brasileiro de Geografia e Estatística*, 01/07/2011, Available from: <http://www.ibge.gov.br/home/estatistica/populacao/censo2010/default_sinopse.shtm>

Juberg P, Schall VT, Barbosa JV, Gatti MJ, Soares MS (1987). Behavior of *Biomphalaria glabrata*, the intermediate host snail of *Schistosoma mansoni*, at different depths in water in laboratory conditions. *Mem Inst Oswaldo Cruz*, Vol. 82, No. pp. 179-208, 0074-0276.

Katz N, Mota E, Oliveira VB, Carvalho EF (1978). *Prevalência da esquistossomose em escolares no estado de Minas Gerais*, Congresso da Sociedade Brasileira de Medicina Tropical 14, ed. SBMT, João Pessoa, PB, pp 102.

Katz N, Carvalho OS (1983). Introdução recente da esquistossomose mansoni no sul do estado de Minas Gerais, Brasil. *Mem Inst Oswaldo Cruz*, Vol. 78, No. 3, pp. 281-284, 0074-0276.

Kawazoe U (1975). *Alguns aspectos de biologia de B. glabrata e B. tenagophila.*, Instituto de Ciências Biológicas Master's thesis, Universidade Federal de Minas Gerais, Belo Horizonte.

Klein HS (2002). As origens Africanas dos Escravos Brasileiros. In *Homo brasilis: aspectos genéticos, linguísticos, históricos e socioantropológicos da formação do povo brasileiro* (ed. PENA, S. D. J. O.), Fundação de Pesquisas Científicas de Ribeirão Preto, Ribeirão Preto, pp 93-112.

Kloos H, Passos LKJ, LoVerde P, Correa Oliveira R, Gazzinelli A (2004). Distribution and *Schistosoma mansoni* infection of *Biomphalaria glabrata* in different habitats in a rural area in the Jequitinhonha Valley, Minas Gerais, Brazil: environmental and epidemiological aspects. *Mem Inst Oswaldo Cruz*, Vol. 99, No. 7, pp. 673-681, 0074-0276.

Lambertucci JR, Rocha RS, Carvalho OS, Katz N (1987). A esquistossomose mansoni em Minas Gerais. *Rev Soc Bras Med Trop*, Vol. 20, No. 1, pp. 47-52, 0037-8682.

Lima e Costa MFF, Guerra HL, Pimenta Júnior FG, Firmo JOA, Uchoa E (1996). Avaliação do programa de controle da esquistossmose (PCE/PCDEN) em municípios situados na Bacia do Rio São Francisco, Minas Gerais, Brasil. *Rev Soc Bras Med Trop*, Vol. 29, No. 2, pp. 117-126, 0037-8682.

Lutz A (1917). Observações sôbre a evolução do *Schistosoma mansoni*. *Rev Soc Brasil Ciências*, Vol. 1, pp. 41-48.

Malone JB, Huh OK, Fehler DP, Wilson PA, Wilensky DE, Holmes RA, Elmagdoub AL (1994). Temperature data from satellite imagery and distribution of schistosomiasis in Egypt. *Am J Trop Med Hyg*, Vol. 51, No. 3, pp. 714-722, 1476-1645.

Martins FT (2008). *Mapeamento do risco da esquistossomose no Estado de Minas Gerais, usando dados ambientais e sociais*. MSc Thesis, Instituto Nacional de Pesquisas Espaciais, São José dos Campos, pp. 144. Retrieved from

< http://www.dpi.inpe.br/geoschisto/publicacoes/Martins_dissertacao.pdf>

Martins-Bedê FT, Freitas CC, Dutra LV, Sandri SA, Fonseca FR, Drummond IN, Guimaraes RJPS, Amaral RS, Carvalho OS (2009a). Risk Mapping of schistosomiasis in Minas Gerais, Brazil, Using MODIS and Socioeconomic Spatial Data. *Geoscience and Remote Sensing, IEEE Transactions on*, Vol. 47, No. 11, pp. 3899-3908, 0196-2892.

Martins-Bedê FT, Godo L, Sandri S, Dutra LV, Freitas CC, Carvalho OS, Guimarães RJPS, Amaral RS (2009b). Classification of schistosomiasis prevalence using fuzzy case-based reasoning. In *Bio-Inspired Systems: Computational and Ambient Intelligence* 5517, Berlin/Heidelberg, pp 8.

Martins-Bedê FT, Dutra LV, Freitas CC, Guimarães RJPS, Amaral RS, Drummond SC, Carvalho OS (2010). Schistosomiasis risk mapping in the state of Minas Gerais, Brazil, using a decision tree approach, remote sensing data and sociological indicators. *Mem Inst Oswaldo Cruz*, Vol. 105, No. 4, pp. 541-548, 0074-0276.

Martins AV, Versiani V (1938). "*Schistosomose mansoni*" no Norte de Minas Gerais. *Brasil-Médico*, Vol. 52, pp. 812-816.

Massara CL (2005). *Integração e análise de estratégias para controle da Esquistossomose: um estudo em área endêmica de Minas Gerais - Brasil*, Biologia parasitária PhD Thesis, Instituto Oswaldo Cruz, Rio de Janeiro, pp 114.

Massara CL, Amaral GL, Caldeira RL, Drummond SC, Enk MJ, Carvalho OS (2008). Esquistossomose em área de ecoturismo do Estado de Minas Gerais, Brasil. *Cadernos de Saúde Pública*, Vol. 24, No. 7, pp. 1709-1712, 0102-311X.

Neter J, Kutner MH, Nachtssheim CJ, Wasserman W (1996). *Applied linear statistical models* (4th), WCB/McGraw-Hill, Boston.

Paraense WL (1955). Self and cross-fertilization in *Australorbis glabratus*. *Mem Inst Oswaldo Cruz*, Vol. 53, No. 2-3-4, pp. 277-291, 0074-0276.

Paraense WL, Deslandes N (1955a). Observations on the morphology of "*Australorbis glabratus*". *Mem Inst Oswaldo Cruz*, Vol. 53, No. 1, pp. 87-103, 0074-0276.

Paraense WL, Deslandes N (1955b). Observations on the morphology of *Australorbis nigricans*. *Mem Inst Oswaldo Cruz*, Vol. 53, No. 1, pp. 121-134, 0074-0276.

Paraense WL, Deslandes N (1959). The renal ridge as a reliable character for separating *Taphius glabratus* from *Taphius tenagophilus*. *Am J Trop Med Hyg*, Vol. 8, No. 4, pp. 456-472, 1476-1645

Paraense WL (1972). Fauna planorbídica do Brasil. In *Introdução à geografia médica do Brasil* (ed. Lacaz, C. S.), Editora Universidade de São Paulo, pp 213-239.

Paraense WL, Correa LR (1973). Susceptibility of *Biomphalaria peregrina* from Brazil and Ecuador to two strains of *Schistosoma mansoni*. *Rev Inst Med Trop São Paulo*, Vol. 15, No. 3, pp. 127-130, 0036-4665.

Paraense WL (1975). Estado atual da sistemática dos planorbídeos brasileiros. *Arq Mus Nac*, Vol. 55, pp. 105-111.

Paraense WL (1981). *Biomphalaria occidentalis* sp. n. from South America (Mollusca Basommatophora Pulmonata). *Mem Inst Oswaldo Cruz*, Vol. 76, No. 2, pp. 199-211, 0074-0276.

Pellegrino J, Salgado AA, Mello RT (1975). Inquérito sorológico para esquistossomose entre escolares no estado de Minas Gerais. *Ciência e Cultura*, Vol. 27, No. 2, pp. 189-196, 0009-6725.

Pellon AB, Teixeira I (1950). *Distribuição geográfica da esquistossomose mansônica no Brasil* Divisão de Organização Sanitária, Rio de Janeiro.

Pellon AB, Teixeira I (1953). *O Inquérito Helmintológico Escolar em cinco estados das regiões Leste, Sul e Centro-Oeste.* Ministério da Educação e Saúde, Departamento Nacional de Saúde, Divisão de Organização Sanitária., Curitiba.

Prado Junior C (1986). *História Econômica do Brasil* Ed. Brasiliense, São Paulo.

Rey L (1956). *Contribuição para o conhecimento da morfologia, biologia e ecologia dos planorbídeos brasileiros transmissores da esquistossomose* Serviço Nacional de Educação Sanitária, Rio de Janeiro.

Rey L (2001). *Parasitologia: parasitos e doenças parasitárias do homem nas Américas e na África* (3), Guanabara Koogan, Rio de Janeiro.

SES (2006). *Análise da situação de saúde,* ed., Secretaria de Estado de Saúde de Minas Gerais - Superintendência de Epidemiologia, Belo Horizonte, 131 pp.

Silva P (1908). Contribuição para o estudo da Schistosomiasis na Bahia. *Brazil-Médico,* Vol. 29, pp. 281-283.

SNIU (2000). Sistema Nacional de Indicadores Urbanos, In: *Ministério das Cidades,* 30/10/2008, Available from: <http://www.cidades.gov.br/secretarias-nacionais/saneamento-ambiental/indicadores/Sniu.zip/view>

Souza CP, Lima LC (1990). *Moluscos de Interesse Parasitológico do Brasil* (2), Fundação Oswaldo Cruz, Centro de Pesquisas René Rachou, Belo Horizonte.

Souza CP, Caldeira RL, Drummond SC, Melo AL, Guimarães CT, Soares DM, Carvalho OS (2001). Geographical distribution of *Biomphalaria* snails in the state of Minas Gerais, Brazil. *Mem Inst Oswaldo Cruz,* Vol. 96, No. 3, pp. 293-302, 0074-0276.

Teixeira MJ (1919). *A schistosomose mansônica na infância em Belo Horizonte,* Faculdade de Medicina, Tese, Imprensa Oficial, Belo Horizonte, 107 pp.

Thomas JD (1995). The snail hosts of schistosomiasis: some evolutionary and ecological perspectives in relation to control. *Mem Inst Oswaldo Cruz,* Vol. 90, No. 2, pp. 195-204, 0074-0276.

Tibiriçá SHC 2008. *Epidemiologia da esquistossomose em três municípios da microrregião de Juiz de Fora, Minas Gerais,* Faculdade de Medicina, PhD Thesis, Universidade Federal de Juiz de Fora, Juiz de Fora, pp. 176.

Tibiriçá SHC, Mittherofhe A, Castro MF, Lima AC, Gonçalves M, Pinheiro IO, Freitas CC, Guimarães RJPS, Carvalho OS, Coimbra ES (2011). Malacological survey of *Biomphalaria* snails in municipalities along the *Estrada Real* in the southeast of the state of Minas Gerais, Brazil. *Rev Soc Bras Med Trop,* Vol. 44, No. 2, pp. 163-167, 0037-8682.

Versiani V, Martins AV, Pena Sobrinho O (1945). Esquistossomose mansoni em Minas Gerais. I Município de Belo Horizonte. *Arquivos do Instituto Químico-Biológico do Estado de Minas Gerais,* Vol. 1, pp. 71-94.

Vidigal THDA, Caldeira RL, Simpson AJG, Carvalho OS (2000). Further studies on the molecular systematics of *Biomphalaria* snails from Brazil. *Mem Inst Oswaldo Cruz*, Vol. 95, No. 1, pp. 57-66, 0074-0276.

WHO (1957). Study Group on the Ecology of Intermediate Snail Hosts of Bilharziasis, *Technical Report Series 120*, World Health Organization, Geneva, pp 120.

The Merits of Urine Color Observation as a Rapid Diagnostic Technique to Estimate *Schistosoma Haematobium* Infection in Two Endemic Areas of Benue State, Nigeria

Robert Houmsou[1], Elizabeth Amuta[2] and Edward Omudu[3]
[1]*Department of Biological Sciences, Taraba State University*
[2]*Department of Biological Sciences, University of Agriculture Makurdi, Benue State*
[3]*Department of Biological Sciences, Benue State University, Makurdi*
Nigeria

1. Introduction

Schistosomiasis is the most prevalent parasitic infection in the world after malaria, with nearly 207 people infected, and 779 million currently at risk in 76 countries of the tropics where the disease is endemic (Steinmann *et al.*, 2006).

In sub-Saharan Africa, about 192 million are found to be infected with schistosomiasis (Hotez and Kamath, 2009).The highest prevalence and intensities of human schistosomiasis occur in school-aged children, adolescents, and young adults who also suffer from the highest morbidity and mortality.

Urinary Schistosomiasis due *Schistosoma haematobium* is a significant cause of clinical morbidity and disability in the endemic countries of Africa and the Middle East, where more than 110 million people are infected (van der Werf and de Vlas, 2001).

In sub-Saharan Africa two-thirds of the schistosomiasis cases are due to *Schistosoma haematobium,* which represents an important cause of severe urinary tract disease (van der Werf *et al.*, 2000). They also estimated that 70 million and 32 million individuals out of 682 million people in sub-Saharan Africa had experienced hematuria and dysuria, respectively, within the last two weeks of their reports. *S. haematobium* produces bladder wall pathology in approximately 18 million people in sub-Saharan Africa, and 10 million people suffer from hydronephrosis (van der Werf *et al.*, 2000). Renal failure accounts for a large percentage of the estimated 150,000 deaths from urinary tract schistosomiasis in sub-Saharan Africa, and significant association was observed between major bladder wall pathology and squamous cell carcinoma (Maxwell, 2008). A significant percentage of women and men with urinary schistosomiasis acquire genital ulcers and other lesions (King and Dangerfield-cha, 2008).

Identification of cases or communities for treatment with *Schistosoma haematobium* infection is usually based on microscopic detection of eggs in urine. Haematuria and proteinuria are recognized clinical features of *S.haematobium* infection (Wilkins, 1977). Many epidemiological studies have been conducted to investigate the characteristics of these methods to measure urinary schistosomiasis; this usually involved comparing the outcomes with intensity of infection.

As part of early and successful control with chemotherapy, rapid, cost-effective and reliable diagnostic tools and assay that will play an important role in assessing cases of infection are needed in the present time. Thus, the study was designed to determine if urine colour can be used as a potential diagnostic tool for rapid screening of urinary schistosomiasis in endemic areas and to compare it with other diagnostic methods such as filtration technique and reagent strip tests.

2. Materials and methods

2.1 Study area

The study was conducted in two contiguous local government areas (Buruku and Katsina-Ala) of Benue State endemic for urinary schistosomiasis (Houmsou *et al.*, 2009). The selection of the areas was based on previous reports from local hospitals, clinics and health centers where cases of urinary schistosomiasis were common particularly among school children. Other parasitic infections like onchocerciasis, malaria and parasites of the gastro-intestinal tract were also reported by health officials. The relative position of the two Local Government Areas in Benue State is about the Middle Eastern part of the State. The areas are drained by streams and rivers among which river Katsina-Ala is the biggest; ponds are also found all over the areas (Figure 1). The areas have a monthly temperature ranging from 27-38°C and 900-1000 mm of rain fall annually with two distinct seasons: the dry season starts in late October and usually ends by March, while the rainy season lasts from mid-April to early October.

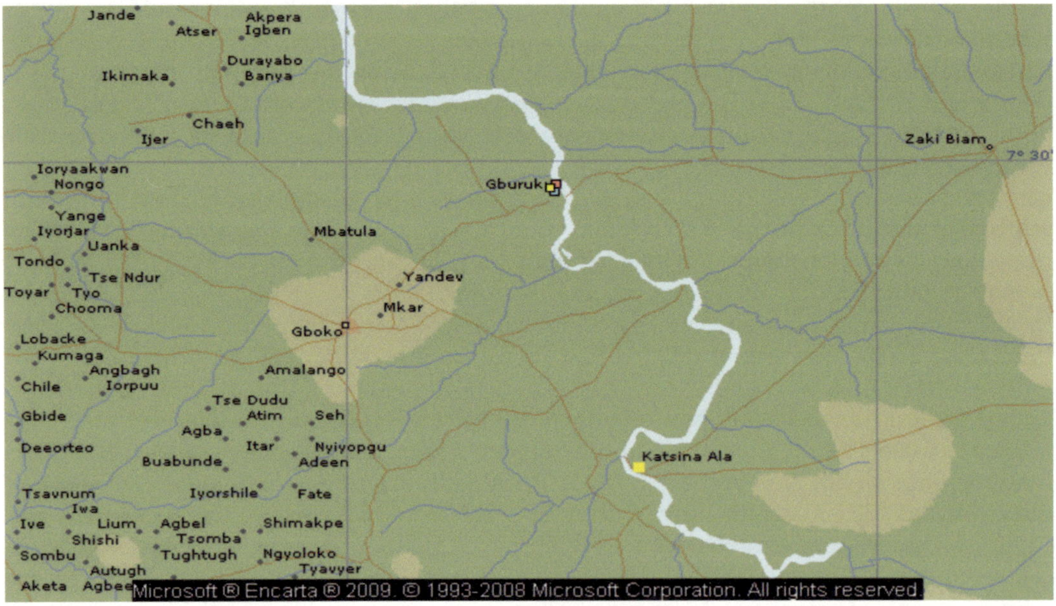

Fig. 1. Physical Map of Buruku and Katsina-Ala LGAs of Benue State, Nigeria (Encarta 2008)

2.2 Study population and samples collection

Prior to the commencement of the research, ethical approval was sought from the Ministry of Health, Benue State and the Local Government Education Authorities of both areas. Parents of the school children were duly informed on the significance of the study.

A total of 1,292 urine specimens were collected from apparently healthy individuals aged 1-30 years, whom were carefully instructed to collect the last part of their urine. About 20 ml of clean-catch, midstream urine samples were collected in a 20 ml capacity autoclaved wide mouthed, leak, proof universal containers. Samples were obtained between 10:00 hrs and 14:00 hrs of the day (Cheesbrough, 2000). Urine specimens were visually inspected for colour and graded, from (1) as urine free of any trace of microhaematuria or proteinuria (light-yellow) to (3) as red urine (blood urine).The specimens were appropriately labeled with identification numbers and placed in a cold box. Where delay in transportation of specimens to laboratory was inevitable, ordinary household bleach was added to the urine samples to preserve any schistosome ova present (Cheesbrough, 2000; W.H.O., 2003).

2.3 Determination of microhaematuria and proteinuria

Reagent strips (Medi-Test Combi 9, Macherey-Nagel GmbH & Co.KG, Germany) were dipped into the urine inside the universal containers. Microhaematuria and proteinuria were evaluated and results were ranked as negative (-ve), trace(+), positive(++), (+++) according to the manufacturer's instructions. Concentrations (Ca) of microhaematuria and proteinuria were measured as erythrocytes/µl (ery/µl) and mg/dl of albumin respectively. The degree of microhaematuria and proteinuria concentrations were graded as follows: 0 (negative), Ca.5-10 (+), Ca.50 (++) and Ca.250 (+++) and 0 (negative), Ca.30 (+), Ca.100 (++) and Ca.500 (+++) respective.

2.4 Egg counts

Eggs were recovered from urine by the filtration technique. Filtration is the most sensitive, rapid, and reproducible technique for detecting and quantifying *S. haematobium* eggs in urine. Using blunt-ended (untoothed) forceps, a polycarbonate membrane filter (13 mm diameter and 13µm porosity) was placed carefully on the filter support of the filter holder (13 mm diameter) and attached to the end of a 10ml Luer syringe. The plunger was removed from the syringe before the syringe is filled to the 10ml mark with well-mixed urine after which the plunger was replaced. Holding the syringe over a beaker the urine was slowly passed through the filter. The filter holder is removed and unscrewed before a blunt-ended forceps is carefully used to remove the membrane filter. This was transferred face upwards (eggs on surface) to a slide before addition of a drop of Lugol's iodine with subsequent covering using a cover glass. Using the 10X objective with the condenser iris closed sufficiently to give good contrast, the entire filter was examined systematically for eggs of *S. haematobium*. The number of eggs are counted and reported as egg per 10ml of urine, 1-49/10 ml urine was considered as light infection and ≥50 eggs/10 ml of urine as heavy infection (W.H.O., 2003).

2.5 Statistical analysis

Microsoft Excel 2007 and PASW (Predictive Analysis software) version 18.0.were used to perform data analysis. Associations between urine colour, microhaematuria, proteinuria and intensity of infection were tested using Spearman correlation (*rho*). The significance level was considered at $p < 0.01$.

2.6 Evaluation of diagnostic performance

The diagnostic performances of urine colour observation, microhaematuria and proteinuria were assessed by calculating sensitivity, specificity, positive and negative predictive values using the following formulae.

- Sensitivity $= \frac{a}{a+b}$ with a = True positive
  b = False negative
- Specificity $= \frac{c}{c+d}$ with c = True negative
  d = False positive
- Positive predictive value (PPV) $= \frac{a}{a+d}$
- Negative predictive value (NPV) $= \frac{c}{c+b}$

2.7 Results

Urine was visually inspected and assigned a number. Figure 2.0 illustrates the urine colour chart related to the presence of proteinuria and microhaematuria. The urine colour chart ranges from 1 to 3, with 1 indicating urine free of any trace of microhaematuria or proteinuria (light-yellow) and 3 corresponding to red urine (blood urine). Whereas number 2 grouped as brown colour corresponds to visually discernable microhaematuria and proteinuria present in the urine.

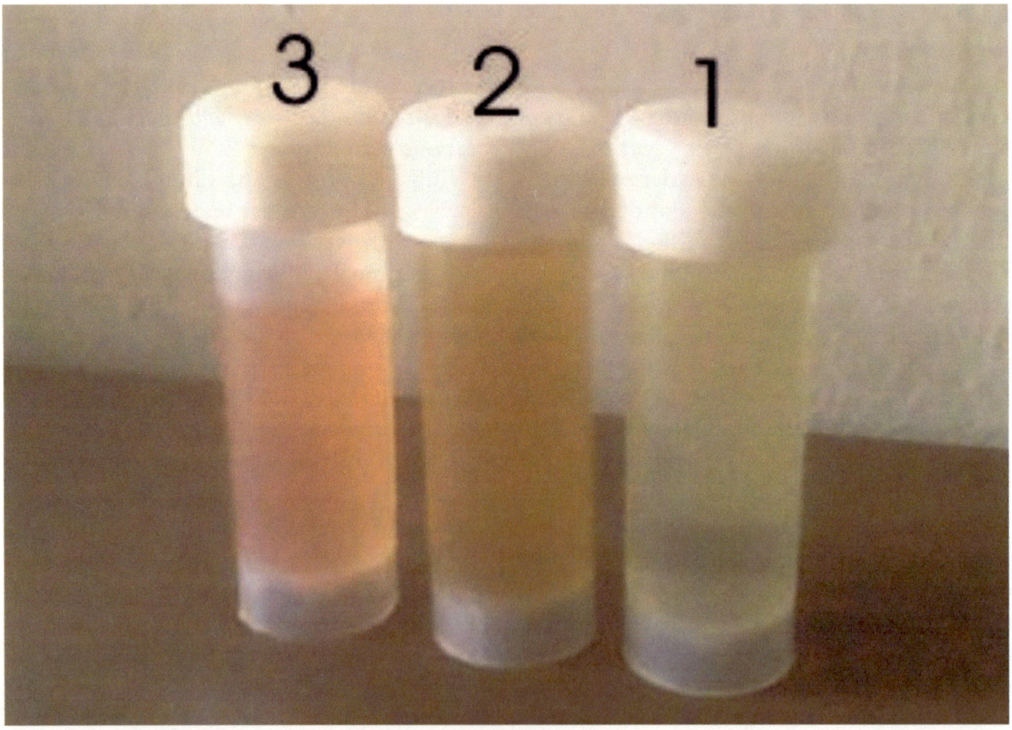

Key: 1 = urine free of any trace of haematuria and proteinuria
2 = urine with presence of haematuria and proteinuria
3 = urine with visible blood

Fig. 1. Urine colour observation

The relationship between urine colour observation and microhaematuria among subjects examined in Buruku and Katsina-Ala LGAs is shown in Fig.3. Of the 666 subjects screened having brown colour, 322(48.3%) had microhaematuria with a breakdown of 21.8%, 10.7% and 15.9% for microhaematuria at Ca.5-10, Ca.50 and Ca.250 respectively. Out of the 48 screened having blood urine, 45(93.8%) had microhaematuria at Ca.250, while 3(6.3%) having light yellow colour of urine had microhaematuria at Ca.5-10. A significant relationship was observed between urine colour observation and microhaematuria (*rho*=0.5, *p<0.01*).

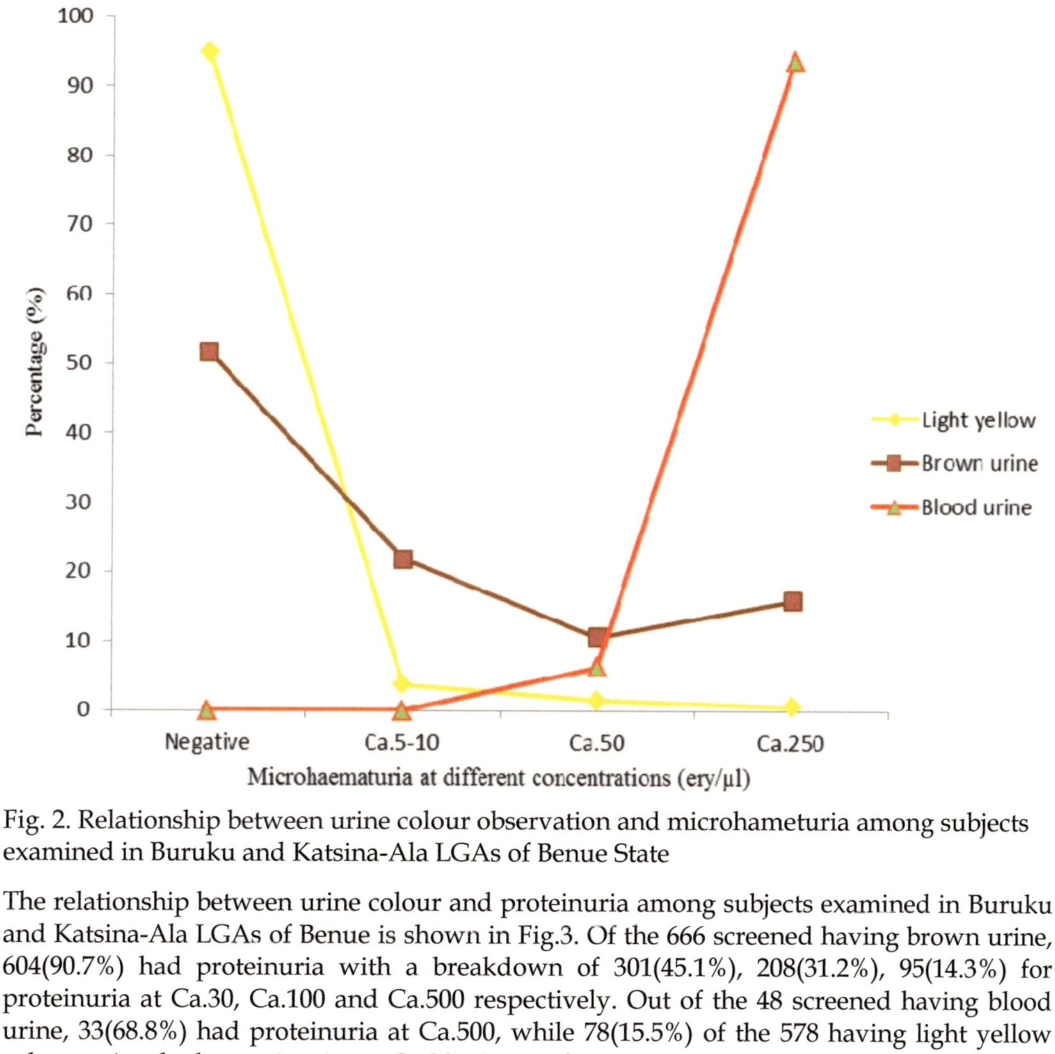

Fig. 2. Relationship between urine colour observation and microhameturia among subjects examined in Buruku and Katsina-Ala LGAs of Benue State

The relationship between urine colour and proteinuria among subjects examined in Buruku and Katsina-Ala LGAs of Benue is shown in Fig.3. Of the 666 screened having brown urine, 604(90.7%) had proteinuria with a breakdown of 301(45.1%), 208(31.2%), 95(14.3%) for proteinuria at Ca.30, Ca.100 and Ca.500 respectively. Out of the 48 screened having blood urine, 33(68.8%) had proteinuria at Ca.500, while 78(15.5%) of the 578 having light yellow colour urine had proteinuria at Ca.30. A significant relationship was observed between urine colour and proteinuria (*rho*=0.7, *p<0.01*).

Figure 4 shows the relationship between urine colour observation and intensity of *Schistosoma haematobium* eggs amongst subjects examined in Buruku and Katsina-Ala LGAs of Benue State. Of the 1,292 subjects screened for urine colour, 578 had light yellow (normal colour) among which 46(8.0%) and 3(0.5%) had 1-49eggs/10ml of urine and ≥50 eggs/10ml respectively. Of the 666 having brown colour urine, 378(56.8%) and 80(12.0%) had 1-49eggs/10ml and ≥50 eggs/10ml of urine respectively. Out of the 48 having blood urine, 38(79.2%) had ≥50eggs/10ml of urine. A significant relationship was found between urine colour and intensity of *Schistosoma haematobium* eggs among participants examined (*rho*=0.6, $p<0.01$).

Table 1.0 compares urine colour observed as an indirect test and the true disease status as determined by filtration technique in Buruku and Katsina-Ala LGAs of Benue State. When Compared to the true disease status, light yellow (normal colour) of urine is considered as negative and this was observed in 529(91.5%) participants having no *S. haematobium* eggs (true negative) and 49(8.5%) having *Schistosoma haematobium* eggs (false negative). Of the 714 participants considered positive (brown + blood urine), 504(70.6%) had *S. haematobium* eggs (true positive), while 210(29.4 %) had no *S. haematobium* eggs (false positive).

Table 2 validates observed urine colour as an indirect test in the screening of urinary schistosomiasis in Buruku and Katsina-Ala LGAs of Benue State. The ability of the observed urine colour to accurately identify all those with the disease (sensitivity) was 91.1%, while its ability to correctly sort out all those without the disease (specificity) was 71.6 %. The positive predictive value (PPV) was (70.6 %), while the Negative Predictive Value (NPV) was 91.5%.

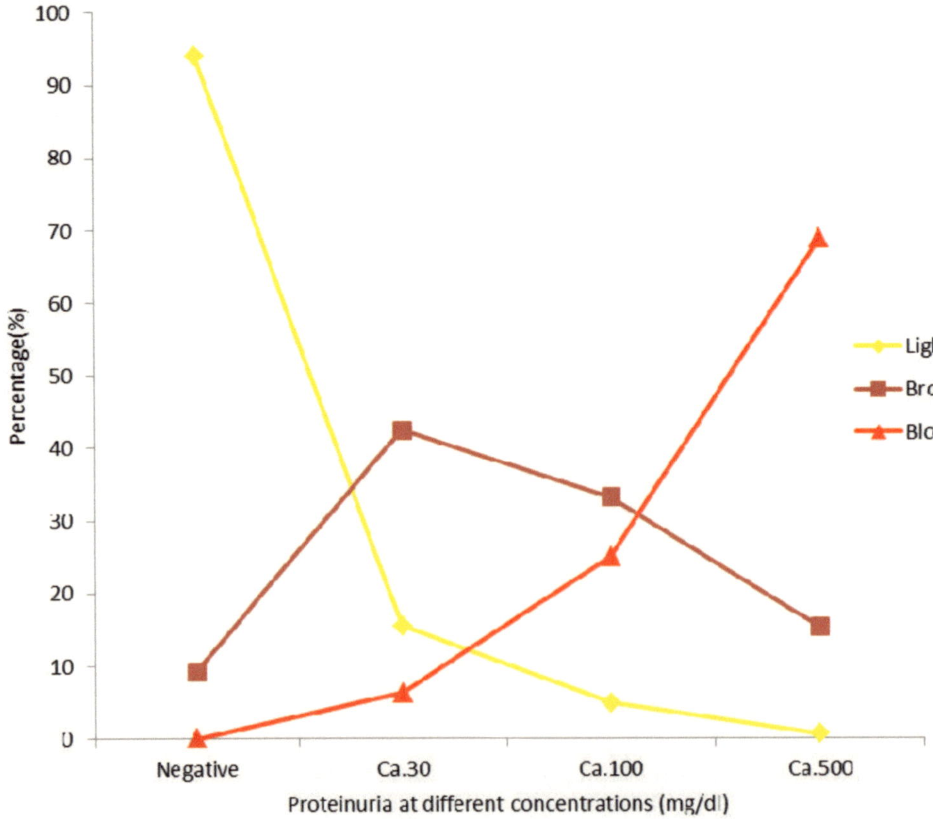

Fig. 3. Relationship between urine colour observation and proteinuria among subjects examined in Buruku and Katsina-Ala LGAs of Benue State, Nigeria

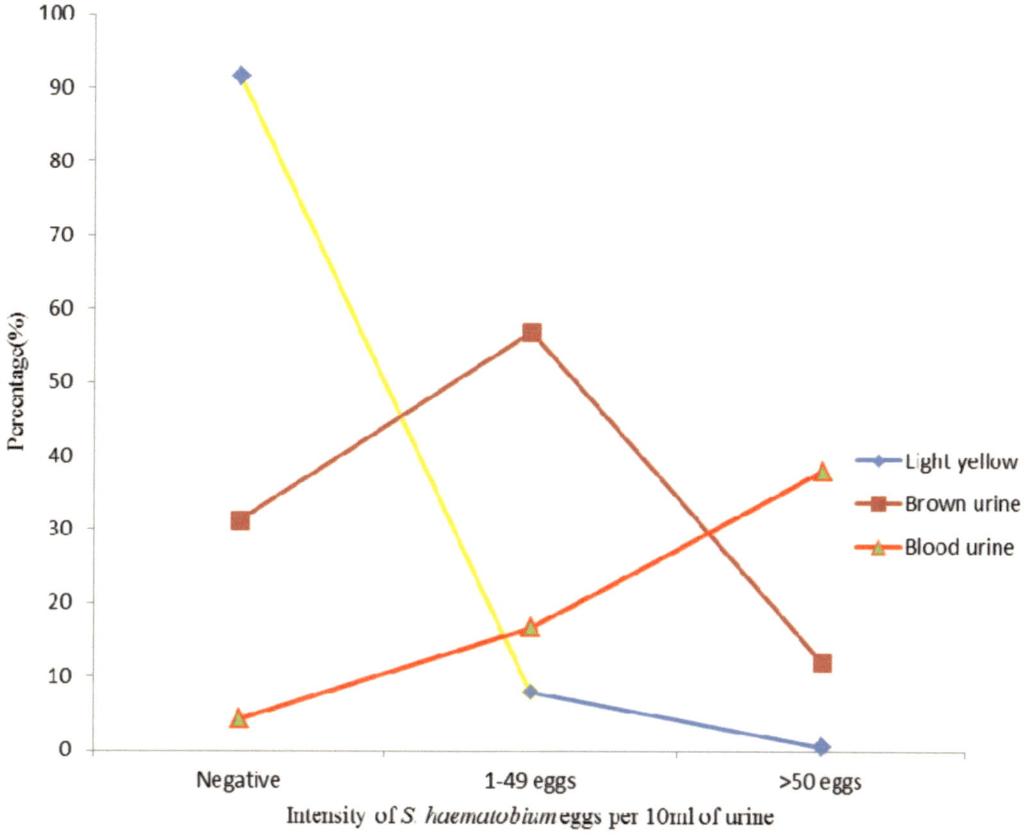

Fig. 4. Relationship between urine colour observation and intensity of *Schistosoma haematobium* eggs among subjects examined in Buruku and Katsina-Ala LGAs of Benue State

	Filtration technique (gold standard method) (%)		
Urine colour	Negative	Positive	**Total**
Negative (light-yellow)	529(91.5)[c]	49(8.4)[b]	**578**
Positive (Brown+Red)	210(29.4)[d]	504(70.6)[a]	**714**
Total	**739**	**553**	**1292**

Key: c= True negative
b= False negative
d= False positive
a= True positive

Table 1. Comparison of urine colour observation as rapid screening test and the true disease status as determined by filtration technique in Buruku and Katsina-Ala LGAs of Benue State

Parameters	Percentage (%)
Sensitivity	91.1
Specificity	71.6
Positive predictive value (PPV)	70.6
Negative predictive value (NPV)	91.5

Table 2. Validation of urine colour as rapid screening test for urinary schistosomiasis in Buruku and Katsina-Ala LGAs of Benue State

3. Discussion

It was demonstrated that assessing urine colour through simple observation significantly estimated the prevalence of infection and correlated with infection intensity as measured by egg counts (Filtration technique) known as the gold standard test. This shows that urine colour observation, if used as rapid screening tool in an endemic area is capable of assessing the endemic community for urinary schistosomiasis prevalence.

In addition to being a useful rapid field diagnostic for *Schistosoma haematobium* infection, urine colour as assessed by observation may also prove to be an indicator of morbidity through proteinuria and microhaematuria. Both proteinuria and microhaematuria correlated well with urine colour, *rho* = 0.7 and *rho* = 0.5 respectively at 0.01 significance level. However, the brown colour of urine should be the result of excreted protein and red blood cells into the urine from the damage of urinary tract and kidney. However, inconclusive evidence suggests that *Schistosoma haematobium* affects the glomeruli, the units of the kidney that function to separate out wastes and extra fluid from the blood. When the glomeruli are damaged, protein and often red blood cells leak into the urine as this might be the case in this study. Although, at the present time the precise origin and clinical significance of the proteinuria observed in *S. haematobium* infection remains unknown (Elissa, 2004). Nonetheless Sabour *et al.* (1972), Ezzat *et al.* (1974 and Ezzat *et al.* (1978) claimed an association between glomerulonephritis, the inflammation of the membrane tissue of the kidney and *S. haematobium* in human. Chugh and Sakuja (1990) reported that glomurelonephritis is highly prevalent in areas of the tropic where urinary schistosomiasis is also common, however its relationship to *S. haematobium* remain unclear. Sobh *et al.* (1991) showed that infected hamsters and not control animals developed significant glomerular damage related to the presence and intensity of *Schistosoma haematobium* infections.

The sensitivity of urine colour for screening test was high (91.1%) and with a specificity of 71.6%. This high sensitivity may be an indication of the predisposition of these rural dwellers to renal complications associated with urinary schistosomiasis. When compared to other indirect tests used in other studies like reagent strips, sensitivity of urine colour observation in this study was higher, but a specificity lower than results obtained by Ugbomoiko *et al.* (2009) who reported sensitivity of 68.3% and specificity of 83.2% using only microhaematuria, and sensitivity of 67.7% and specificity of 79.6% using only proteinuria respectively as indirect tests. However, variation in sensitivity and specificity of indirect tests during *Schistosoma haematobium* infection has been reported in several studies conducted in different African settings. They have been reported to vary from 41.0 % to 93 % and from 67 % to 99 % for sensitivity and specificity respectively (Anosike *et al*, 2001;

Takougang *et al.*, 2004; Brooker and Utzinger, 2007; Robinson *et al.*, 2009; French *et al.*, 2009; Ugbomoiko *et al.*, 2009).

The results obtained, however, agree with preliminary reports undertaken earlier to find its possibility as a rapid screening method in endemic areas (Houmsou *et al.*, 2009). Futhermore it is recommended that additional researches should be conducted in order to elucidate its feasibility in other endemic areas.

4. References

Anosike, J.C., Nwoke, B.E.B. & Njoku, A.J. (2001). Validity of haematuria in the community diagnosis of urinary schistosomiasis infection. *Journal of Helminthology*, 75: 223-225.

Brooker, S. & Utzinger, J. (2007). Integrated disease mapping in polyparasitic world. *Geospatial Health*, 1: 141-146.

Cheesbrough, M.(2000). District Laboratory Practice in Tropical Countries, part 1 Cambridge Press, London, 454pp.

Chugh, K.S. & Sakhuja, V. (1990). Glomerular diseases in the tropics. *American Journal of Nephrology*, 10(6): 437-450.

Elissa, K.V. (2004). Measuring micro-albuminuria: An innovative approach to estimating intensity of *Schistosoma haematobium* infection in zanzibari school children. *Working Paper Series*, 14(5). Havard Center for Population and Development Studies, Havard, School of Public Health, 41pp.

Ezzat, E., Osman, R.A., & Ahmet, K.Y. (1974). The association between *Schistosoma haematobium* infection and heavy proteinuria. *Transactions of the Royal Society of Tropical Medicine and Hygiene*, 68: 315-318.

Ezzat, E., Tohamy, M. & El-sherif, A. (1978). Immunopathological study of glomerulonephritis associated with *Schistosoma haematobium* infection. *Proceedings of the International Conference on schistosomiasis*, 2: 625-628.

French, M.D., Rollinson, D., Basáñez, M.G., Mgeni, A.F., Khami, I.S. & Stothard, J.R. (2009) School-based control of urinary schistosomiasis on Zanzibar, Tanzania: monitoring microhaematuria with reagent strips as a rapid urological assessment. *Journal of Pediatrics Urology*, 3:364-368.

Hotez, P.J. & Kamath, A. (2009). Neglected tropical diseases in sub-Saharan Africa: review of their prevalence, distribution and disease burden. *PLoS Neglected Tropical Diseases*, 3. e412.

Houmsou, R.S., Kela, S.L., Suleiman, M.M. & Ogidi, J.A. (2009). Urine colour as a rapid indicator of urine schistosomiasis in Katsina-Ala and Buruku LGAs of Benue State, Nigeria. *The Internet Journal of Tropical Medicine*, 6(1). www.ispub.com.

King C.H. & Dangerfield-Cha, M. (2008). The unacknowledged impact of chronic schistosomiasis. Chronic Illness 4(1): 65–79.

Maxwell, P.D. (2008). The global burden of urinary bladder cancer. *Scandinav Journal of Urology and Nephrology*. 1–9. 10.1080/03008880802285032.

Robinson, E., Picon, D., Sturrock, H.J., Sabasio, A., Lado, M., Kolaczinski, J. *et al.* (2009). The performance of haematuria reagent strips for the rapid mapping of urinary schistosomiasis: field experience from southern Sudan. *Tropical Medicine and International Health*, 14(12): 1484-1487.

Sobh, M.A., Moustapha, F.E., Ramzy, R.M., Deelder, A.M. & Ghoreim, M.A. (1991). *Schistosoma haematobium*-induced glomerular disease: and experimental study in the golden hamster. *Nephron*, 57(2): 216-224.

Steinmann, P., Keiser, J., Bos, R., Tanner, M. & Utzinger, J. (2006). Schistosomiasis and water resources development: systematic review meta-analysis and estimates of people at risk. The *Lancet Infectious Diseases*, 6(7): 411-425.

Takougang, I., Meli, J., Fotso, S., Angwafo III, F., Kamajeu, R. & Ndumbe, P.M. (2004). Haematuria and dysuria in the self diagnosis of urinary schistosomiasis among school children in Northern Cameroon. *African Journal of Health Sciences*, 11(3&4): 121-127.

Ugmoboiko, U.S., Dalumo, V., Ariaza, L., Bezerra, F.S.M. & Heukelbach, J. (2009). A simple approach improving the performance of urine reagent strips for rapid diagnosis of urinary schistosomiasis in Nigerian school children. *Memorias Instituto Oswaldo Cruz*, 104(3):456-461.

van der Werf, M.J., de Vlas SJ, Brooker S, Looman CW, Nagelkerke NJ, *et al.* (2003) Quantification of clinical morbidity associated with schistosome infection in sub-Saharan Africa. *Acta Tropica*, 86(2–3): 125–139.

van der Werf, M.J. & de Vlas, S.J. (2001). Morbidity and infection with schistosome or soil transmitted helminths. *Rotterdam Erasmus University*, 1-103.

Wilkins, H.A. (1977). *Schistosoma haematobium* in a Gambian community. The intensity and prevalence of infection. *Annals of Tropical Medicine and Parasitology*, 71(1): 53-58.

World Health Organization. (2003). Manual of basic techniques for a health laboratory, 2nd edition. World Health Organization, Geneva, 126pp.

Part 6

Malacology

15

Pattern of Genetic Divergence of Mitochondrial DNA Sequences in *Biomphalaria tenagophila* Complex Species Based on Barcode and Morphological Analysis

Roseli Tuan, Fernanda Pires Ohlweiler, Raquel Gardini Sanches Palasio, Ricardo Dalla Zanna and Marisa Cristina De Almeida Guimarães

Superintendência de Controle de Endemias, São Paulo
Brazil

1. Introduction

Neotropical region has a high diversity of *Biomphalaria* (Pulmonata: Basommatophora: Planorbidae) fauna with at least twenty-six of the world's estimated thirty- seven species recorded (Carvalho,2008). Nearly one –third of these species occur in freshwater ecosystems related to the main drainage river basins in Brazil (Estrada et al.,2006; Teodoro,2010),where *Biomphalaria glabrata* (Say,1818),*Biomphalaria tenagophila (*Orbigny,1835) and *Biomphalaria straminea (*Dunker,1848) have serious impact on human health for these species host *Schistosoma mansoni* Sambon 1907 (Figure 1).

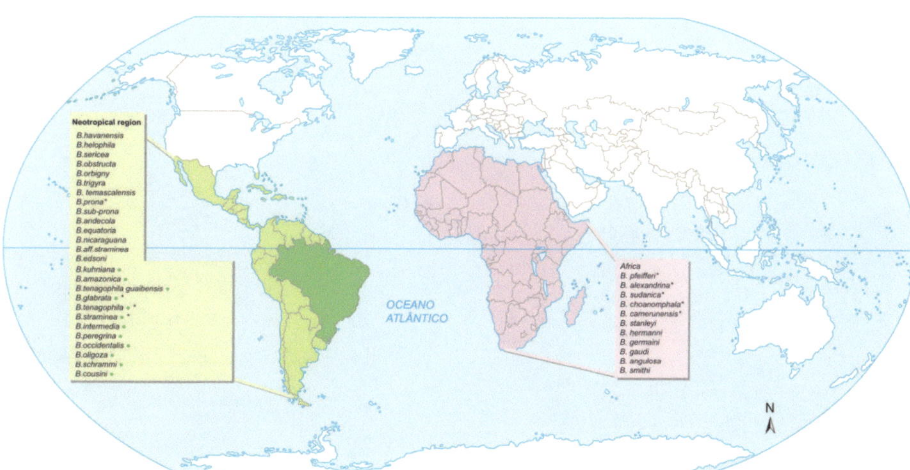

Fig. 1. Map (according Palasio, R.G.S., 2011) showing the worldwide distribution of the 37 *Biomphalaria* species, the 26 neotropical *Biomphalaria* species and the 11 species and 1 subspecies naturally described in Brazil (•) (Brasil,Ministério da Saúde 2007; Carvalho et al., 2008; Teodoro et al.,2010). An asterisk indicates *Schistosoma mansoni* host species (Palasio, RGS, 2011).

B. tenagophila is the nominal member of a species complex of freshwater snails distributed widespread in the neotropical region (Figure 2). *B. tenagophila* is the main host of *S. mansoni* in the southeastern Brazil. (Paraense & Corrêa,1978).As currently defined,the *B. tenagophila* complex includes a sub-species *B. tenagophila guaibensis* (Paraense,1984) and a species *B. occidentalis* (Paraense,1981).

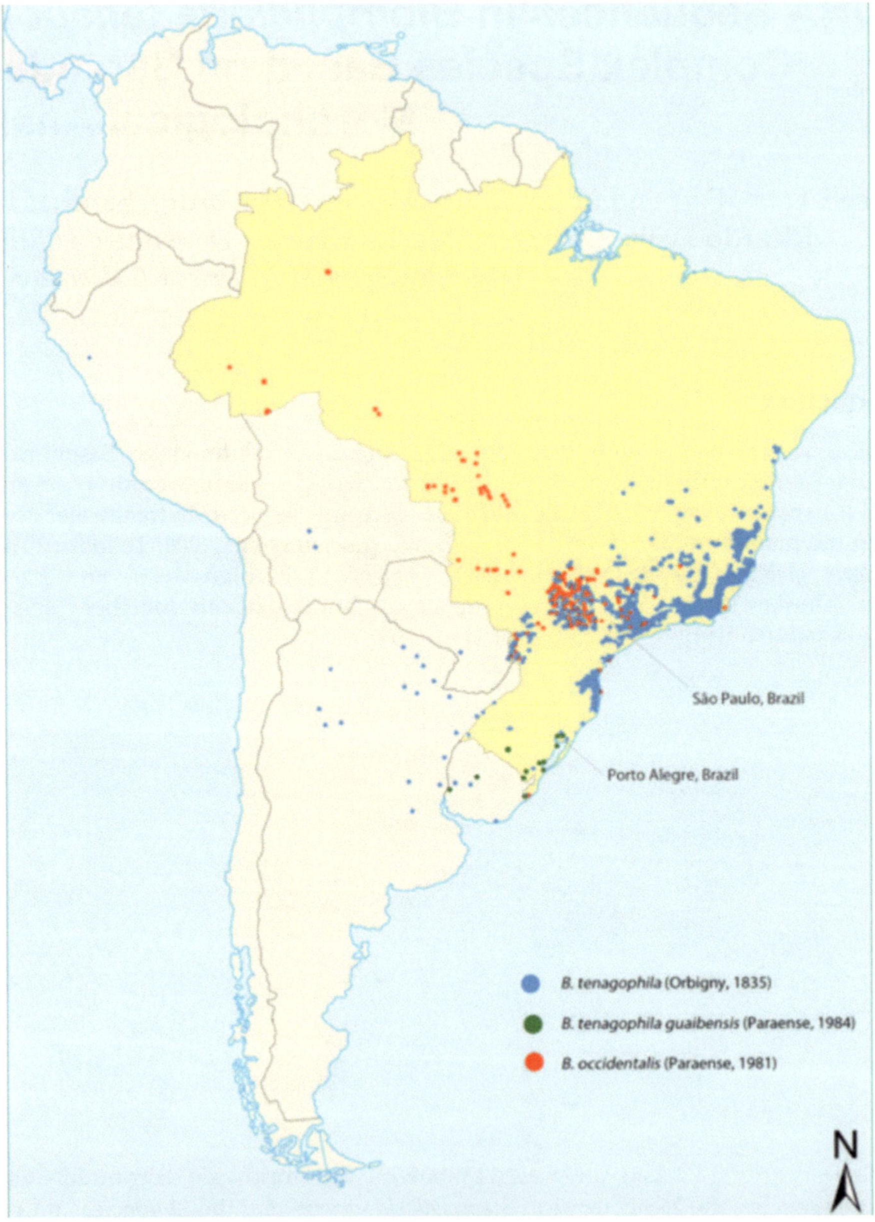

Fig. 2. Geographic distribution of *Biomphalaria tenagophila* complex in the southeastern Brazil. (R.G.S. Palasio & R. Tuan based on illustrations in Lima et al.,1993; Paraense 1984, 2001; Carvalho & Caldeira,2004).

The morphological characters of the genital organs employed by the malacologist WL Paraense permits all of us to correctly identify the taxonomic units of the *tenagophila* complex. But,in fact,identifying *Biomphalaria* species solely on morphological characters leads to a less precise identification of these taxonomical groups,which are found to be difficult to diagnose in a malacological work routine.

The following examples may illustrate how morphological or technical variations can lead to erroneous species identification with serious epidemiological consequences.

Example 1: Within the species of planorbid described in Brazil,a *B. glabrata* is the only species to feature pigmented renal ridge (Paraense and Deslandes 1959). This character is known to be the only to set the difference between *B. glabrata* (the most important host species of *S. mansoni* in the Americas) and *B. tenagophila*,responsible for the transmission of schistosomiasis in the southeastern region of Brazil. Pepe et al. (2009) reports that a pigmentation-like may appear associated to the renal ridge in *B. t. guaibensis*,as a result from an intraspecies variation. Such diagnosis would trigger an unnecessary alert once *B.t.guaibensis* is not an intermediary host of *S. mansoni.*

Variation in the pattern of the pigmentation of the renal ridge may also reflect the influences of the freshwater substrate types leading us to an erroneous identification of all *Biomphalaria* species.

Here we exemplified the two major aggravating factors in a morphological identification system: morph variation within the species and variation caused by interaction of the organism with the environment.

Example 2: According to Paraense (1984) an essential condition for a clear distinction of *B.tenagophila* from the subspecies *B. t. guaibensis "is that the animal body is preserved for dissection in a well relaxed condition"*,that is,for the identification of the subspecies,more rigorous laboratorial methods of looseness need to be used instead of the methods utilized in the current identification of mollusks. If the *B.t. guaibensis* subspecies were dispersed,it would be difficult to have a morphological differential diagnosis of these subspecies.

The intrinsic difficulties to the system of morphological identification of organisms limit the description of taxonomic discreet units,although they lead to the development of auxiliary molecular techniques to overcome these difficulties (Estrada et al.,2006; Carvalho,2008).

Species of planorbid snails belonging to the genus *Biomphalaria* have received increasing attention in molecular systematic and phylogeographic studies in recent years (Vidigal et al. 2000,2004; Carvalho et al. 2001; DeJong et al. 2001,2003; Mavárez et al. 2002a,b; Morgan et al. 2002; Pointier et al. 2005; Tuan and Santos,2007). The development of genetic markers and the databases generated in such studies can be further used for multiple purposes,of both theoretical and applied interest: species identification,analysis of population genetic structure and speciation patterns,inference of common/independent origins of susceptibility to *Schistosoma*,detection of natural hybridization,tracking of geographical expansions and biological invasions,evaluation of genetic differentiation between phenotypic variants and/or geographic isolates,amongst others. Genetic markers used in *Biomphalaria* studies include mitochondrial DNA (Spatz et al. 1999; DeJong et al. 2001,2003; Mavárez et al. 2002b; Pointier et al. 2005). The latter is especially useful for species identification.

The dispersal and colonizing ability of *B. tenagophila* highlights the need to monitor the spread of this species within and outside the neotropical region. The identification of *B. tenagophila* in Kinshasa,Africa (Pointier,2005) and Romania (Majoros et al. 2008) certainly caused great concern to public health authorities.

For *Biomphlalaria* species two important characteristics play an important role to successfully establish snail populations in a environment outside the native range of the species: self-fertilization and desiccation. *B.tenagophila* species are simultaneous hermaphrodites snails with the possibility of both self and cross-fertilization (Paraense,1955; Tuan & Simões,1989; Guimarães,2003). Such a complex mode of reproduction might probably increase colonization since new populations can arise from just one snail by self-fertilization.

On the other hand reproduction alone is not enough to establish a species because snails still must be able to survive conditions outside their native range. One important aspect to *B. tenagophila* survival it is the ability to withstand desiccation in response to water shortage (Tuan & Simões,1989; Ohlweiler & Kawano,2002) that greatly increases the possibility of recolonization after a population crash or colonization of new environments. These must be a major source of genetic diversity amongst the same species creating patchily distributed populations that can be easily distinguished by molecular markers.

In this study,we obtained mitochondrial COI and 16SrRNA sequences from *B. tenagophila,B. t. guaibensis*,and *B. occidentalis* specimens collected in the São Paulo state,and Rio Grande do Sul state,Brazil to estimate the divergence of each species amongst the three members of the *tenagophila* complex and evaluate the potential of COI and 16S rRNA mitochondrial genes for identification of closely related species.

2. Materials and methods

2.1 Molecular analysis

B. tenagophila and *B. occidentallis* snails were collected along the banks of different streams of Paranapanema,Ribeira do Iguape,Paraíba do Sul,Tietê,and Litoral Basins at São Paulo,Brazil. *B.t. guaibensis* specimens were collected at Rio Grande do Sul,Brazil (Table 1). Two samples from Argentina were also analyzed. A total of 66 specimens were used in this study. Prior to molecular analysis snails were identified through morphological analysis,according to Deslandes (1959) and Paraense (1975,1981,and 1984).

Total genomic DNA was extracted from foot tissue of individual snails using DNeasy Tissue Kits (Qiagen®) and was preserved as DNA vouchers specimens in the DNA voucher collection of the Laboratory of Molecular Biology and Biochemical at SUCEN. Amplification of COI gene was attempted using LCO-1490 and HCO-2198 (Folmer et al.,1994). Amplifications (in 50µl of total volume) consisted of 10-100 ng of DNA,0.2 mM of each dNTP,0.10 µM of each primer and 1 U of *Taq* DNA polymerase (BioLabs) with the supplied buffer. The following PCR temperature profile was used: a initial 3 min step at 95°C for denaturation,25 iterations of 1 min at 95°C,1 min at 47°C and 1 min 30 sec at 72°C,and a final extension step for 7 min at 72°C. The amplification profile of 16SrRNA fragment included an initial denaturation step at 94°C for 2 min. and 35 cycles of 30 sec at 94°C,30 sec at 54°C and 1 minute at 72°C,and a final step at 72°C for 5 minutes. Amplification of 16S gene was attempted using a Palumbi forward and reverse primer (Palumbi, 1996).

PCR products were checked by agarose gel electrophoresis,cleaned using QIAquick PCR Purification Kits (Qiagen®). Cycle-sequencing of PCR products were carried out using terminal primers given above and the BigDye Terminator v3.1 kit of Applied Biosystems (ABI),purified using DyeEx-Kit (Qiagen®) according to the modified protocol and sequenced on an ABI 310 automated sequencer.

Species/Locality	Code	Geographical coordinates
B. tenagophila		
Ourinhos (SP),Brazil	*Btt_Our1 -6*	22°58′02″S 49°52″25″ W
Ipauçu (SP),Brazil	*Btt_Juq1-8*	23°02′54″S 49°34′41″W
Taubaté (SP),Brazil	*Btt_Tau1-3*	23°01'35"S 45°33'21"W
Pindamonhangaba (SP),Brazil	*Btt_Pin1-2*	22°53'30"S 45°28'09"W
Caraguatatuba (SP),Brazil	*Btt_Car1-7*	23°37'31"S 45°24'44"W
São Sebastião (SP),Brazil	*Btt_SSe1*	23°47′08″S 45°33′22″W
Campinas (SP),Brazil	*Btt_Cam1-4*	23°02'13"S 47°06'21"W
Sorocaba (SP),Brazil	*Btt_Sor1-5*	23°29'56"S 47°27'30"W
Registro (SP),Brazil	*Btt_Reg1-3*	24°29'20"S 47°51'06″W
Juquiá (SP),Brazil	*Btt_Juq1-8*	24°19'33″S 47°38'22"W
Araraquara (SP),Brazil	*Btt_Ara1*	23°01'35"S 45°33'21"W
Rio da Prata,Argentina	*Btt_Arg1-2*	NA
B. t. guaibensis		
Porto Alegre (RS),Brazil	*Btg_POA1-4*	29°59′52. 3′′S 51°15′38.6′′W
B. occidentalis		
Ourinhos (SP),Brazil	*Boc_Our 1-5*	22°58′02″S 49°52′25″W
Martinópolis (SP),Brazil	*Boc_Mar1-2*	22°14′04″S 51°09′36″W
Presidente Prudente (SP),Brazil	*Boc_PPr1*	22°10′12″S 51°22′34″W
Candido Mota (SP),Brazil	*Boc_CMo1*	22°44'52"S 50°23'08"W

NA,Not Available.

Table 1. Collecting data,code and geographical identification of the specimen used in molecular study.

Sequences were corrected using Chromas (Technelysium Pty Ltd.),aligned in ClustalX 1.8 (Thompson et al. 1997). The alignments of COI datasets comprised sequences with no gaps or indels. The alignments were subsequently adjusted by eye using BioEdit 7.0 (Hall, 1999). Phylogenetic and molecular evolutionary analyses were conducted using *MEGA* version 5 (Tamura,Peterson,Stecher,Nei,Kumar 2011). Sequence divergence between species was estimated with Kimura 2 parameter model (K2P) (Kimura, 1980). The Neighbor-Joining (Saitou and Nei 1987) trees were obtained using K2P model and the support for the nodes was calculated using 1000 bootstrap replicates (Felsenstein, 1985). Nucleotide diversity (pi,Nei,1987,equations 10.5 or 10.6 and 10.7); and nucleotide divergence between sequence groups (D_{xy},Nei,1987,equation 10.20 using Jukes and Cantor correction) were calculated using DnaSP v.5 (Librado and Rozas,2009). F*st* was estimated following Hudson et al. 1992.

2.2 Morphology analysis

The morphological analysis was based on 10 dissected specimens *B. tenagophila* from Arambaré,Rio Grande do Sul (lot DPE 9011); 13 dissected specimens *B. t. guaibensis* from Porto Alegre,Rio Grande do Sul (lot DPE 9008,Figure 3) and 31 dissected specimens *B. occidentalis* from Tremembé,São Paulo (lot DPE 9028). Only large and adult specimens were used for dissection and anatomic study.

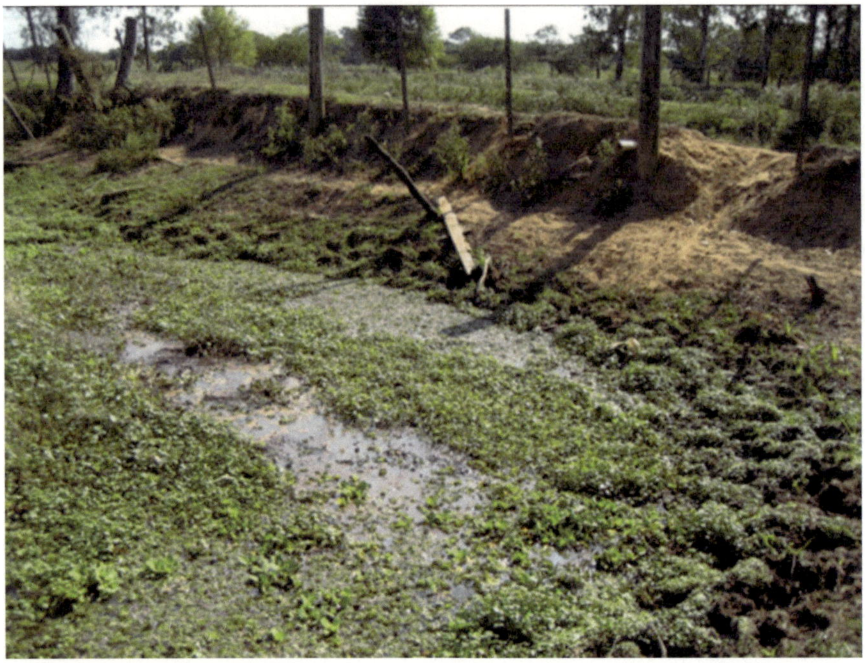

Fig. 3. A natural freshwater habitat at Porto Alegre where *B. tenagophila guaibensis* were collected. 29° 59′ 52 3′′S, 51° 15′ 38. 6′ W.

Snails were identified according to Paraense (1975). Soft parts were preserved under fixation as vouchers. The identification of the mollusks was done under the stereomicroscopy (Leica MZ 95) and was photographed with the image Program IMS 50. We took into consideration the morphology of the shell and soft parts,especially the reproductive system.
Three radulae and three jaws of the *B. occidentalis,B. tenagophila* and *B. t. guaibensis* were extracted and examined under a Scanning Electron Microscope LEO 440 at the Museum of the Zoology,São Paulo University (MZUSP).

3. Results

3.1 Molecular analysis

The evolutionary relationships of *tenagophila* complex were inferred using Neighbor-Joining method for COI and 16SrRNA mitochondrial genes (Figure 4). The evolutionary distances depicted as branch lengths were computed using the Kimura 2p method using 550 nucleotides positions for the COI dataset and 314 nucleotide positions for the 16S rRNA dataset. The *tenagophila* complex sequences were retrieved in two well distinct and bootstrap supported branches: one with *B. occidentalis* clustering with *B. t. guaibensis*,and another distinct branch with the nominal *B.tenagophila* sequences.
For each component that belongs to *tenagophila* complex we obtained intraspecific identical sequences that support morphological taxonomy.
Two distinct groups of *B. tenagophila* were recovered in each analysis (COI and rRNA16S).
The estimates of genetic divergence (Table2) under Kimura 2p model over the COI and 16S between sequences pairs of the taxa analyzed show that *B. t. guaibensis* are more closely related with *B. occidentallis* than with *B. tenagophila*.

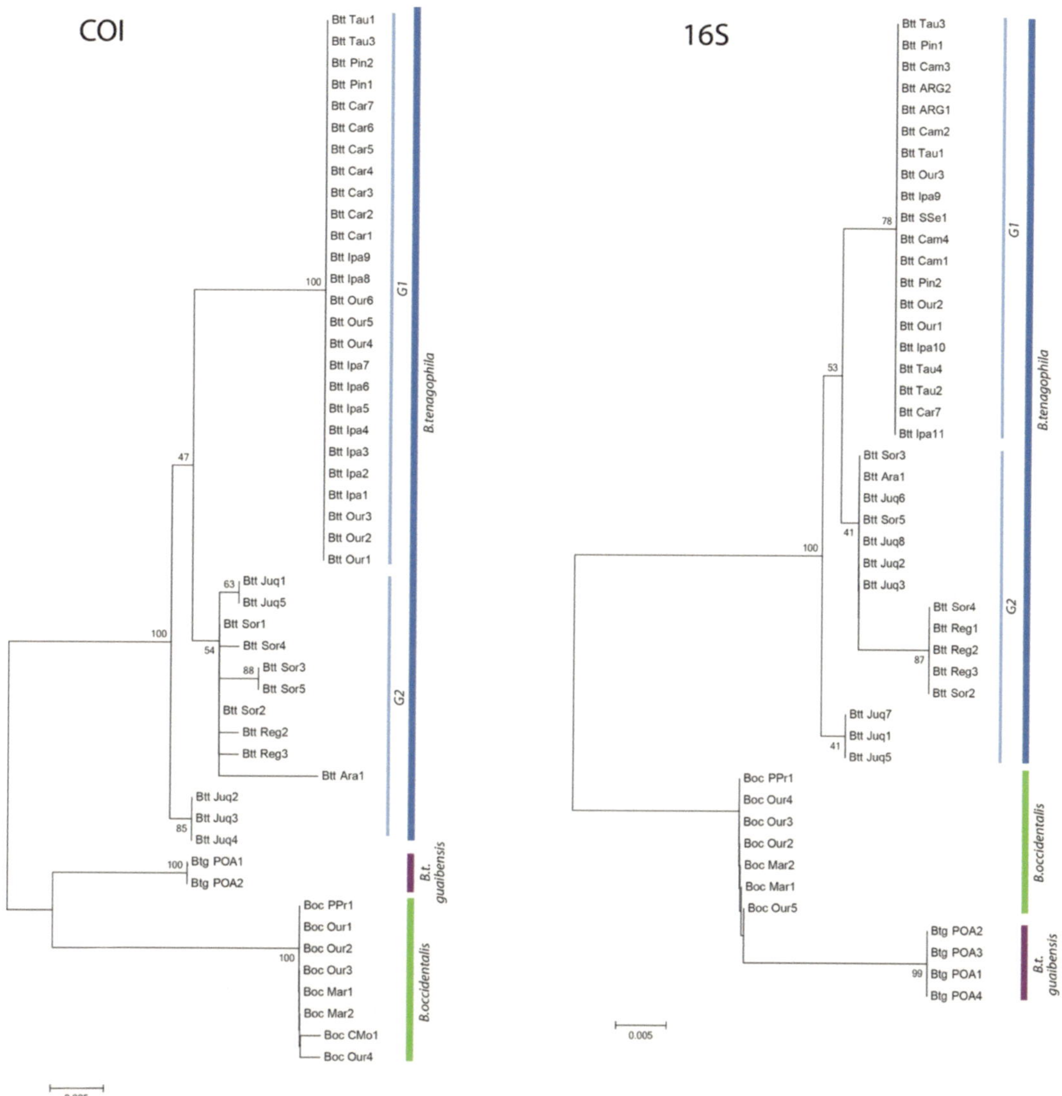

Fig. 4. Optimal trees inferred for a 550 fragment COI mtDNA(A),sum of branch length= 0.09775397,and for a 314 nucleotides 16SrRNA,sum of branch length= 0.07712277. Bootstrap values (1000 replicates) are shown next to the branches.

Species 1	Species 2	COI	16S
B.tenagophila	*B.t.guaibensis*	0.0436	0.0668
B.tenagophila	*B.occidentalis*	0.0546	0.0478
B.t.guaibensis	*B.occidentalis*	0.0362	0.0178

Table 2. Mean Pairwise distance values calculated under Kimura´s 2 -parameter model (K2P) for 49 COI sequences and 46 16SrRNA sequences.

The Figure 5 shows that no overlap exists between intraspecific and interspecific distribution distance calculated under Kimura 2P. Indeed,the distributions of the COI and 16S genetic distances are very similar (Figure 5).

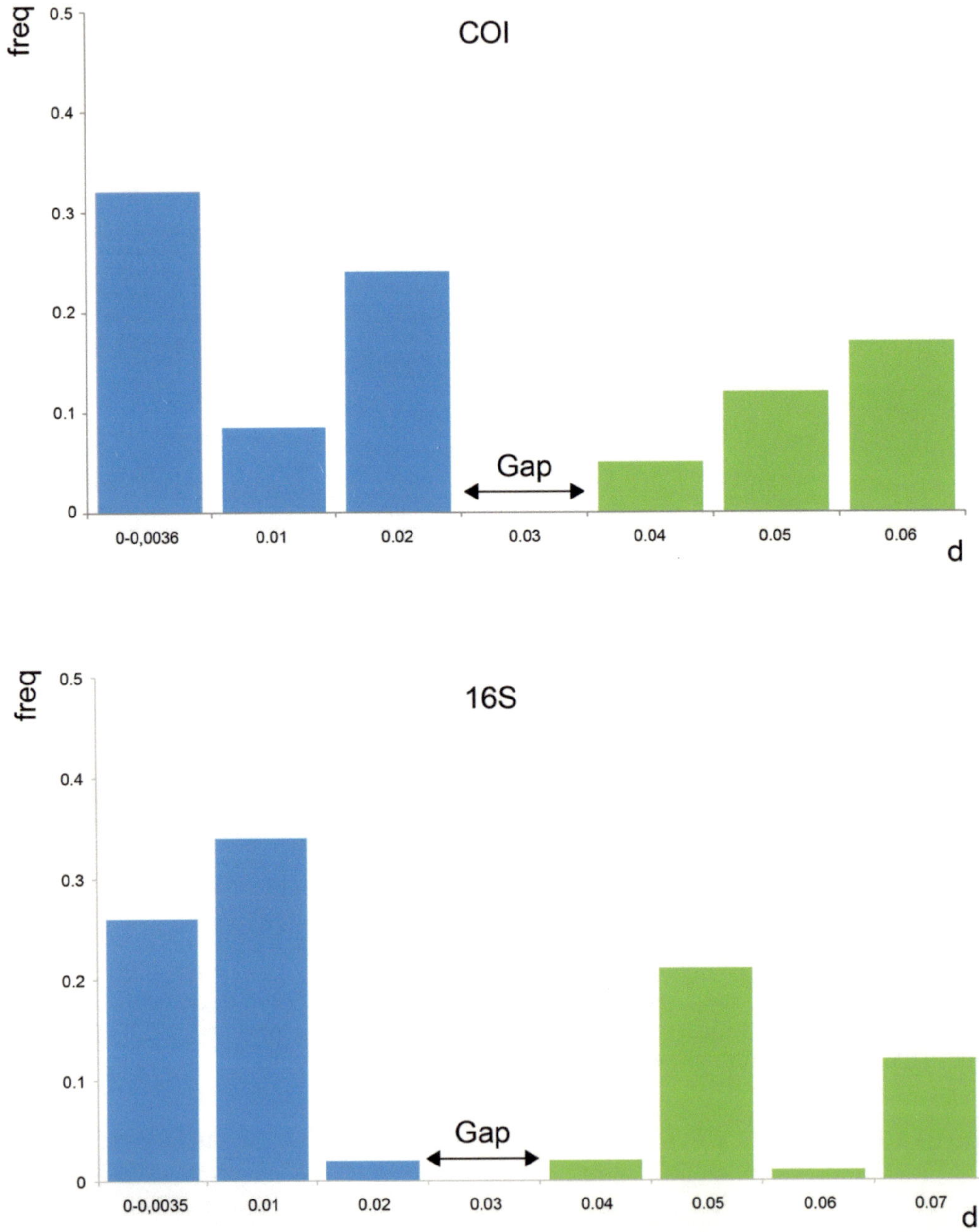

Fig. 5. Distribution of intraspecific variation genetic distance (in blue bars),and interspecific distance (in green bars) estimated by Kimura´s 2 -parameter model (K2P) for all the species studied

In order to examine the ability of the barcoding methodology to identify the three *Biomphalaria* taxa we plotted the intra and interspecific divergence of COI and 16S using a threshold of 3% minimum interspecific genetic variation and 3% maximum intraspecific genetic variation (Figure 6).

According the 3% threshold value for within and between species variation four quadrants are defined. Species on quadrant I (dark grey) are well-defined species. Groups on quadrant II (white colored) are composite species. Species on quadrant III (medium grey) are recent divergent species,and species on quadrant IV (light grey) are misidentified species.

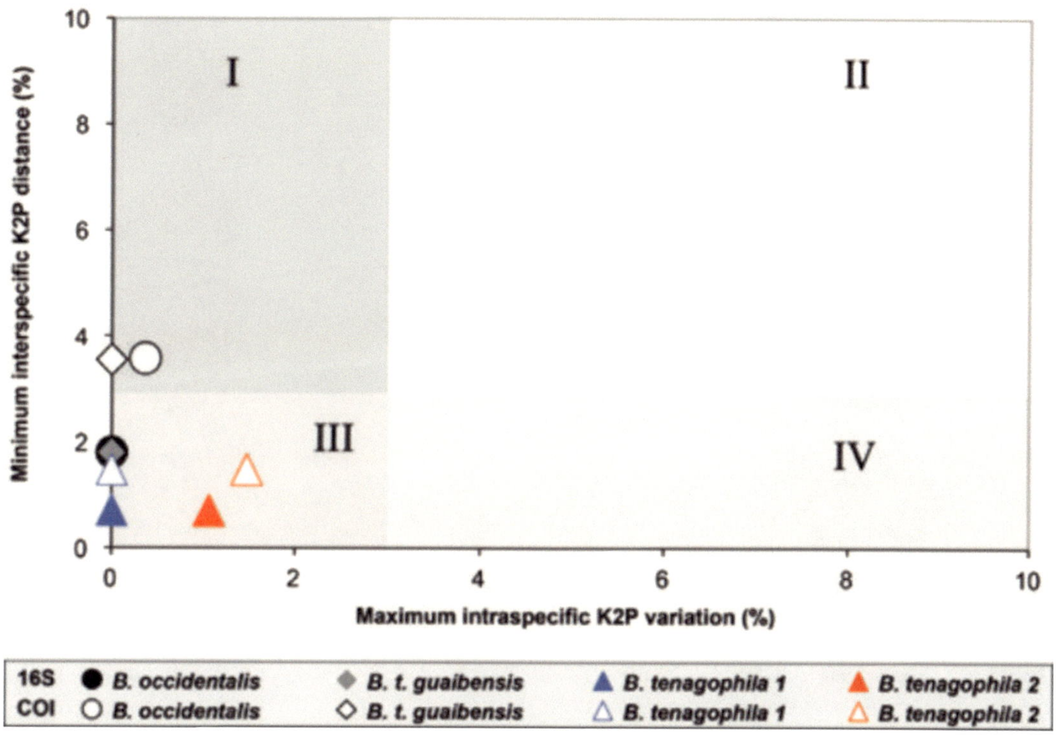

Fig. 6. Minimum Interspecific distances versus Maximum intraspecific distances of COI and 16S sequences for *B. tenagophila,B. occidentalis* and *B. t. guaibensis* (according Ballard et al.,2009).

3.2 Comparative analysis of shell,reproductive system and radula

B. tenagophila,B.t. guaibensis and B. occidentalis had no significant differences among the number of whorls. The species had typically six to eight whorls. Otherwise,the shell aperture would be shorter and narrower in *B.t guaibensis* than in the other two species analyzed (Figure 7).

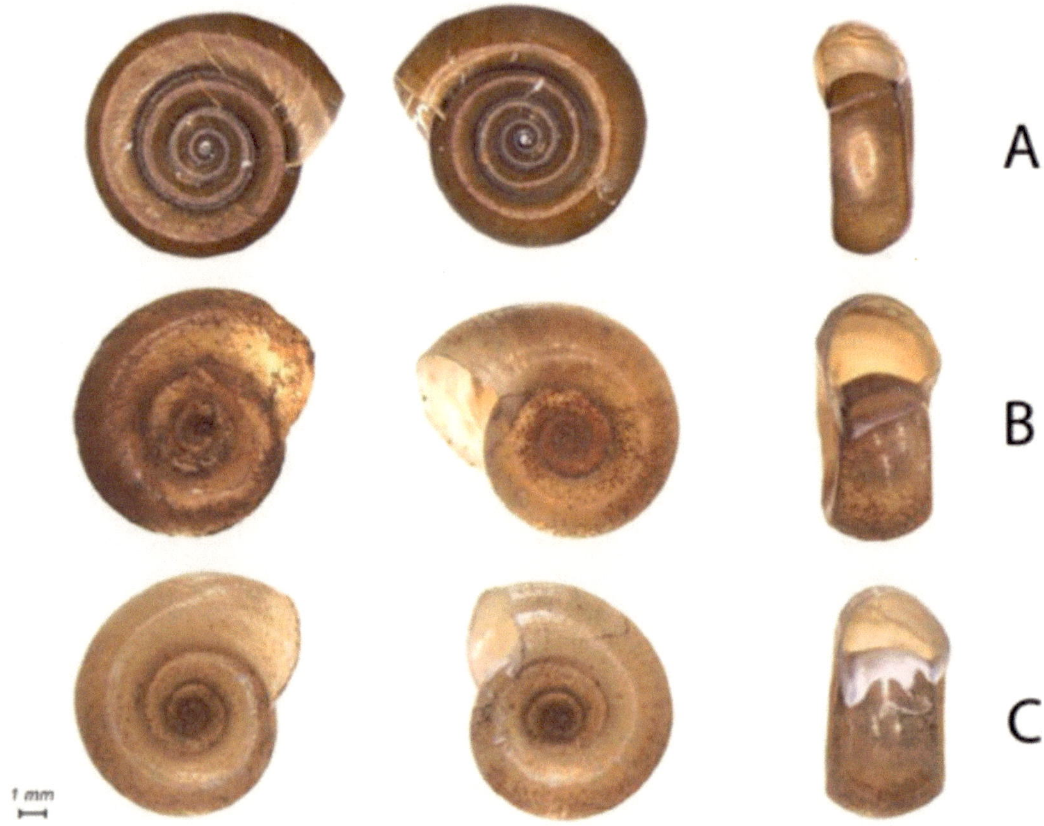

Fig. 7. Shell. A: *B. t. guaibensis Biomphalaria tenagophila,* C: *B. occidentalis*

Biomphalaria snails can be distinguished based on differences in the shape and size of their male and female internal organs as described in Figure 8.

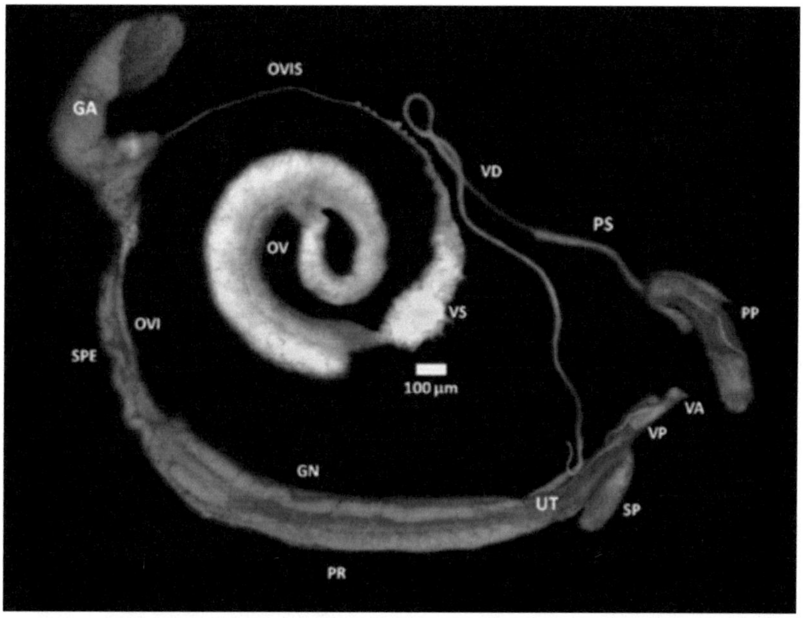

Fig. 8. Reproductive System from *Biomphalaria tenagophila*. GA: albumen gland,GN: nidamental gland,OV: ovotestis,OVI: oviduct,OVIS: ovispermiduct,PP: prepuce,PR: prostate,PS: penial sheath,SP: spermatheca,SPE: spermiduct,UT: uterus,VA: vagina,VD: vas deferens,VP: vaginal pouch, VS: seminal vesicle.

The hermaphrodite part did not present differences between *B.tenagophila,B.t. guaibensis* and *B. occidentalis*.
The differences between the species were mainly found in the male and female systems. The anatomical characters that clearly groups *B.tenagophila* and *B. t. guaibensis* in a same taxon is a well developed vaginal pouch located in the vaginal wall of this species,and also the shape and size of the prepuce and the volume of prostata (Table 5,Figure 9).

	Biomphalaria tenagophila	*Biomphalaria tenagophila guaibensis*	*Biomphalaria occidentalis*
Vagina	short	Long and slender	Long and slender
Vaginal pouch	Well developed	Well developed	absent
penis	thick	Long and slender	Long and slender
prepuce	Wider at the free end of the prepuce	Wider at the free end of the prepuce	Same diameter along the prepuce
Penis sheath	Shorter and slenderer than the prepuce	Shorter and slenderer than the prepuce	Shorter and slenderer than the prepuce
Próstata	Robust with a great number of diverticula	Robust with a great number of diverticula	Refined with a small number of diverticula
spermatheca	large	small	small

Table 5. Differences among *B. tenagophila* species complex based on reproductive parameters

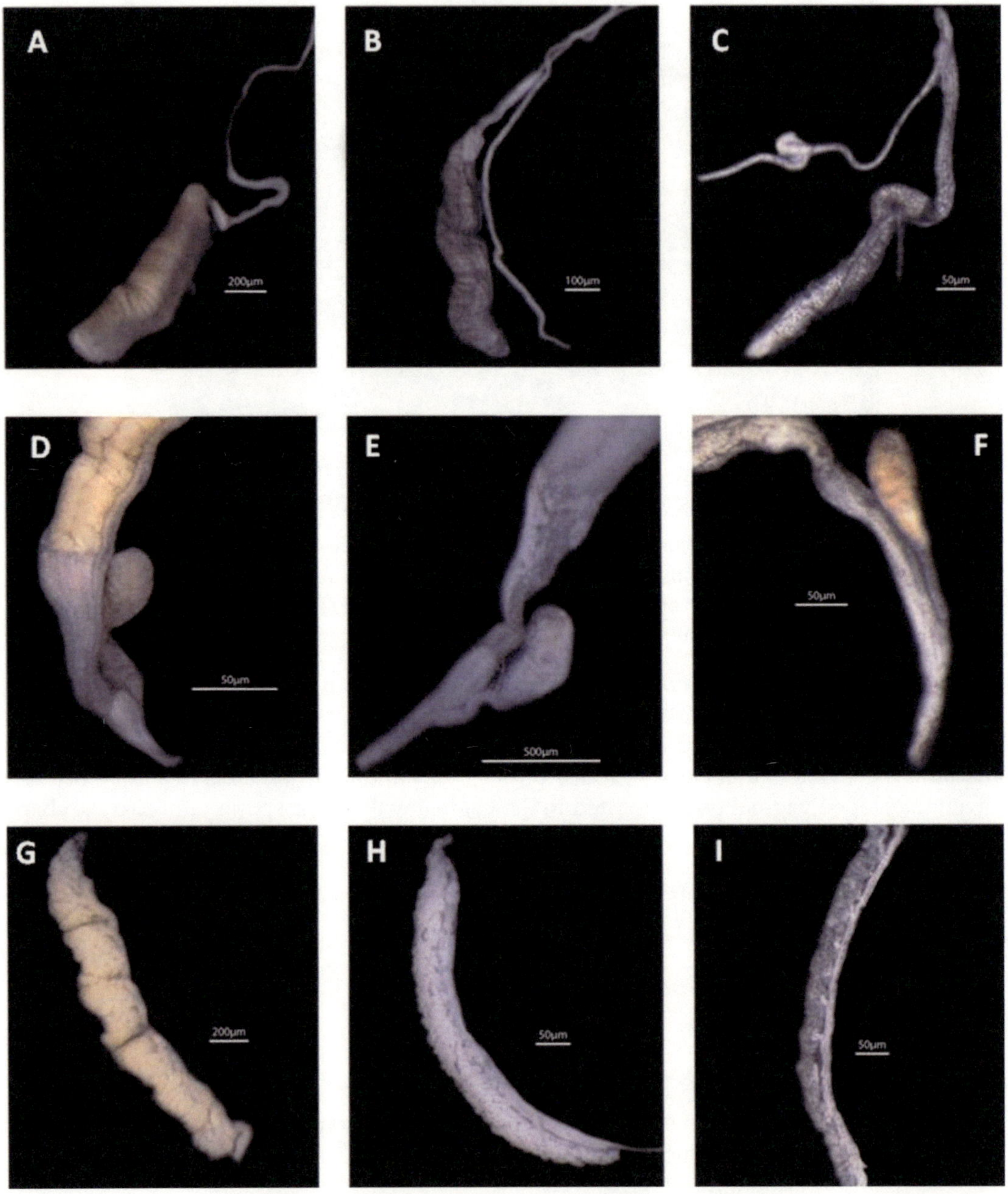

Fig. 9. Detail of reproductive system. A,D and G: *B. tenagophila*,B,E and H: *B. t. guaibensis*,C,F and I: *B. occidentalis*. A,B and C: Penis; D,E and F: Vaginal complex; G,H and I: Prostate

The radulae of *B tenagophila,B. t. guaibensis and B. occidentalis* consisted of a fused jaw (Figure 10) to which the teeth are attached.

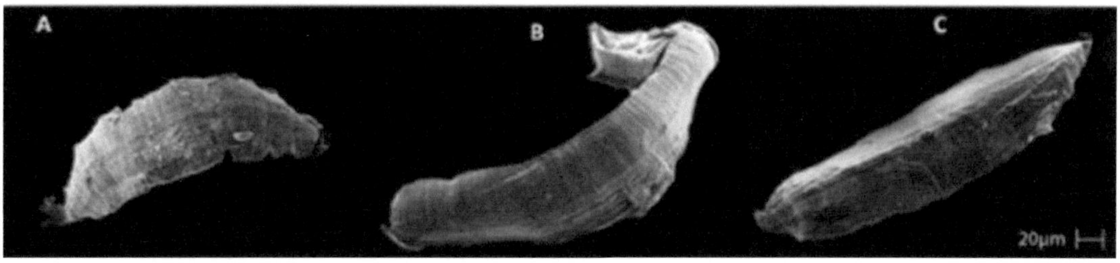

Fig. 10. Mandíbula. A.: *B. tenagophila,B.: B.t. guaibensis,C: B. occidentalis.*

In all the species analyzed there was only one central tooth with two cusps and several lateral teeth at each side of the central tooth. In *B.t. guaibensis* the central tooth showed variations that affected the inner and outer faces of the cuspids (Figure 11).

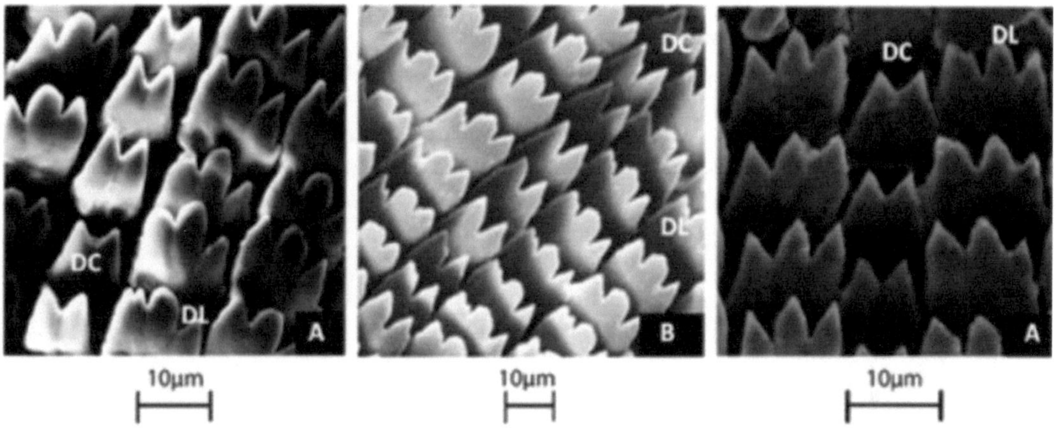

Fig. 11. Radula. A: *B. tenagophila*,B: *B.t. guaibensis*,C: *B. occidentalis*. DC: central tooth,DL: lateral teeth.

In all the three species the lateral were characterized with three cuspids. Small subcusps appear on lateral teeth near the margins given a serrated appearance for the radulae. (Figure 12)

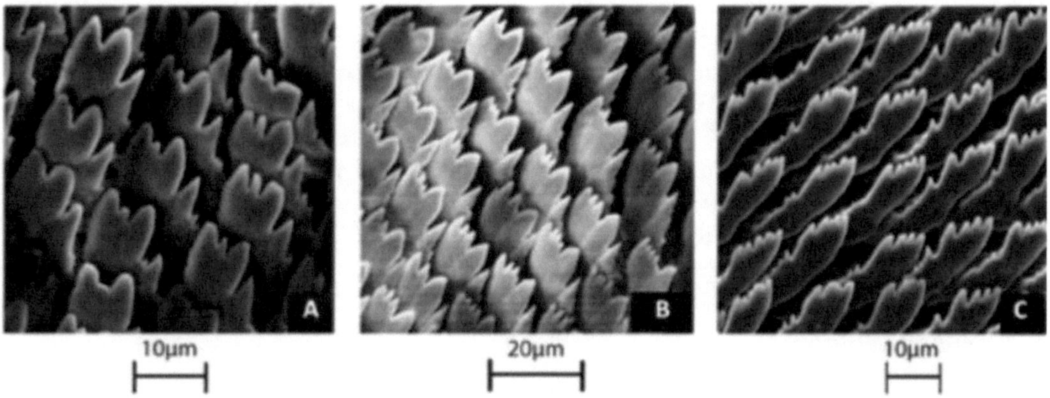

Fig. 12. Marginal teeth of the radula. A: *B. tenagophila*,B: *B.t. guaibensis*,C: *B. occidentalis*.

4. Discussion

Phylogenetic analysis using short sequences of the mitochondrial COI and 16SrRNA genes resulted in trees with high support values morphologycally pairs of species *B. tenagophila* and the subspecies *B. t. guaibensis*,and the *B. occidentalis* and *B. t guaibensis*,assigned as *tenagophila* species complex (Figure 4).

The molecular evidence thus strongly suggests that *B. occidentalis* and *B.t. guaibensis* are part of a clade of closely related species with a minimal genetical divergence between them (Table 2).

The result obtained here is in perfect agreement with our observations with respect to the resemblance between *guaibensis* and *occidentalis* morphology,both thin and elongated species when compared to *tenagophila* species. For taxonomically purposes,the vaginal pouch places *B. tenagophila* and *B.t. guaibensis* closer to each other (Paraense,1984). The vaginal pouch represents a character easy to score unambiguously (1 for presence 0 for absence) but instead of inferring a close relationship between *B.tenagophila* and *B.t guaibensis*,the vaginal pouch could also be considered a case of homoplasy and might not have great confidence and definition for such a complex taxonomic groups as in other gastropod groups (Collin,2003). To sustain such hypothesis,further additional sequences from other sites are clearly required.

Our sequence data (COI,16S) revealed significant intraspecific variation for *B. tenagophila*. Two major branches were resolved by phylogenetic analysis,one of which -G1- with very low internal variation (pi=0.0000 for COI and 16S) and a second branch -G2- with a significant degree of internal genetic differentiation amongst sequences (pi=0.00587 for COI and pi= 0.00995 for 16S).

The extremely low levels of genetic variation in G1 branch exists amongst populations across a broad geographic range area,including Ourinhos,Pindamonhangaba and Taubate. All these sites presented were in the past active areas of transmission of schistosomiasis (Piza,1972; Silva,1985),subjected to intensive use of moluscicide measure that resulted in cycles of extinction followed by recolonization of *B. tenagophila* (Tuan,1996).

Whereas G1 population occurs in historical unstable sites,G2 population inhabits freshwater sites at São Paulo (Registro,Juquia) with fragments of the Brazilian Atlantic Rain Forest,one of the most important hot- spots of genetic diversity in the world (Carnaval et al. 2009). The significant differentiation between G1 and G2 *B. tenagophila* populations (Fst COI= 0.82; Fst 16S=0.77) and the retention of even a small genetic diversity in G2 populations could be due to historical signatures since Atlantic coastal regions played an important role as a climatic refugee during the last Pleistocene (Pfenninger and Posada,2009). A taxonomist working with a series of snails of this species collected over a broad geographical range certainly would not recognize any significant morphological variation. This shows the lack of resolution of morphology and that DNA barcoding data can direct us to what we need to look further into: biodiversity.

According to Moritz and Cicero (2004) "accurate diagnosis" by a short COI DNA sequence,"depends on low intraspecific variation compared with that between species" So we can conclude that COI and 16S may be used for detection of species in *B. tenagophila* complex species (Figure 5). Furthermore,mtDNA lineages found in B. *tenagophila* may help explain heterogeneous patterns of schistosomiasis transmission.

5. Acknowledgments

We thank Lucia MZ Richinitti from PUCRS for collecting specimens in RS,Brazil,and Dr. Eliana Zanotti-Magalhães from UNICAMP for donating snails from Rio da Prata used in this study. This work was supported by FAPESP (Fundação de Amparo a Pesquisa do Estado de São Paulo) Grant 2007/03458-7 for Roseli Tuan and 2008/57792-8 for Fernanda Pires Ohlweiler.

6. References

Ballard, J. W. O.; Puslednik, L.; Wolff, J. N.; Russell, R. C. (2009). Variation Under Nature: A Sesquicentennial DNA Barcoding Perspective. *Chiang Mai J. Sci.* Vol. 36, No. 2, pp.188-199, ISSN 0125-2526

Brasil. Ministério da Saúde. (2007). Vigiláncia e Controlde de Moluscos de iImportáncia Epidemiológica: diretrizes técnicas: Programa de Vigilância e Controle da Esquistossomose (PCE). Ministério da Saúde (Ed.), Brasilia, 178p. ISBN 978-85-334-1438-9

Carnaval, A. C.; Moritz, C.; Hickerson, M.; Haddad, C.; Rodrigues, M. (2009). Stability predicts diversity in the Brazilian Atlantic Forest hotspot. *Science*, Vol. 323, No. 5915, pp.785-789, ISSN 0036-8075

Carvalho, O. S.; Amaral R. S.; Dutra, L. V.; Scholz, R. G. C.; Guerra, M. A. M. (2008). Distribuição Espacial de *Biomphalaria glabrata, B. straminea* e *B. tenagophila*, Hospedeiros Intermediários do *Schistosoma mansoni* no Brasil. In: *Schistosoma mansoni* e esquistossomose: uma visão multidisciplinar, Fiocruz, (Ed.), , Rio de Janeiro, Brasil, pp.393-418, ISBN: 978-857541-150-6

Carvalho, O. S.; Caldeira R. L.; Simpson, A. J.; Vidigal, T. H. (2001). Genetic variability and molecular identification of Brazilian *Biomphalaria* species (Mollusca: Planorbidae). *Parasitology*, Vol. 123, pp.197-209, ISSN 0031-1820

Carvalho, O. S.; Caldeira, R. L. Identificação morfologica de Biomphalaria glabrata, B. tenagophila e B. straminea hospedeirosintermediários do Schistoma mansoni. Belo Horizonte: Centro depesquisas René Rachou/Fiocruz, 2004. 1 CD. (Série Esquistossomose; n.6).

Collin, R. (2003). The utility of morphological characters in gastropod phylogenetics: an example from the Calyptraeidae. *Biological Journal of the Linnean Society*, Vol 78, No. 4, pp.541-593, ISSN 1095-8312

DeJong, R. J.; Morgan, J. A.; Paraense, W. L.; Pointier, J. P.; Amarista, M.; Ayeh-Kumi, P. F.; Babiker, A.; Barbosa, C. S.; Bremond, P.; Pedro Canese A.; Souza, C. P. de.; Dominguez, C.; File, S.; Gutierrez, A.; Incani, R. N.; Kawano, T.; Kazibwe, F.; Kpikpi, J.; Lwambo, N. J.; Mimpfoundi, R.; Njiokou, F.; Noel Poda, J.; Sene, M.; Velasquez, L. E.; Yong, M.; Adema, C. M.; Hofkin, B. V.; Mkoji, G. M.; Loker, E. S. (2001). Evolutionary relationships and biogeography of *Biomphalaria* (Gastropoda: Planorbidae) with implications regarding its role as host of the human bloodfluke, *Schistosoma mansoni*. *Mol Biol Evol.* Vol. 18, No. 12, pp. 2225-2239, ISSN 0737-4038

DeJong, R. J.; Morgan, J. A.; Wilson, W. D.; Al-Jaser, M. H.; Appleton, C. C.; Coulibaly, G.; D'Andrea, P. S.; Doenhoff, M. J.; Haas W.; Idris, M. A.; Magalhaes, L. A.; Mone, H.; Mouahid, G.; Mubila, L.; Pointier, J. P.; Webster, J. P.; Zanotti-Magalhaes, E. M.; Paraense, W. L.; Mkoji, G. M.; Loker, E. S. (2003). Phylogeography of *Biomphalaria glabrata* and *B. pfeifferi*, important intermediate hosts of *Schistosoma mansoni* in the New and Old World tropics. *Mol Ecol.* Vol. 12, No. 11, pp. 3041-3056, ISSN 1365-294X

Deslandes, N. 1959. Técnica de dissecção e exame de planorbídeos. *Rev. Serv. Espec. Saúde Publica* Vol.4, pp. 371-382

Estrada, E. V. E.; Velásquez, L. E.; Caldeira, R. L.; Bejarano, E. E.; Rojas, W.; Carvalho, O. M. (2006). Phylogenetics of South American Biomphalaria and description of a new species (Gastropoda: Planorbidae). *J. Mollus. Stud*, Vol. 72, No.3, pp. 221-228, ISSN 0260-1230

Felsenstein J. (1985). Confidence limits on phylogenies: An approach using the bootstrap. *Evolution,* Vol. 39, No. 4, pp. 783-791

Folmer, O.; Black, M.; Hoeh, W.; Lutz, R.; Vrijenhoek, R. (1994). DNA primers for amplification of mitochondrial cytochrome c oxidase subunit I from diverse metazoan invertebrates. Molecular *Marine Biology and Biotechnology.*Vol. 3, No.5, pp. 294-299, ISSN 1053-6426

Guimarães, M. C. A. (2003). Estudo comparativo dos aspectos reprodutivos de duas populações de *B. tenagophila* (Orbigny 1835) de áreas com e sem transmissão de esquistossomose no estado de São Paulo. Dissertação de Mestrado em Epidemiologia da Faculdade de Saúde Pública, Universidade de São Paulo, USP, Brasil.

Hall, T. A. (1999). BioEdit: a user-friendly biological sequence alignment editor and analysis program for Windows 95/98/NT. *Nucl Acids Symp Ser.* Vol. 41, pp. 95-98

Hudson, R. R.; Slatkin, M; Maddison, W. P. (1992). Estimation of levels of gene flow from DNA sequence data. *Genetics,* Vol.132, pp. 583-589, ISSN 0016-673

Kimura, M. (1980). A simple method for estimating evolutionary rate of base substitutions through comparative studies of nucleotide sequences. *Journal of Molecular Evolution,* Vol. 16, pp. 111-120, ISSN 0022-2844

Librado, P.; Rozas, J. (2009). DnaSP v5: software for comprehensive analysis of DNA polymorphism data. *Bioinformatics,* Vol.25, No. 11, pp. 1451-1452, ISSN 1367-4803

Lima, L. C.; Soares, D. M.; Guimarães, C. T. (1993).Biomphalaria occidentalis paraense, 1981 in the state of Minas Gerais, Brazil. *Mem. Inst. Oswaldo Cruz,* vol.88, No.2, pp.289-292, ISSN 0074-0276

Majoros, G.; Fehér, Z.; Deli T; Földvári, G. (2008). Establishment of *Biomphalaria tenagophila* Snails in Europe. *Emerging Infectious Dis*ease Vol.14, No. 11 (Nov 2008), pp.1812–1814, ISSN 1080-6059

Mavárez, J.; Pointier, J-P.; David, P.; Delay, B.; Jarne, P. (2002). Genetic differentiation, dispersal and mating system in the schistosome-transmiting freshwater snail *Biomphalaria glabrata. Heredity,* Vol.89, No. 4, pp.258-265, INSS 0018-067X

Mavárez, J.; Steiner C.; Pointier, J-P.; Jarne, P. (2002). Evolutionary history and phylogeography of the schistosome-vector freshwater snail *Biomphalaria glabrata* based on nuclear and mitochondrial DNA sequences. *Heredity,* Vol.89, No. 4, pp. 266-272, INSS 0018-067X.

Morgan, J.A., DeJong, R. J., Jung Y., Khallaayoune, K.; Kock S; Mkoji, G. M.; Loker, E. S. (2002).A phylogeny of planorbid snails, with implications for the evolution of *Schistosoma* parasites. *Moecular Phylogenetics Evolution.*Vol. 25, No. 3, pp. 477-488. ISSN 1055-7903

Moritz, C. & Cicero, C. (2004). DNA Barcoding: Promise and Pitfalls. *PLos Biology,* Vol. 2, No. 10, pp. 1529-1531

Nei, M. (1987). Molecular Evolutionary Genetics. Columbia University Press, New York, USA, 448p.

Ohlweiler, F. P.; Kawano, T. (2002) *Biomphalaria tenagophila* (Orbigny, 1835) (Mollusca): adaptation to desiccation and susceptibility to infection with *Schistosoma mansoni* Sambon, 1907. *Rev. Inst. Med. Trop. S. Paulo,* Vol. 44, No. 4, pp. 191-201. ISSN 0036-4665

Palasio, R.G.S. (2011). Estudo da variabilidade genética e morfológica de *Biomphalaria tenagophila* Orbigny 1835 (Gastropda, Planorbidae) procedente do Vale do Rio Ribeira do Iguape e do Litoral Norte do Estado de Sao Paulo. Projeto de Mestrado, UNICAMP, São Paulo, 32p

Palumbi, S. R. (1996). Nucleic acids II: the polymerase chain reaction. In: *Molecular Systematics,* Hillis DM, Moritz C, Mable BK (Eds.), pp. 205 - 247, Sinauer & Associates Inc., ISBN 0-87893-282-8, Sunderland, Massachusetts.

Paraense, W. L. (1955). Autofecundação e fecundação cruzada em *Australorbis glabratus. Mem. Inst. Oswaldo Cruz.* Vol.53, Nos. 2-3-4, (Jun/Dec 1955) pp. 277-291. ISSN 0074-0276.

Paraense, W. L. (1975). Estado atual da sistemática dos planorbídeos brasileiros. *Arq. Mus. Nac. Rio de Janeiro.* Vol. *55* (1975), pp. 105-128.

Paraense, W. L. (1981). *Biomphalaria occidentalis* SP.N. from South America (Mollusca: Basommatophora: Pulmonata). *Mem Inst Oswaldo Cruz,* Vol. 76, No. 2, (Apr/Jun 1981)2, pp. 199- 211, ISSN 0074-0276

Paraense, W. L. (1984). *Biomphalaria tenagophila guaibensis* ssp. n. from southern Brazil and Uruguay (Pulmonata: Planorbidae). I. Morphology. *Mem Inst Oswaldo Cruz,* Vol. 79, No. 4 (oct./dec 1984), pp. 465-469, ISSN 0074-0276.

Paraense, W.L. (2001) The schistosome vectors in the Americas. *Mem. Inst.Oswaldo Cruz.* vol. 96, pp. 7-16

Paraense, W. L., Deslandes N. (1959). The renal ridge as a reliable character for separating *Taphius glabratus* from *Taphius tenagophilus. Am J Trop Med Hyg,* Vol. *8,* (Jul 1959) pp. 456-472, INSS 0002-9637.

Paraense, W. L. & Correa L.R. (1978). Differencial susceptibility of *Biomphalaria tenagophila* populations to infection with a strain of *Schistosoma mansoni. J Parasitol,* Vol. 64, No. 5, pp. 822-826

Pepe, M. S.; Caldeira R. L.; Carvalho O. S.; Muller G.; Jannotti-Passos, L. K.; Rodrigues A. P.; Amaral H. L.; Berne M. E. A. (2009). *Biomphalaria* molluscs (Gastropoda: Planorbidae) in Rio Grande do Sul, Brazil. *Mem Inst Oswaldo Cruz,* Rio de Janeiro, Vol. 104, No. 5, pp. 783-786, INSS 0074-0276

Pfenninger M. & Posada D.(2002). Phylogeographic history of the land snail candidula unifasciata (Helicellinae, Stylommatophora): Fragmentation, corridor migration, and secondary contact. *Evolution,* Vol.56, No. 9, pp. 1776–1788

Piza, J.T., Ramos, A.S., Moraes, L.V.C., Correa, R.R., Takaku, L. & Pinto, A.C.M. (1972). Carta Planorbídica do Estado de São Paulo. Secretaria da Saúde do Estado de São Paulo, São Paulo. Campanha de Combate à Esquistossomose.

Pointier, J-P.; DeJong, R. J.; Tchuem Tchuenté, L. A.; Kristensen, T. K.; Loker, E. S. (2005). A neotropical snail host of *Schistosoma mansoni* introduced into Africa and consequences for the schistosomiasis transmission: *Biomphalaria tenagophila* in

Kinshasa (Democratic Republic of Congo). *Acta Tropica* Vol. *93*, No. 2, pp.191-199, ISSN 0001-706X

Saitou N. & Nei M. (1987). The neighbor-joining method: a new method for reconstructing phylogenetic trees. *Mol Biol Evol,* Vol. 4, No. 4, pp. 406-425, ISSN 0737-4038

Silva L. J. (1985). Urban growth and disease: schistosomiasis in the municipality of S. Paulo (Brazil). *Rev. Saúde Pública,* Vol. 19, No. 1, pp. 1-7, ISSN 0034-8910

Spatz L.; Vidigal, T. H. D. A.; Caldeira, R.L.; Dias Neto, E.; Cappa, S. M. G.; Carvalho, O. S. (1999). Study of *Biomphalaria tenagophila tenagophila, B. t. guaibensis* and *B. occidentalis* by polymerase chain reaction amplification and restriction enzyme digestion of the ribosomal RNA intergenic spacer regions. *Journal Molluscan Studies.*, Vol. *65*, No. 2, pp. 143-149, ISSN 0260-1230

Tamura K.; Peterson, D.; Peterson, N.; Stecher, G.; Nei, M.; Kumar, S. (2011). Mega5: Molecular Evolutionary Genetics Analysis using Maximum Likelihood, Evolutionary Distance, and Maximum Parsimony Methods. *Molecular Biology and Evolution*. (to be submitted).

Teodoro, T. M.; Janotti-Passos, L. K.; Carvalho, O. S.; Caldeira, R. L. (2010). Occurrence of *Biomphalaria cousini* (Mollusca: Gastropoda) in Brazil and its susceptibility to *Schistosoma mansoni* (Platyhelminths: Trematoda), *Molecular Phylogenetics and Evolution,* Vol. 57, No. 1, pp. 144-151, ISSN 1055-7903

Thompson, J. D.; Gibson, T. J.; Plewniak, F.; Jeanmougin, F.; Higgins, D. G. (1997). The Clustal X windows interface: flexible strategies for multiple sequence alignment aided by quality analysis tools. *Nucleic Acids Res.* Vol. *25*, No. 24, pp. 4876-4882. ISSN 0305-1048

Tuan, R. & Santos, P. dos. (2007). ITS2 variability of *Biomphalaria* (Mollusca, Planorbidae) species from the Paranapanema Valley (São Paulo State, Brazil): Diversity patterns, population structure, and phylogenetic relationships. *Genetics and Molecular Biology,* Vol. *30,* No. 1, pp. 139-144, ISSN 1415-4757

Tuan, R. & Simões, L. C. G. (1989). Effect of self-fertilization on *Biomphalaria tenagophila* (Orbigny, 1835) (Pulmonata: Planorbidae). *Genet. Mol. Biol.* Vol. 21, No. 4, pp. 477-478, ISSN 1415-4757

Tuan, R. (1996). Biologia de *Biomphalaria tenagophila* (Pulmonata:Planorbidae) em relação ao uso do moluscicida químico Bayluscide (Bayer): implicações para o controle. *Tese de Doutorado* em Ciências Biológicas (Biologia Genética), Universidade de São Paulo, USP, Brasil.

Tuan, R. & Simões L. C. G. (1989). Spermatogenesis and desiccation in *Biomphalaria tenagophila* (Orbigny, 1985) (Gastropoda, Planorbidae). *Braz J Genetic,* Vol.12, No. 4, pp. 881-5

Vidigal, T. H.; Spatz, L.; Kissinger, J. C.; Redondo, R. A.; Pires, E. C.; Simpson, A. J.; Carvalho, O. S. (2004). Analysis of the first and second internal transcribed spacer sequences of the ribosomal DNA in *Biomphalaria tenagophila* complex (Mollusca: Planorbidae). *Mem Inst Oswaldo Cruz,* Rio de Janeiro, Vol. 99, No. 2, pp. 153-158, ISSN 0074-0276

Vidigal, T. H. D. A.; Kissinger, J. C.; Caldeira, R. L.; Pires, E. C. R.; Monteiro, E.; Simpson, A. J. G.; Carvalho, O. S. (2000). Phylogenetic relationships among Brazilian *Biomphalaria* species (Mollusca: Planorbidae) based upon analysis of ribosomal ITS2 sequences. *Parasitology,* Vol. 121, No. 6, pp. 611-620, ISSN 0031-1820